The Renal Papilla and Hypertension

The Renal Papilla and Hypertension

Edited by
Anil K. Mandal, M.D., F.A.C.P.
Veterans Administration Medical Center and
University of Oklahoma College of Medicine
Oklahoma City, Oklahoma

and
Sven-Olof Bohman, M.D.
Karolinska Institute
Stockholm, Sweden

PLENUM MEDICAL BOOK COMPANY
New York and London

Library of Congress Cataloging in Publication Data

Main entry under title:

The Renal papilla and hypertension.

Includes bibliographical references and index.
1. Renal hypertension. 2. Renal papilla. I. Mandal, Anil K. II. Bohman, Sven-Olof. [DNLM: 1. Hypertension. 2. Kidney medulla. WG340 R393]
RC918.R38R46   616.6′1   80-15989
ISBN 978-1-4684-8117-4   ISBN 978-1-4684-8115-0 (eBook)
DOI 10.1007/978-1-4684-8115-0

© 1980 Plenum Publishing Corporation
Softcover reprint of the hardcover 1st edition 1980

227 West 17th Street, New York, N.Y. 10011

Plenum Medical Book Company is an imprint of Plenum Publishing Corporation

This book is dedicated to our beloved wives and children for their gracious cooperation, which encouraged us in our venture.

This book was facilitated in large part through the support of the
Medical Research Service of the Veterans Administration, Washington, D. C.,
and by the Medical Service, Veterans Administration Medical Center, and the
Department of Medicine, University of Oklahoma at Oklahoma City, Oklahoma.

Contributors

SVEN-OLOF BOHMAN • Department of Pathology, Karolinska Institute, Huddinge Hospital, S-141 86 Huddinge, Sweden

INGE NORBY BOJESEN • Institute of Experimental Hormone Research, University of Copenhagen, DK-2100 Copenhagen, Denmark

MUKUL C. GANGULI • Hypertension Section, Department of Internal Medicine, University of Minnesota Hospital and School of Medicine, Minneapolis, Minnesota 55455

CATHERINE LIMAS • Department of Pathology, Veterans Administration Hospital, and Departments of Laboratory Medicine and Pathology, University of Minnesota School of Medicine, Minneapolis, Minnesota 55455

ANIL K. MANDAL • Department of Medicine, Veterans Administration Medical Center and University of Oklahoma College of Medicine, Oklahoma City, Oklahoma 73104

BASAB K. MOOKERJEE • State University of New York at Buffalo, Buffalo, New York 14215, and Medical Research Service, Veterans Administration Medical Center, Buffalo, New York 14218

ROBERT C. MUEHRCKE • Department of Medicine, West Suburban Hospital, Oak Park, Illinois 60302

E. E. MUIRHEAD • University of Tennessee Center for the Health Sciences and Baptist Memorial Hospital, Memphis, Tennessee 38146

JOHN A. NORDQUIST • Renal Electron Microscopy Laboratory, Veterans Administration Medical Center, Oklahoma City, Oklahoma 73104

RAM V. PATAK • University of Kansas Medical Center, Kansas City, Kansas 66103, and Medical Research Service, Veterans Administration Medical Center, Kansas City, Missouri 64128

J. A. PITCOCK • University of Tennessee Center for the Health Sciences and Baptist Memorial Hospital, Memphis, Tennessee 38146

WOLFGANG SIESS • Department of Internal Medicine, University Hospital, D-8000 Munich 2, West Germany

DINKO SUŠIĆ • Institute for Medical Research, 1101 Belgrade, Yugoslavia

LOUIS TOBIAN • Hypertension Division, University of Minnesota College of Medicine, Minneapolis, Minnesota 55455

PETER C. WEBER • Department of Internal Medicine, University Hospital, D-8000 Munich 2, West Germany

RANDALL MARK ZUSMAN • Harvard Medical School, Boston, Massachusetts 02115, and Cardiac and Hypertension Units, Medical Services, Massachusetts General Hospital, Boston, Massachusetts 02114

Foreword

LOUIS TOBIAN

There are many reasons for suspecting that the medulla of the kidney is involved in the pathogenesis of hypertension. Although our present knowledge does not permit the assignment of a precise and exact role for the medulla, there are so many indications of its involvement that this is an appropriate time for the subject to be thoroughly reviewed, as Drs. Mandal and Bohman have done in this volume.

The involvement of the renal medulla in hypertension was first strongly indicated by the studies of Eric Muirhead. Studying renoprival hypertension, he demonstrated that the injection of extracts of renal medulla could prevent this type of hypertension in the dog, rabbit, and rat. Subsequently, a number of experiments showed that implants of renal medulla could not only prevent renoprival hypertension but also greatly reduce the level of blood pressure in Goldblatt hypertension in the rat and rabbit. It was later noted that the majority of the surviving cells in these medullary implants were interstitial cells. Pitcock and Muirhead were able to culture these interstitial cells, and implants of the cultured cells lowered blood pressure in renoprival hypertension and Goldblatt hypertension, particularly in the rat. We were able to confirm these general observations by employing implants of medulla in "postsalt" hypertension. The medullary implants did indeed bring the blood pressure down. The belief that the implants themselves were the effective agent was strengthened even further by the finding that when they were removed, their antihypertensive effect would disappear and the blood pressure would rise again.

The interstitial cells secrete some interesting substances with vasoactive properties. They have definitely been shown to secrete prostaglandins E_2 and $F_{2\alpha}$, which of course are very powerful vasoactive agents, and they also

LOUIS TOBIAN • Hypertension Division, University of Minnesota College of Medicine, Minneapolis, Minnesota 55455.

secrete a neutral lipid material with strong antihypertensive properties. Moreover, another cell in the renal medulla—the collecting duct cell—also has a rich supply of the enzyme that can convert arachidonic acid into prostaglandins. There are thus two types of cells in the renal medulla that are able to synthesize prostaglandins, making the renal medulla one of the tissues in the body with the richest supply of prostaglandin cyclooxygenase, equaled only by the seminal vesicles themselves. One can therefore look upon the renal medulla as potentially a very active prostaglandin factory. The renal medulla also contains the collecting ducts, which, as the last bit of renal tubule that the urine passes through before emerging into the renal pelvis, have "the last word" with regard to the ultimate excretion of sodium in the urine. Since sodium handling is so intimately involved with the process of hypertension, this particular medullary structure could be of pivotal importance in the hypertensive process from the sodium standpoint alone. Of course, the ascending limb of the loop of Henle also has an extremely active sodium transport system, and this provides the driving force for the countercurrent multiplier system that produces a concentration gradient for NaCl and urea from the tip of the papilla toward the cortex. The very high concentration of NaCl and urea in the papilla is a key element in the conservation of body water.

It is now quite definitely known that the prostaglandins have a profound influence on the concentration of NaCl in the papilla of the kidney. The administration of prostaglandin synthesis inhibitors, such as indomethacin or meclofenamate, can cause a doubling of the sodium concentration in the renal papilla. It is thought that this is primarily the result of enhancement of sodium transport out of the ascending limb and the collecting tubules or ducts after a profound inhibition of prostaglandin synthesis. These are two more examples in which the level of prostaglandin E_2 in the papilla and the level of sodium in the papilla appear to go in opposite directions. This may turn out to be a common physiological relationship and indicates that prostaglandin levels have a very profound governing influence on the concentration of NaCl in the papilla.

One might question what the concentrations of Na and Cl in the papilla have to do with hypertension. First of all, such concentrations would influence the conservation of water in the body. Furthermore, we have observed repeatedly that all forms of experimental hypertension appear to be characterized by an abnormally low concentration of sodium in the papilla. The precise reason for the relationship between the sodium concentration in the renal papilla and the presence of hypertension has not been clearly elucidated, but the low sodium concentration in this region appears to be a part of the general hypertensive process. An alteration in prostaglandin content may be related to this lowering of papillary sodium concentration. Moreover, in earlier studies, it was noted that the number of lipid granules in the cytoplasm of the interstitial cells was also greatly reduced, and that this reduction correlated very strongly with the reduction of sodium concentration in the renal papilla. This general picture of low lipid granules in the interstitial cells and low sodium concentration in the papilla was observed in four distinct forms of experimental hypertension.

It has also been pointed out by Moffat that the descending vasa recta are invested with smooth muscle cells and could therefore undergo vasoconstriction or vasodilation. Originally, in an effort to study the process of autoregulation in a papilla from a hypertensive rat, the plasma flow to the renal papilla was measured in various types of experimental rat hypertension. It was found that all forms of experimental rat hypertension could be characterized by reduced plasma flow to the renal papilla, even though the flow to virtually every other organ was at normal levels, implying a disproportionate amount of vasoconstriction in the vessels supplying the papilla. This would suggest that the circulation to the papilla was involved in the hypertensive diathesis to a greater extent than was the circulation to all other vascular beds. This conclusion is suggested by the fact that the papillary vascular resistance increased enough to actually reduce blood flow, whereas in all other vascular beds the resistance also increases, but not sufficiently to actually bring blood flow to lower than normal levels.

One can thus find a myriad of abnormalities in the renal papilla in various forms of experimental hypertension. These findings suggest a definite involvement of the renal papilla in the hypertensive process and imply that a number of papillary functions are distinctly abnormal during hypertension.

Preface

In spite of intensive research, the pathogenesis of most forms of hypertension—in particular essential hypertension—is far from clear. Although a vast amount of data has been accumulated to support a vasodepressor or antihypertensive property of the kidney in man and animals as a distinct entity, the exact *in vivo* action of this renal property in modifying hypertension is not understood. There is substantial evidence to indicate that the renal papilla (medulla) is the site of the antihypertensive property of the kidney. Among many documented studies the strongest support for this belief is offered by the isolation of the neutral lipid (antihypertensive substance) and acid lipids (prostaglandins) from renal papilla and by the demonstration in abundant number of a secretory type of cell called the renal interstitial cell in the renal papillary (medullary) interstitium. There is a growing tendency to implicate renal interstitial cells as a new endocrine cell type.

Much research has now been done using physiological, biochemical, morphological, and other techniques in attempting to define the role of the renal papilla in hypertension. In this vast field of investigation, it has up to now been difficult for scientists studying individual aspects of the problem to obtain a complete overview, for no books and few reviews are available to survey and clarify its many facets.

The aim of these chapters is to compile the available data and provide an authoritative and critical survey of accomplishments in renal papilla and hypertension research. Our contributors attempt throughout to substantiate important findings, relate their application to medical practice, and bring out clearly the controversial aspects of the field. This book should thus provide a good background for both established investigators and freshman researchers. It should also prove useful to clinicians, pathologists, and medical postgraduates as a comprehensive medium for updating knowledge about the intimate role of the kidney in protection against hypertension.

Anil K. Mandal
Sven-Olof Bohman

Acknowledgments

First of all, I would like to acknowledge my deep gratitude to Dr. Robert C. Muehrcke, who taught me much about the renal papillary interstitial cell. This initial teaching from Dr. Muehrcke contributed significantly to the materialization of my idea for and the successful completion of this volume. I am also very grateful to Dr. Sheldon C. Sommers for his continuous encouragement during the editing of this book and to my co-editor, Dr. Sven-Olof Bohman, for supporting my idea and working very diligently toward completion of this project. Dr. Bohman and I are most thankful to all the contributors for their time, effort, and prompt cooperation in writing and rewriting their individual chapters, and to Dr. Louis Tobian for his willingness to write the Foreword. We extend our appreciation to Carolyn Clay and Glenda Huff (both from the Veterans Administration Medical Center and the University of Oklahoma Health Sciences Center) for their secretarial assistance. Finally, we are very pleased to offer our thanks to Hilary Evans and Peter Strupp of Plenum for their encouragement and support.

Anil K. Mandal

Contents

CHAPTER 3

Studies on the Mechanism of the Renomedullary Hypertensive Action

DINKO SUŠIĆ

CHAPTER 4

Vasodepressor Substances Extractable from Kidney Tissue

BASAB K. MOOKERJEE and RAM V. PATAK

CHAPTER 5

Renal Prostaglandin Synthesis and Metabolism in Normal and Hypertensive States

CATHERINE LIMAS

CHAPTER 6

Fatty Acid Composition and Depot Function of Lipid Droplet Triacylglycerols in Renomedullary Interstitial Cells

INGE NORBY BOJESEN

CHAPTER 7

Alterations in the Renal Medullary and Papillary Interstitial Cells in Experimental
and Spontaneous (Essential) Hypertension

ANIL K. MANDAL and JOHN A. NORDQUIST

CHAPTER 8

Regulation of Plasma Flow and Other Functions of the Renal Papilla in
Hypertension

MUKUL C. GANGULI

CHAPTER 9

Prostaglandin E₂ Biosynthesis by Renomedullary Interstitial Cells: *In Vitro* Studies and Patholphysiological Correlations

RANDALL MARK ZUSMAN

CHAPTER 10

Influence of Renal Prostaglandins on Renin Release

PETER C. WEBER and WOLFGANG SIESS

Introduction

ANIL K. MANDAL and ROBERT C. MUEHRCKE

A variety of pathological states, e.g., acute interstitial nephritis, chronic interstitial nephritis, and papillary necrosis, involve the renal papilla. Although its existence has been known for several decades (Councilman, 1898), only since 1960 has the renal interstitium constituted an increasingly important subject for discussion among clinicians. This interest has been warranted in part by the frequent use of drugs such a methicillin in combating staphylococcal infections, often leading to an undesirable reaction affecting the renal interstitum—acute interstitial nephritis.

Despite our increasing awareness concerning disease processes of the renal interstitium, the anatomy of this compartment remained poorly defined until the mid-1960s. With the use of electron microscopy techniques, Muehrcke and associates (1965) and, soon thereafter, Osvaldo and Latta (1966) published elaborative studies of the renal interstitium and renal interstitial cells. These studies have established that the renal interstitium is a clearly discernible space in the renal papillae and medullae and is enriched with a uniform type of very conspicuous cells called renomedullary interstitial cells (RIC). The anatomical definition of RIC immediately raised the question of their physiological function and stimulated researchers to reinvestigate the antihypertensive function of the kidney and to attempt to identify the specific site in the kidney producing the so-called "antihypertensive" substance.

It is unclear exactly how, when, and by whom the groundwork for investigations of the antihypertensive function of the kidney was laid. Historically, it appears that a hypotensive function of the kidney was suspected almost a century ago by two separate groups of individuals (Brown-Sequard

ANIL K. MANDAL • Department of Medicine, Veterans Administration Medical Center and University of Oklahoma College of Medicine, Oklahoma City, Oklahoma 73104. ROBERT C. MUEHRCKE • Department of Medicine, West Suburban Hospital, Oak Park, Illinois 60302.

1

and d'Arsonval, 1892, Meyer, 1893). These authors reported that nephrectomized animals were "improved" by the crude extract of their kidneys; interestingly enough, this observation was made a few years before the discovery of the prohypertensive property of the kidney (Tigerstedt and Bergman, 1898). There was no further expansion of knowledge in this area for the 40 years, until it was found that a substance recovered from renal venous blood, as well as an extract of the kidney, produces diuresis (Tokumitsu, 1934).

The basic observations concerning the potential antihypertensive action of the kidney were first made by Chanutin and Ferris (1932) and later confirmed by Wood and Ethridge (1933), all of whom noted increased blood pressure after subtotal nephrectomy. Shortly thereafter, Braun-Menendez and von Euler (1947) and Grollman et al. (1949) observed that after total bilateral nephrectomy blood pressure increased significantly in the dog, they called this form of hypertension *renoprival hypertension*. In our opinion the era of understanding of the antihypertensive function of the kidney really dawned when Grollman et al. (1949) reported no rise of blood pressure in animals with one ureter implanted into small intestine or vena cava and the contralateral kidney removed. Furthermore, transplantation of the normal kidney reversed renoprival hypertension despite the maintenance of an expanded extracellular volume (Kolff and Page, 1954; Kolff, 1957; Muirhead et al., 1956). All these studies unequivocally established that the presence of normal renal tissue is essential to maintain a normotensive state. Also, the vasodepressor (or antihypertensive) substance appeared to be nonexcretory in nature.

The immediate goal than was to unravel the site of the antihypertensive function within the kidney. The results of two separate investigations published in the early 1960s provided some insights concerning this question: (1) Muirhead and colleagues (1960) reported that intravenous injection of renomedullary extract lowered blood pressure in dog, and (2) Muehrcke and associates (1965) demonstrated the presence in large number of a type of RIC in the inner medullary and papillary interstitium that appeared to have secretory characterisics: the presence of abundant rough-sufaced endoplasmic reticulum, a moderate number of mitochondria, and a large number of conspicuous homogeneous granules (lipid droplets). These two findings suggested that RIC might be the potential source of the renal medullary vasodepressor substance. This concept was strengthened by the finding of reduced RIC granularity in various forms of experimental hypertensions (Mandal et al., 1967; Muehrcke et al., 1969; Tobian et al., 1969; Ishii and Tobian, 1969).

At almost the same time, Lee et al. (1967) and Daniels et al. (1967) isolated prostaglandins (PG) from renal medulla and identified them as PGE_2, $PGF_{2\alpha}$, and PGA_2. As PGE_2 and PGA_2 demonstrate pharmacological properties consistent with those of the vasodepressor substances, this study confirmed the previous observations concerning renal medulla as the site of production of prostaglandins.

Further substantiation was provided by the experiments of Muirhead and colleagues (1970) who observed a persistent fall of blood pressure in hypertensive animals by explantation of live histocompatible renal medulla. While transient fall of blood pressure was observed after explantation of histoincompatible renal medulla, no fall in blood pressure was noted after transplantation of dead medulla or renal cortex.

Thus far, three major types of vasoactive substances have been isolated from the renal medulla: (1) Muirhead's antihypertensive neutral renomedullary lipid (ANRL), (2) polar lipid (Prewitt et al., 1979), and (3) PGE_2 and PGA_2. Transplantation of pure RIC from tissue culture is found to lower blood pressure in various forms of experimental hypertension (Muirhead et al., 1975). The results of experiments using transplantation of renal medulla or pure RIC have led Muirhead and colleagues (1975) to propose that the medulla of the kidney exerts an endocrine-type antihypertensive action. This is supported by the observations of Bohman (personal communication, 1979). In addition, Zusman and Keiser (1977a,b, 1980) have demonstrated synthesis and inhibition of synthesis of PGE_2 in the RIC by tissue culture techniques. These experiments are a direct proof that RIC is the site of production of renal papillary (medullary) prostaglandins.

The source of vasoactive substances in the RIC is still controversial, although the striking ultrastructural appearance of the granules (lipid droplets) within RIC and in the free interstitium has tempted investigators to implicate these granules as the secretory source of vasoactive substances. Chemical analysis of isolated fractions from homogenized papillae tend to deny this notion (Änggård et al., 1972), but the implication cannot be ignored, especially since ultrastructural alterations in both number and appearance of the granules have been observed following inhibition of prostaglandin synthesis by indomethacin (Limas et al., 1976; Pitcock et al., 1976). Thus, the specific constituent of RIC that is involved in the production of vasodepressor substances remains to be identified. Furthermore, although many investigators claim interstitial cells to be the major source of PGE_2, Bohman (1977) has shown by direct histochemical techniques that the collecting tubule is also a site of prostaglandin production. It seems reasonable to state that both RIC and collecting tubules contribute in the synthesis of renomedullary vasoactive substances.

Although investigations in vitro have contributed significantly to our understanding of the anatomy of the renal medulla and the function of its contents, especially the vasoactive substances, the exact functions of renal medulla in the regulation of blood pressure in vivo still remain to be determined. Theoretically, it is possible that excessive amounts of prostaglandins and ANRL, potent naturally occurring antihypertensive substances (or hormones), normally tend to mitigate against rises in blood pressure and that absence or deficiency of these substances (either genetic or acquired) could result in hypertension (Lee, 1969). Thus far, however, there is no direct evidence to support this contention.

Quantitative studies of RIC granularity in the spontaneously hypertensive rat (SHR), a rat model of essential hypertension, have provided some insight into the primary or secondary role of RIC in hypertension (Mandal *et al.*, 1974, 1975). Limas and Limas (1977) have demonstrated significantly higher renal prostaglandin synthetase activity in young (10-week) SHR than in age-matched normotensive Wistar Kyoto rats. However, Okamoto–Aoki SHR become progressively hypertensive despite increased prostaglandin synthesis by their kidneys. High blood pressure occurring *pari passu* with increased renal synthesis of vasodilator substances (PGE_2) appears to be contradictory but is not impossible. The practical aspect of this condition is supported by an earlier study in which increased secretion of prostaglandins was demonstrated in rats with experimentally induced hypertension (Tobian and Azar, 1971). As human kidney possesses RIC resembling those in rat or dog and because RIC granularity is found to be decreased in the malignant hypertensive kidney (Muehrcke *et al.*, 1970), a similar condition may be hypothesized in the human. Further isolation and purification of vasodepressor substances may clarify the biochemical nature of the antihypertensive substances of the human kidney.

Although the existence of vasodepressor or antihypertensive factors in the renal papilla (or medulla) seems unequivocal, little is known about the physiological role of these substances in normal man or animals. Surely further investigation is necessary to determine the function *in vivo* of the renal papilla in modifying blood pressure control in normotensive and hypertensive states.

REFERENCES

Änggård, E., Bohman, S.-O., Griffin, J. E., Larsson, C., and Maunsbach, A. B., 1972, Subcellular localization of the prostaglandin system in the rabbit renal papilla, *Acta Physiol. Scand.* **84**:231.

Bohman, S. O., 1977, Demonstration of prostaglandin synthesis in collecting duct cells and other cell types of the rabbit renal medulla, *Prostaglandins* **14**:729.

Braun-Menendez, E., and von Euler, V. S., 1947, Hypertension after bilateral nephrectomy in the rat, *Nature* **160**:905.

Brown-Sequard and d'Arsonval, 1892, *C. R. Acad. Sci.* **114**:400. [Quoted in Grollman *et al.* (1940).]

Chanutin, A., and Ferris, E., 1932, Experimental renal insufficiency produced by partial nephrectomy, *Arch. Intern. Med.* **49**:767.

Councilman, W. T., 1898, Acute interstitial nephritis, *J. Exp. Med.* **3**:4.

Daniels, E. G., Hinman, J. W., Leach, B. E., and Muirhead, E. E., 1967, Identification of prostaglandin E_2 as the principal vasodepressor lipid of rabbit renal medulla, *Nature* **215**:1298.

Grollman, A., Williams, J. R., and Harrison, T. R., 1940, Reduction of elevated blood pressure by administration of renal extracts, *J. Am. Med. Assoc.* **115**:1169.

Grollman, A., Muirhead, E. E., and Vanatta, J., 1949, Role of the kidney in pathogenesis of hypertension as determined by a study of the effects of bilateral nephrectomy and other experimental procedures on the blood pressure of the dog, *Am. J. Physiol.* **157**:21.

Ishii, M., and Tobian, L., 1969, Interstitial cell granules in renal papilla and the solute composition of renal tissue in rats with Goldblatt hypertension, *J. Lab. Clin. Med.* **74**:47.

Kolff, W. J., 1957, Reduction of experimental renal hypertension by kidney perfusion, *Univ. Mich. Med. Bull.* **23**:238.

Kolff, W. J., and Page, I. H., 1954, Blood pressure reducing function of the kidney: Reduction of renoprival hypertension by kidney perfusion, *Am. J. Physiol.* **178**:75.

Lee, J. B., 1969, Hypertension, natriuresis, and the renal prostaglandins (an editorial), *Ann. Intern. Med.* **70**:1033.

Lee, J. B., Crowshaw, B. H., Takman, B. H., and Attrep, K. A., 1967, The identification of prostaglandins E_2, $F_{2\alpha}$ and A_2 from rabbit kidney medulla, *Biochem. J.* **105**:1251.

Limas, C., Limas, C. J., and Gessell, M. S., 1976, Effects of indomethacin on reno-medullary interstitial cells, *Lab. Invest.* **34**:522.

Limas, C. J., and Limas, C., 1977, Prostaglandin metabolism in the kidneys of spontaneously hypertensive rats, *Am. J. Physiol.* **233**(1):H87.

Mandal, A. K., Muehrcke, R. C., Epstein, M., and Volini, F. I., 1967, Relationship of the renomedullary interstitial cells to experimental hypertension, *J. Lab. Clin. Med.* **70**:872.

Mandal, A. K., Frohlich, E. D., Chrysant, K., Pfeffer, M. A., Yunice, A. A., and Nordquist, J. A., 1974, Ultrastructural analysis of renal papillary interstitial cell of spontaneously hypertensive rat, *J. Lab. Clin. Med.* **83**:256.

Mandal, A. K., Frohlich, E. D., Chrysant, K., Nordquist, J., Pfeffer, M. A., and Clifford, M., 1975, A morphological study of the renal papillary granule analysis in the interstitial cell and in the interstitium, *J. Lab. Clin. Med.* **85**:120.

Meyer, E., 1893, *Arch. Physiol. Norm. Pathol.*, p. 760. [Quoted in Grollman *et al.* (1940).]

Muehrcke, R. C., Rosen, S., and Volini, F. I., 1965, The interstitial cells of the renal papilla: Light and electron miscroscopic studies in: *Progress in Pyelonephritis* (E. H. Kass, ed.), F. A. Davis, Philadelphia, p. 422.

Muehrcke, R. C., Mandal, A. K., Epstein, M., and Volini, F. E., 1969, Cytoplasmic granularity of the renal medullary interstitial cells in experimental hypertension, *J. Lab. Clin. Med.* **73**:299.

Muehrcke, R. C., Mandal, A. K., and Volini, F. I., 1970, Renal interstitial cells: Prostaglandins and hypertension, *Circ. Res.* (Suppl. 1) **26–27**:109.

Muirhead, E. E., Stirman, J. A., Lesch, W., and Jones, F., 1956, The reduction of postnephrectomy hypertension by renal homotransplants, *Surg. Gynecol. Obstet.* **103**:673.

Muirhead, E. E., Jones, F., and Stirman, J. A., 1960, Antihypertensive property in renoprival hypertension of extract from renal medulla, *J. Lab. Clin. Med.* **65**:176.

Muirhead, E. E., Brown, G. B., Germain, G. S., and Leach, B. E., 1970, The renal medulla as an antihypertensive organ, *J. Lab. Clin. Med.* **76**:641.

Muirhead, E. E., Germain, G. S., Armstrong, F. B., Brooks, B., Leach, B. E., Byers, L. W., Pitcock, J. A., and Brown, P., 1975, Endocrine type antihypertensive function of renomedullary interstitial cells, *Kidney Int.* **8** (Suppl):271.

Osvaldo, L. and Latta, H., 1966, Intersitial cells of the renal medulla, *J. Ultrastruct. Res.* **15**:589.

Pitcock, J. A., Rightsel, W. A., Brown, P., Brooks, B., and Muirhead, E. E., 1976, Functional–morphological correlates of renomedullary interstitial cells, *Clin. Sci. Mol. Med.* **51** (Suppl.):291.

Prewitt, R., Leach, B. E., Byers, L. W., Brooks, B., Lands, W. E. M., and Muirhead, E. E., 1979, Antihypertensive polar renomedullary lipid, a semi-synthetic vasodilator, *Hypertension* **1**:299.

Tigerstedt, R., and Bergman, P. G., 1898, *Skand. Arch. Physiol.* **8**:223. [Quoted in Grollman *et al.* (1940).]

Tobian, L., and Azar, S., 1971, Antihypertensive and other functions of the renal papilla, *Trans. Assoc. Am. Phys.* **84**:281

Tobian, L., Ishii, M., and Duke, M., 1969, Relationship of cytoplasmic granules in renal papillary interstitial cells to "post-salt" hypertension, *J. Lab. Clin. Med.* **73**:309.

Tokumitsu, Y., 1934, *Folia Endocrinol. Jpn, Tr. Jpn. Pathol. Soc.* **24**:444. [Quoted in Grollman *et al.* (1940).]

Wood, J. E., Jr., and Ethridge, C., 1933, Hypertension with arteriolar and glomerular changes in the albino rat following subtotal nephrectomy, *Proc. Soc. Exp. Biol. Med.* **30**:1039.

Zusman, R. M., and Keiser, H. R., 1977a, Prostaglandin biosynthesis by rabbit renomedullary interstitial cells in tissue culture: Stimulation by angiotensin II, bradykinin and arginine vasopressin, *J. Clin. Invest.* **60**:215.

Zusman, R. M., and Keiser, H. R., 1977b, Prostaglandin E_2 biosynthesis by rabbit renomedullary interstitial cells in tissue culture: Mechanism of stimulation by angiotensin II, bradykinin, and arginine vasopressin, *J. Biol. Chem.* **252**:2069.

Zusman, R. M., and Keiser, H. R., 1980, Regulation of prostaglandin E_2 biosynthesis by rabbit renomedullary interstitial cells in tissue culture: Effects of potassium, osmolality, corticosteroids, arachidonic acid and protein synthesis inhibition, *Kidney Int.* **17**:277.

CHAPTER 1

The Ultrastructure of the Renal
Medulla and the Interstitial Cells

SVEN-OLOF BOHMAN

1. INTRODUCTION

During recent years, the theory has evolved that the kidney, similar to several other organs such as the gonads and the thyroid gland, contains an interstitial cell type with endocrine functions. The cells implicated are the interstitial cells of the renal medulla, which are characterized by their content of abundant cytoplasmic lipid inclusions. The secretory product is believed to be a lipid and appears to have potent antihypertensive properties (see later chapters of this volume).

Although described in some detail long ago (Schweigger-Seidel, 1865; Renaut and Dubreuil, 1907) the interstitial cells of the renal medulla did not become the subject of much study until the last 10–15 years. Early ultrastructural studies of the renal medulla (Novikoff, 1960; Muehrcke *et al.*, 1965; Gloor and Neiditsch-Halff, 1965; Osvaldo and Latta, 1966*b*; Bulger and Trump, 1966), as well as the experimental studies by Nissen (1968*a,b*) and Mandal and co-workers (1967), which showed variations in the number of interstitial cell lipid inclusions during various physiological and pathological conditions, stimulated much research in this field. The main basis for the theory about the endocrine function of the interstitial cells, however, is the work of Muirhead's group (Muirhead *et al.*, 1975). They first showed that the renal medullary tissue (but not cortex) can exert an endocrinelike antihypertensive action (Muirhead *et al.*, 1960, 1968, 1970) and, later, that this effect may be ascribed to the lipid-containing interstitial cells (Muirhead *et al.*, 1972, 1975).

SVEN-OLOF BOHMAN • Department of Pathology, Karolinska Institute, Huddinge Hospital, S-141 86 Huddinge, Sweden.

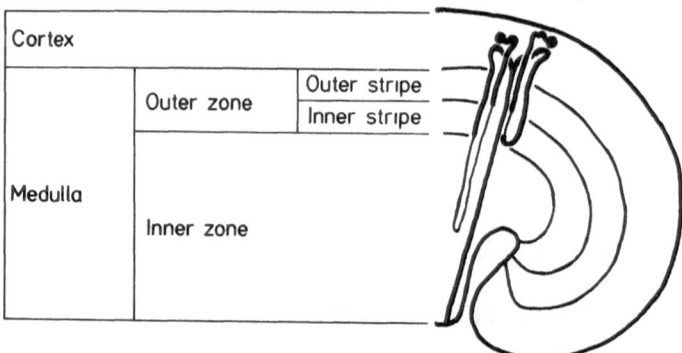

FIGURE 1. Schematic drawing showing the different layers of the kidney. The nomenclature for the layers used in this chapter is indicated to the left. The locations of a superficial (right) and a juxtamedullary (left) nephron as well as a collecting duct are indicated in the drawing.

As can be seen from this volume, much work has recently been done with morphological, biochemical, physiological, and other experimental techniques to elucidate the endocrine antihypertensive properties of the kidney and the role of the interstitial cells therein. In this chapter the structural basis for these studies will be described. Emphasis will be laid on the structure of the inner zone of the renal medulla and in particular the interstitial cells, which are most abundant in this part of the medulla.

2. THE RENAL MEDULLA

2.1. Subdivision and Nomenclature

In the unipapillary kidney of rodents, a rather clear-cut macroscopic subdivision into different zones can be seen due to the very precise alignment of the different parts of the nephrons. This is illustrated schematically in Fig. 1, in which a recommended nomenclature for the different zones is also indicated. The multipapillary kidney, such as that of humans, is less rigidly organized and the different regions are less clearly delineated.

The papilla, in a strict sense, is the more or less conical part of the medulla that has a free surface facing the renal sinus, i.e. corresponding to the major part of the inner zone. Often however, the term *papilla* is used synonymously with *inner zone of the medulla*.

The *outer stripe of the outer zone* (Fig. 2*) contains the straight parts of the proximal and distal tubules from both superficial and juxtamedullary nephrons. Collecting ducts descend from the cortex in the medullary rays, which are not sharply demarcated from the rest of the outer stripe. The

* Figures 2–18 appear on the insert facing this page.

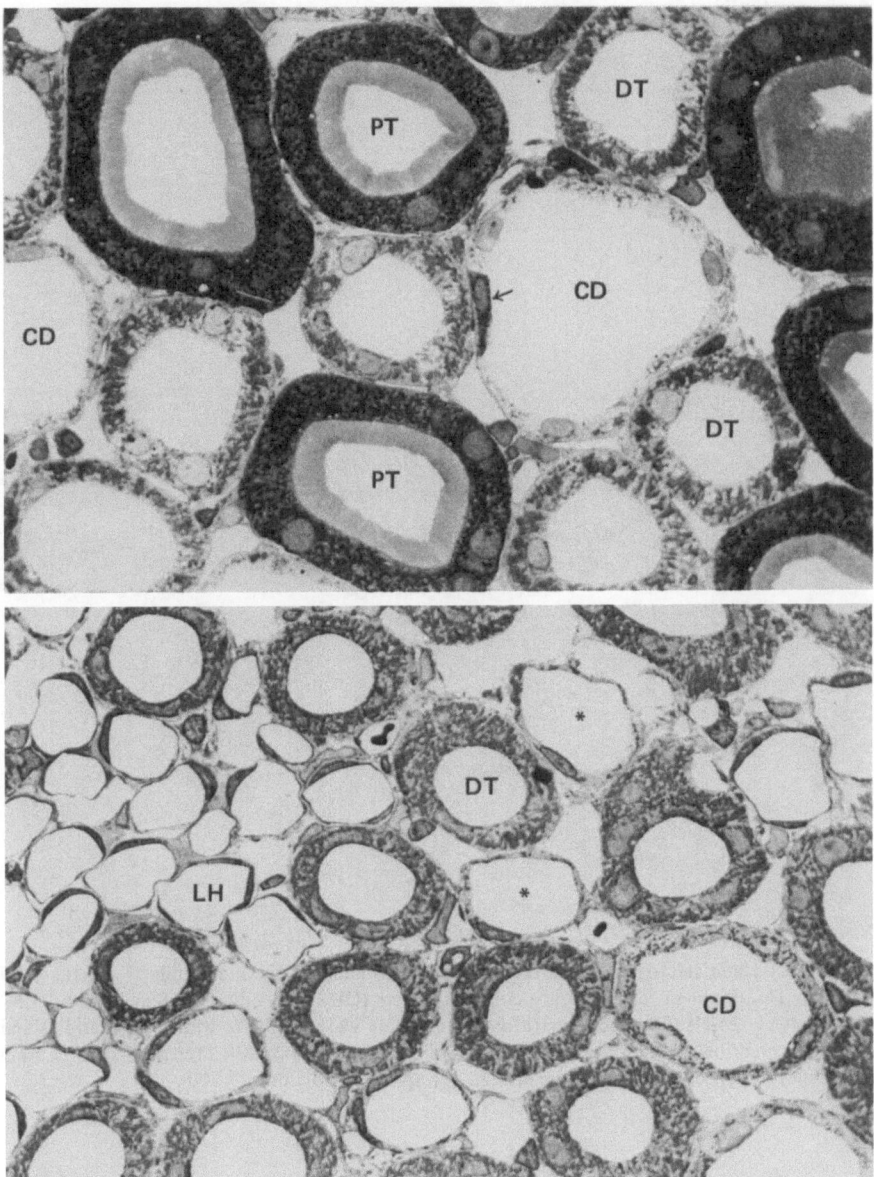

FIGURE 2. Light micrograph of a section from the outer stripe of the outer zone of the rat renal medulla. The third segments (pars recta) of the proximal tubules (PT) are characterized *inter alia* by a very tall brush border. Distal tubules (DT) as well as collecting ducts (CD) are also seen. The latter consist of light and dark (arrow) cells (1-μm plastic section, toluidine blue, $\times$700).

FIGURE 3. Light micrograph of a section from the inner stripe of the outer zone of the rat renal medulla. Numerous straight parts of distal tubules (DT) are seen as are collecting ducts (CD) and part of a vascular bundle (left) which contains vasa recta and thin limbs of Henle's loops (LH). The thin limbs of juxtamedullary nephrons are located at some distance from the vascular bundle (asterisks) (1-μm plastic section, toluidine blue, $\times$700).

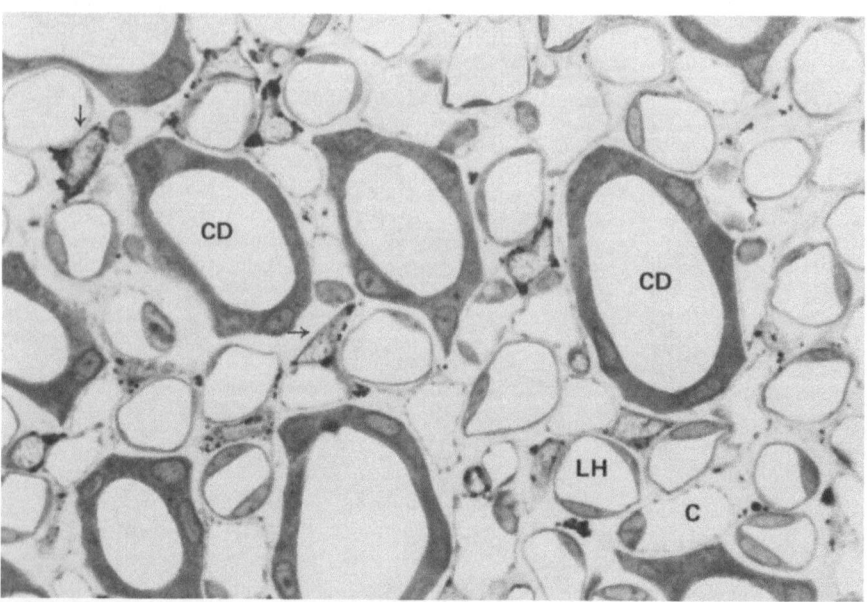

FIGURE 4. Light micrograph of a section from the middle of the inner zone of the rat renal medulla. The dominant elements are collecting ducts (CD), thin limbs of Henle's loops (LH) and capillary vessels (C). The interstitium is relatively wide (compare with Figs. 2 and 3) and contains numerous interstitial cells of different shapes (arrows). All interstitial cells contain abundant lipid droplets (1-μm plastic section, paraphenylenediamine, ×700).

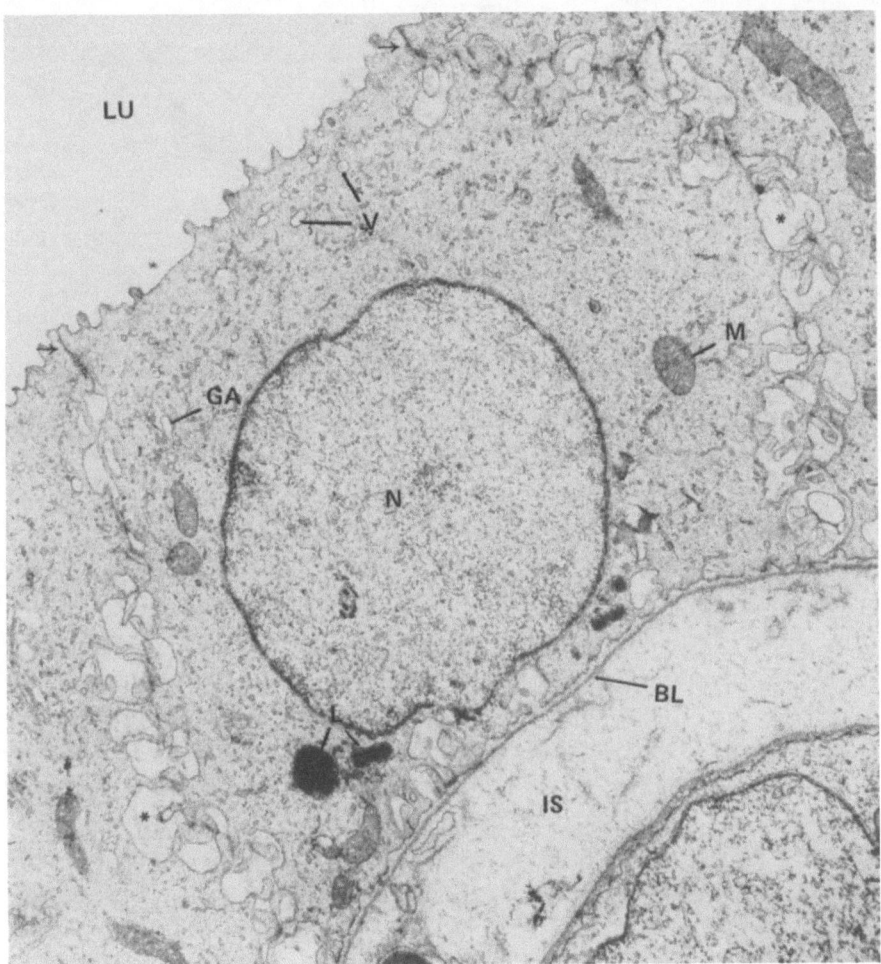

FIGURE 5. Electron micrograph of a collecting duct cell from the apical part of the rat renal papilla. Cell shape is cuboidal and adjacent cells are separated by an irregularly shaped intercellular space (asterisks) except at the most luminal part where the lumen (LU) is sealed off from the intercellular space by a tight junction (arrows). In the cytoplasm there are a few mitochondria (M), small apical vacuoles (V), a Golgi apparatus (GA) and, in the basal part, lysosomes (L). There are some free ribosomes but very sparse endoplasmic reticulum. The plasma membrane forms a number of basal infoldings. BL, basal lamina; IS, interstitial space (×16,000).

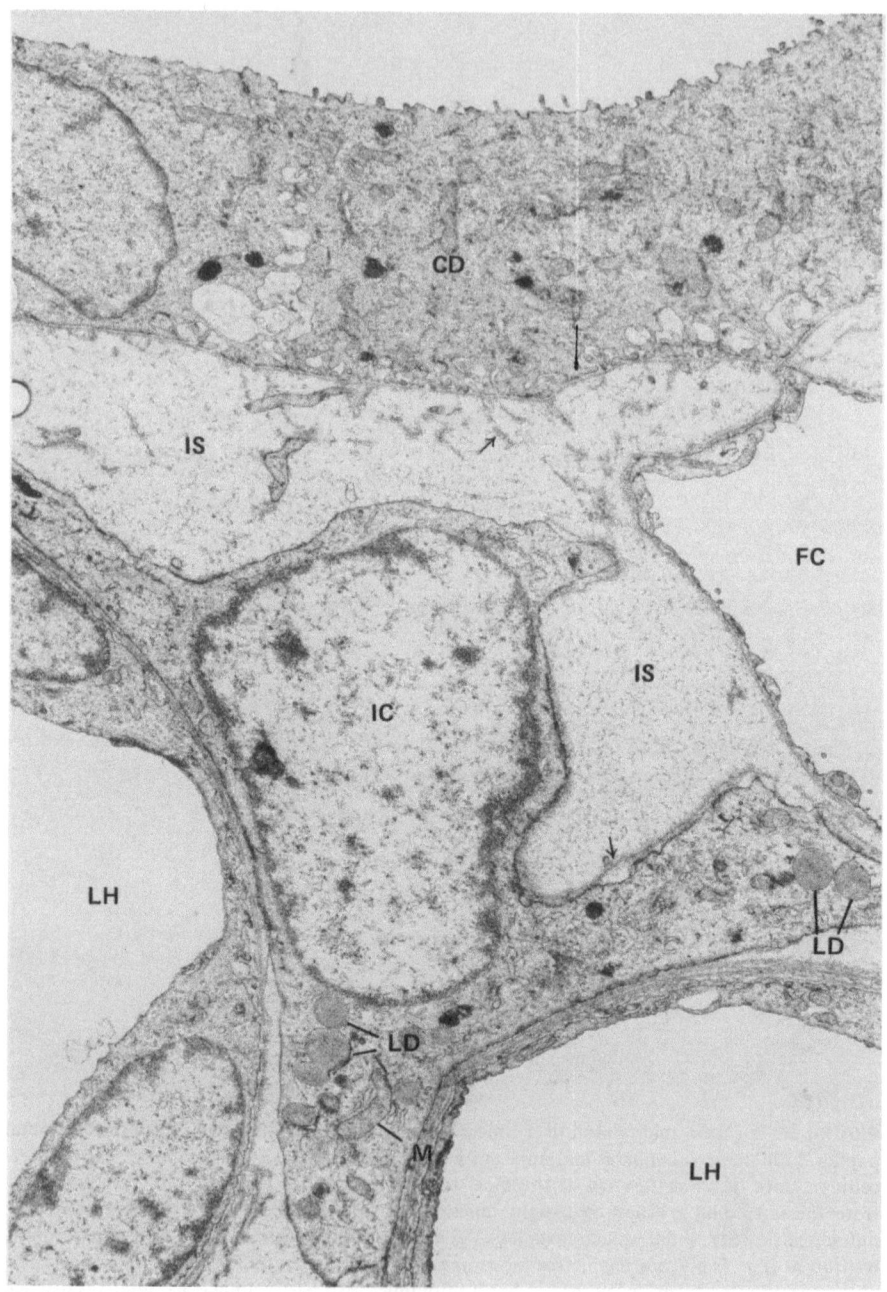

FIGURE 6. Electron micrograph showing a Type 1 interstitial cell (IC) in the inner zone of the rat renal papilla. The cell has several cytoplasmic projections, which are close to thin limbs of Henle's loop (LH) and a capillary (FC). The latter is of the fenestrated type. Numerous lipid droplets (LD) are seen in the cytoplasm of the interstitial cell. In the interstitial space (IS) there is an evenly distributed flocculent material and numerous strands of basement-membrane-like material (arrows), some of which are close to the surface of the interstitial cell. CD, collecting duct cell; M, mitochondrion (×8800).

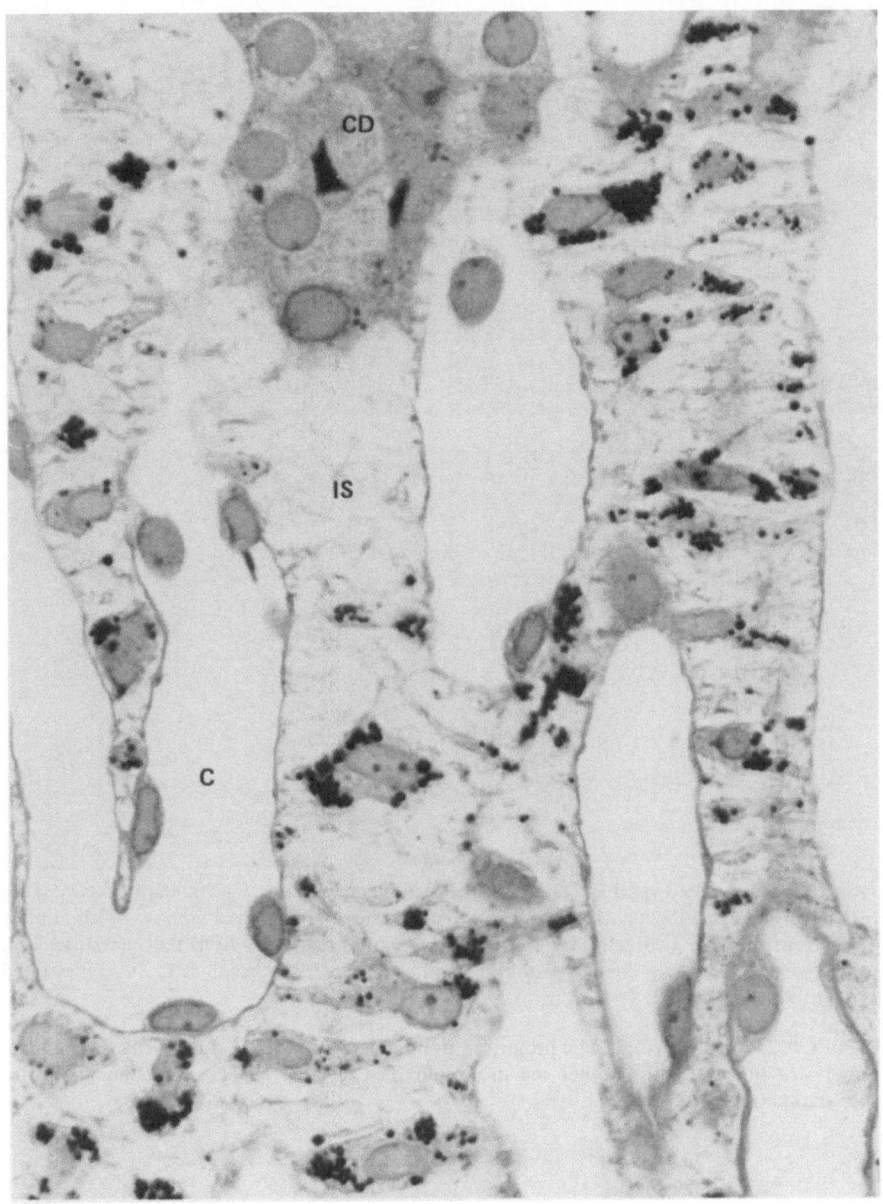

FIGURE 7. Longitudinal light microscopic section from the inner zone of the medulla of a water-loaded (5 hr) rat, illustrating the distribution and the flattened shape of many of the interstitial cells. The lipid droplets are particularly abundant in water-loaded rats. C, capillary; CD, collecting duct cell; IS, interstitial space (1-μm plastic section, paraphenylenediamine, ×1000).

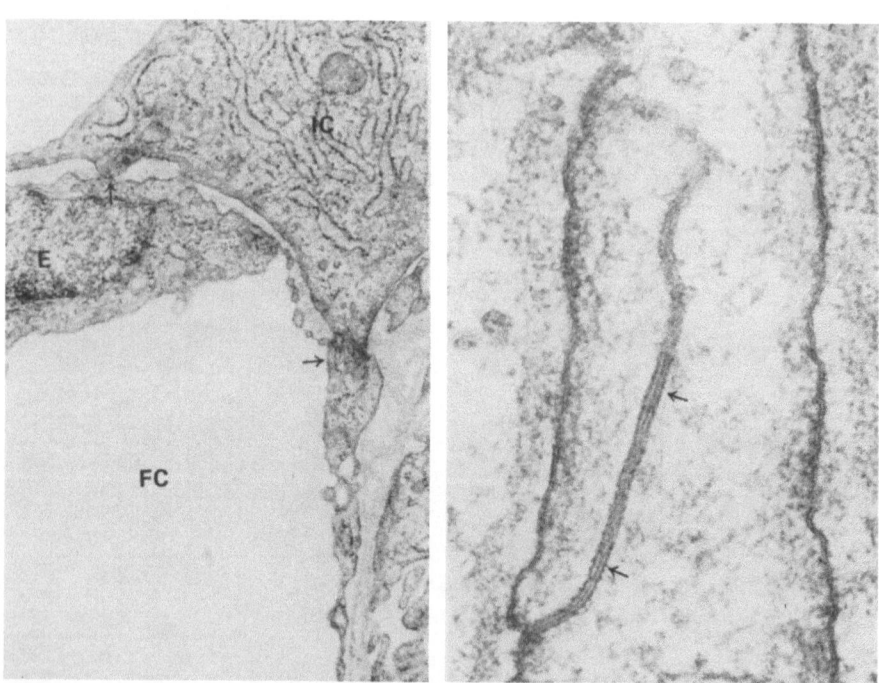

FIGURE 8. Part of a Type 1 interstitial cell (IC) in the inner stripe. The interstitial cell is close to a fenestrated endothelial cell (E) and in two places (arrows) the basal lamina, which in most places separates the two cells, is interrupted by short projections from the interstitial cell, which comes into close contact with the surface of the endothelial cell. FC, fenestrated capillary (rat, ×21,000).

FIGURE 9. Part of a cytoplasmic projection from an interstitial cell, which forms a long junctional area (arrows) with another cell projection. The junction appears pentalaminar in this preparation (rat, ×100,000).

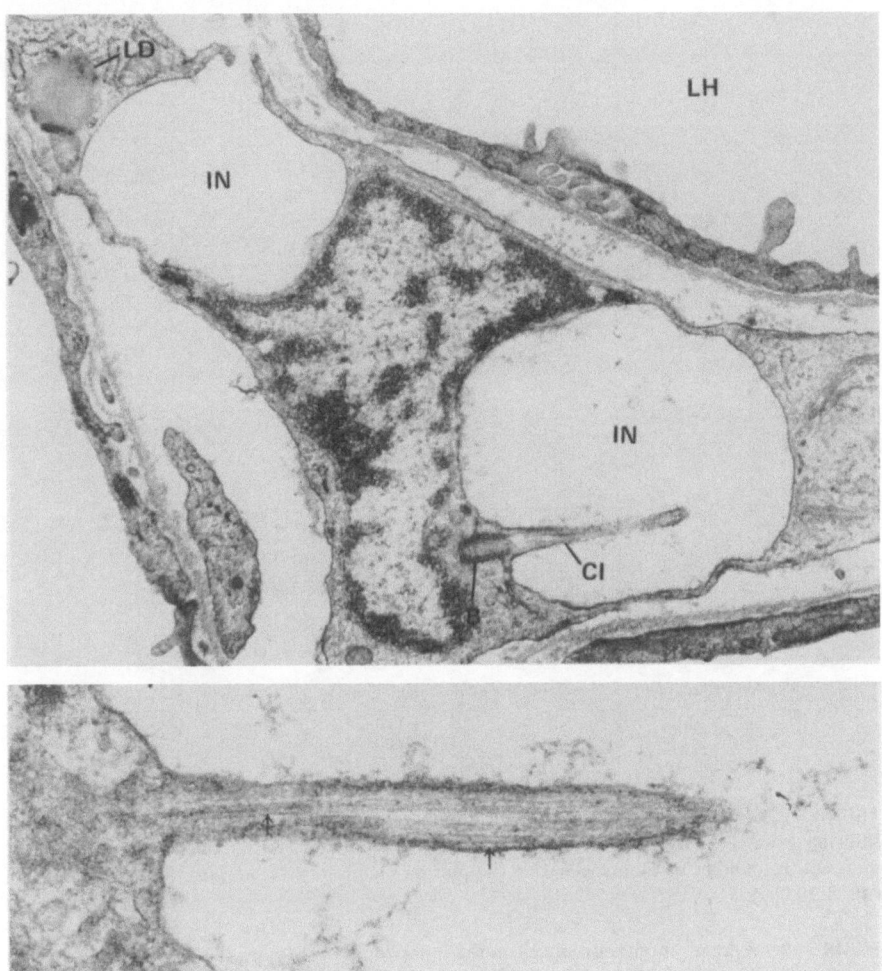

FIGURE 10. Interstitial cell in the inner stripe of the outer zone. The cell has two large invaginations (IN) and into one of these a cilium (CI) projects from the cell surface. In the cytoplasm the basal body (B) of the cilium is seen. LD, lipid droplet; LH, loop of Henle (rat, ×18,000).

FIGURE 11. Higher magnification of a section adjacent to that in Fig. 10, showing the cilium and the microtubular elements of the axoneme (arrows) (×65,000).

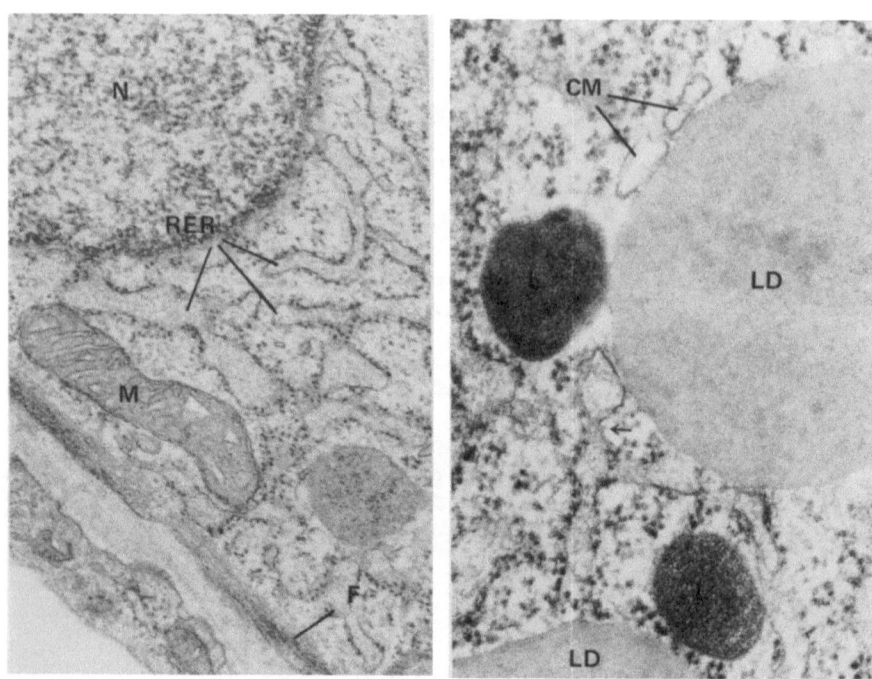

FIGURE 12. Part of the cytoplasm of an interstitial cell in the inner stripe of the outer zone showing expanded cisternae of rough endoplasmic reticulum (RER) filled with a flocculent material. F, bundles of filaments inside the plasma membrane; N, nucleus; M, mitochondrion (rat, ×34,000).

FIGURE 13. Part of an interstitial cell in the inner zone. Lysosomes (L) have a triple-layered membrane while the lipid droplets (LD) are devoid of a surrounding membrane. However, small vesicular profiles of smooth cytoplasmic membranes (CM) are close to the lipid droplet surface. In one place continuity between a smooth vesicular profile and the rough endoplasmic reticulum is suggested (arrow) (rat, ×67,000).

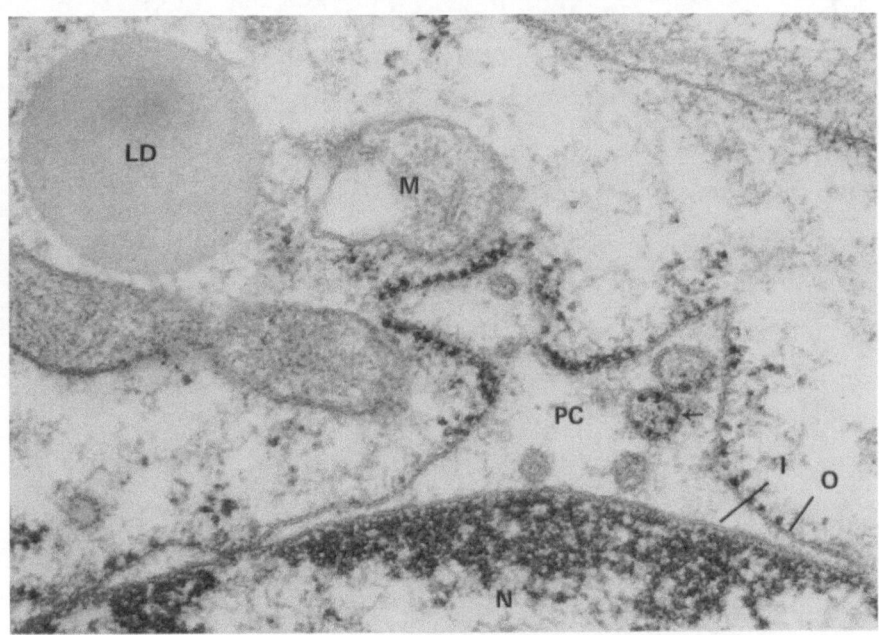

FIGURE 14. Part of an interstitial cell in the inner zone after perfusion fixation with a fixative with too low an osmolality (350 mOsm/kg). The perinuclear cisterna (PC), i.e., the space between the inner (I) and outer (O) nuclear membranes, is dilated. The outer nuclear membrane is here studded with ribosomes and within the expanded perinuclear cisterna peculiar cisternae of endoplasmic reticulum are present that seem to have ribosomes on the *inside* of the membrane (arrow). This cell also shows other signs of poor fixation, such as swollen mitochondria (M). LD, lipid droplet; N, nucleus (rat, ×80,000).

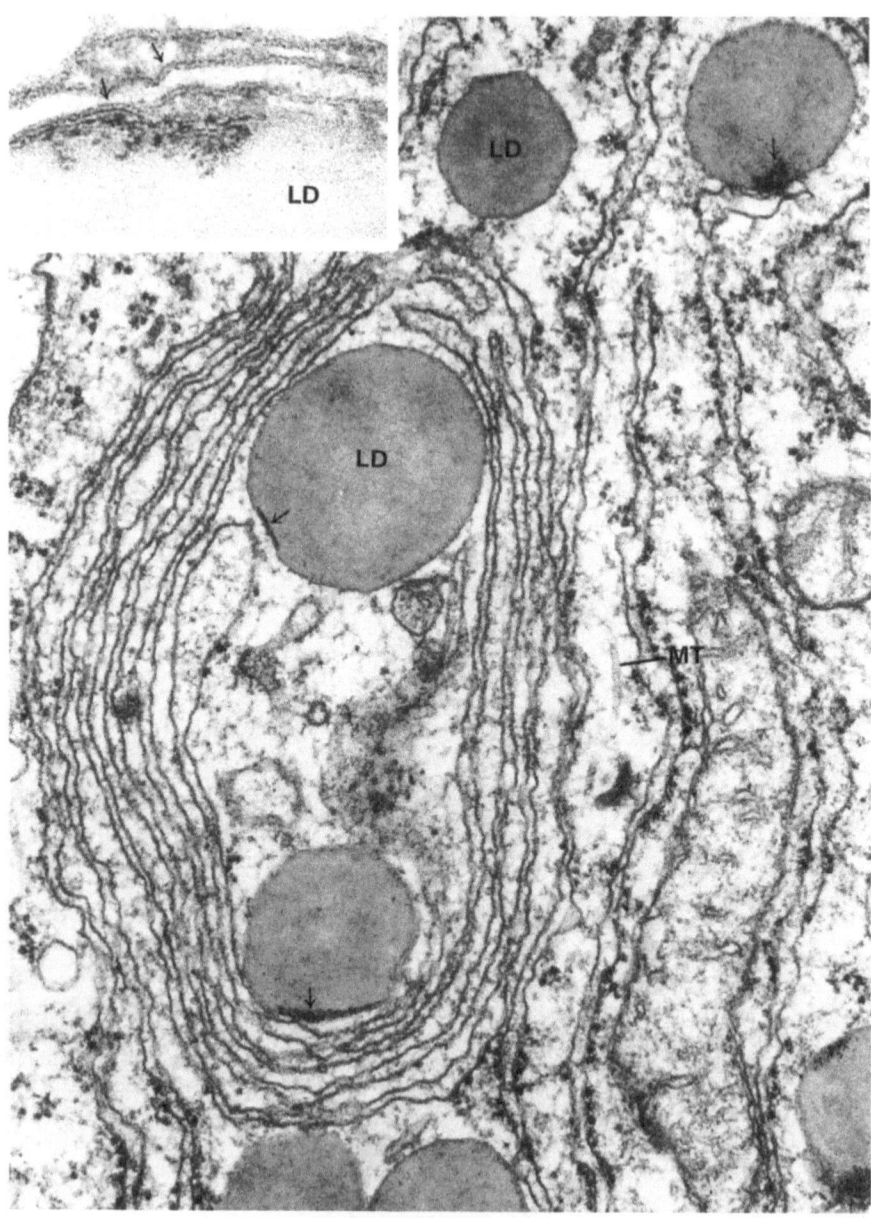

FIGURE 15. Part of an interstitial cell in the inner zone with numerous lipid droplets (LD), some of which are surrounded by a "whorl" of concentric smooth cytoplasmic membranes. The latter are in some places (lower left) continuous with the rough endoplasmic reticulum. In many areas where a smooth membrane is close to a lipid droplet, accumulations of an electron-dense material are seen within the droplet (arrows). MT, microtubule (rat, ×65,000). Inset: High-magnification of peripheral part of a lipid droplet (LD) with adjacent smooth membranes (arrows). The latter have a thickness of about 60 Å. Close to the smooth membrane the lipid droplet shows a peripheral accumulation of a highly electron-dense, granular material (×190,000).

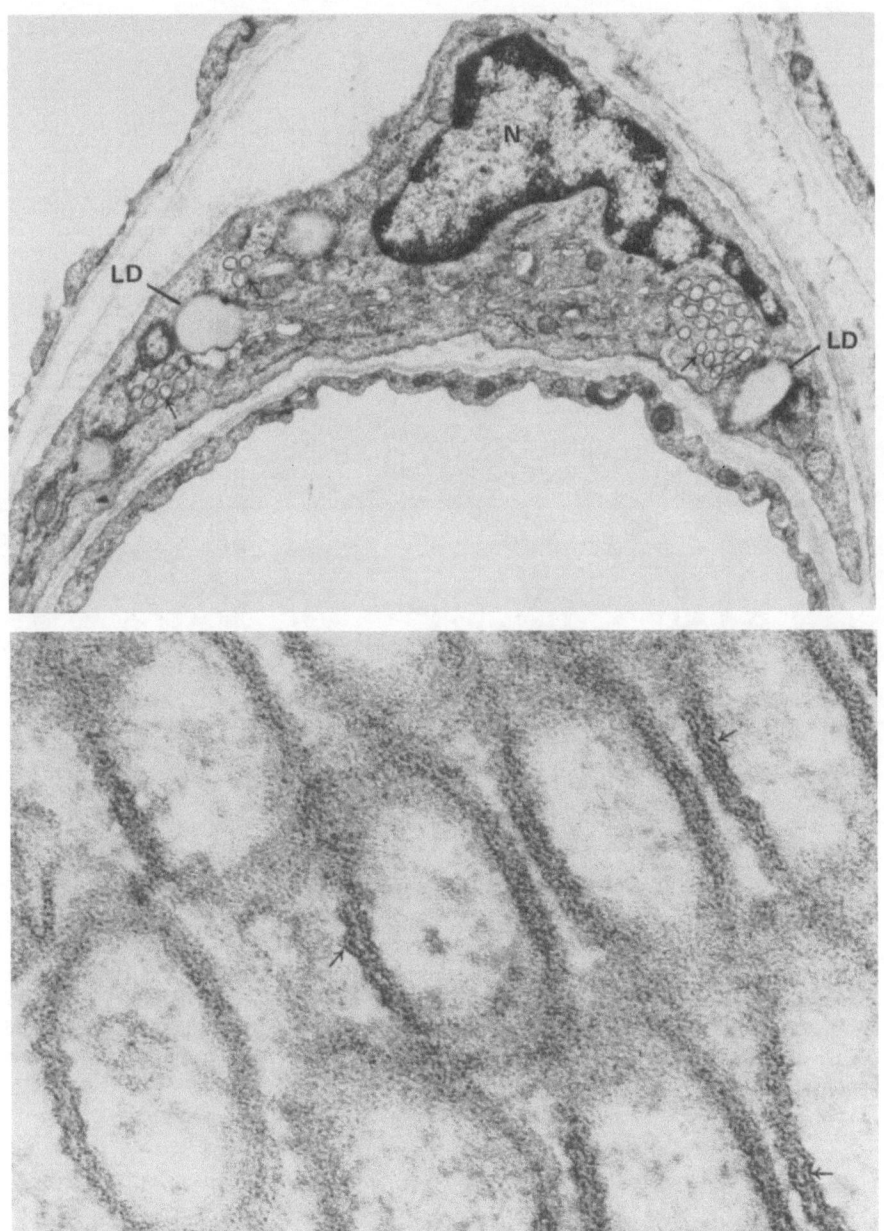

FIGURE 16. Interstitial cell in the inner zone showing three groups of cylindrical bodies that have been cut at right angles (arrows). LD, lipid droplets; N, nucleus (rat, ×16,000).

FIGURE 17. A group of cylindrical bodies in high magnification. In this slightly oblique section the wall of the cylinders in many places is seen to consist of two somewhat wavy, triple-layered membranes, each with a thickness of about 60 Å (arrows). Between these two membrane layers there is an electron-lucent layer about 20 Å thick, and the whole thickness of the wall is about 140 Å (rat, ×250,000).

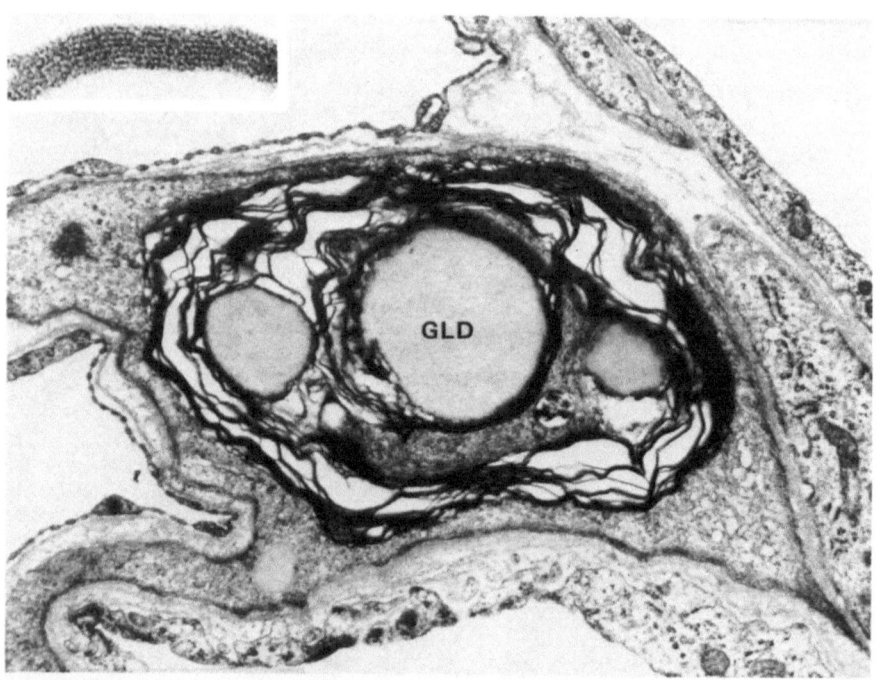

FIGURE 18. Interstitial cell in the inner zone of the gerbil renal medulla. A large part of the cytoplasm is occupied by a group of very large, "giant" lipid droplets (GLD) with a surrounding electron-dense, irregularly multilayered material (×19,000). Inset: Higher magnification of the electron-dense material surrounding the lipid droplets. A lamellar substructure with a periodicity of about 40 Å is seen (×170,000).

outer stripe is also characterized by the vascular bundles. The interstitium is narrow and contains sparse interstitial cells, which are similar to those of the cortex and do not include the lipid-laden interstitial cells typical of the rest of the medulla.

The *inner stripe of the outer zone* (Fig. 3) contains the vascular bundles, in which there are arterial and venous vasa recta. Around the vascular bundles are the thin descending limbs of Henle's loop, the straight part of the distal tubule (thick ascending limb of Henle's loop), and collecting ducts. The precise orientation of the different nephron segments in relation to the vascular bundle varies among species. The interstitium of the inner stripe is narrow.

The *inner zone* of the medulla (Fig. 4) contains the thin limbs of Henle's loop (descending and ascending), collecting ducts, and blood vessels. The latter are mainly of the capillary type since toward the inner zone the descending vasa recta break up into a capillary network that is drained by the ascending vasa recta. The pattern of vascular bundles as well as that of medullary rays is dissolved in the outer levels of the inner zone. The interstitium increases gradually in size toward the papillary tip.

2.2. Preparation Problems

Before discussing the ultrastructure of the different structural elements of the renal medulla it seems relevant to mention briefly the technical problems encountered in the preparation of this tissue for ultrastructural studies.

Most investigators in this field (Pease, 1964; Osvaldo and Latta 1966a,b; Bulger and Trump, 1966; Moffat, 1967a, Dieterich, 1968) have agreed that it has been difficult to obtain what could be considered a good quality of fixation of the renal medulla, even with perfusion fixation. The main reason for this difficulty is the very special osmotic conditions prevailing in this tissue.

Fixation solutions with an osmolality slightly above isotonicity with plasma, which are suitable for the fixation of other tissues including the renal cortex, under most circumstances create a very pronounced swelling of all cell types in the renal medulla (Bohman, 1974). Swelling is also evident with perfusion fixation and in fact if such fixation solutions are used, immersion fixation may have the slight advantage that the slow diffusion allows more time for osmotic equilibration between the fixative solution and the tissue fluid in the deep parts of the specimen. However, if a good quality of fixation is to be obtained, the osmolality of the fixative solution has to be adjusted to the high osmolality of the medullary tissue fluid by the addition of solutes (Bohman, 1974). Since an osmotic gradient is present in the medulla, the fixative osmolality has to be chosen according to the layer of the medulla to be studied. If 3% glutaraldehyde is used as a fixative, the optimal buffer osmolalities for the inner stripe, middle level of the inner zone, and papilla tip of the rat renal medulla are about 400, 1000, and 1500 mOsm/kg H_2O, respectively (Bohman, 1974).

Unfortunately, different species of animals as well as different states of diuresis present different osmotic gradients in the medulla, which all require differently tailored fixation solutions. This variability tends to make the performance of detailed and reliable ultrastructural studies of the renal medulla a rather tedious task. Some guidance with respect to the required osmolality of the fixative can be obtained by urine osmolality determinations.

Thus, particular attention to the fixation method is of decisive importance in order to obtain useful and reliable ultrastructural data from the renal medullary tissue. In my opinion, several erroneous concepts regarding the ultrastructure of the interstitial cells have arisen as a result of interpretations of fixation artifacts (Bohman, 1974), e.g., that the interstitial cells have a "vacuolated" cytoplasm with widely expanded, empty-looking cisternae of endoplasmic reticulum as well as dilated perinuclear cisternae, and that intact lipid droplets are released through the plasma membrane into the interstitium.

2.3. The Structural Elements of the Inner Zone of the Medulla

2.3.1. *The Collecting Ducts*

While the cortical and outer medullary collecting ducts are made up of two distinct cell types, the principal or light cells and the intercalated or dark cells, the inner medullary collecting ducts consist of only principal cells. These cells gradually increase in height, from flattened cuboidal in the outer part of the inner zone to truly cuboidal (Fig. 5) toward the apical part. In some species, like the rabbit (Kaissling and Kriz, 1979), they become very tall columnar cells close to the papilla tip.

The luminal surface of the collecting duct cells has a number of blunt microvilluslike projections and a relatively thick surface coat (Fig. 5). Close to the luminal surface, neighboring cells are connected by a tight junction, which is about 0.3 μm deep. Below this, there is an intermediate junction and in some places desmosomes can be seen (Kaissling and Kriz, 1979). The lateral surfaces of the cells possesses a moderate number of short projections, which may interdigitate with neighboring cells (Fig. 5). The lateral intercellular spaces vary in width, and this may reflect the route of water flow across this epithelium in response to antidiuretic hormone (ADH) (Tisher, 1976). The basal surface of the cells shows a number of moderately deep invaginations forming a small "basal labyrinth" (Fig. 5). The surface area of the basolateral cell membrane of collecting duct cells, at least in the cortex, is under the influence of different physiological factors, such as hormones, and variations in the surface amplification occur concomitantly with changes in ion transport capacity (Wade et al., 1979).

The cytoplasm contains a small or moderate number of organelles. There are a moderate number of rounded or elongated mitochondria, which show no obvious orientation in relation to the plasma membrane (Fig. 5). Endoplasmic reticulum is sparse but free ribosomes are relatively numerous. The inner medullary collecting duct cells contain rather abundant Golgi complexes and lysosomes compared to the principal cells of the cortical and outer medullary collecting ducts (Kaissling and Kriz, 1979). Many of the lysosomes are of the "lipofuscin granule" type (Bulger and Trump, 1966; Bohman and Maunsbach, 1972), while others are multivesicular bodies (Bulger and Trump, 1966). In the apical part of the cytoplasm small (0.2–0.3 μm) vesicles are seen, some of which have an outer "coat." Small (0.2–0.4 μm) lipid inclusions may be found in the basal part of the cytoplasm (Bohman and Jensen, 1976). Microtubules and filaments have been observed, but in spite of the increasing amount of evidence that they are specifically involved in the response to ADH (Dousa and Barnes, 1974) ultrastructural information about these organelles in the collecting duct cells is very sparse.

The nucleus is oriented basally in the cell. In several studies, the cytoplasm of the collecting duct cells has been reported to be unusually "clear" or "pale" and the nucleus has been depicted as spherical with a very homogeneous distribution of the chromatin. However, this appearance may partly be due to swelling of the cells during fixation with fixatives of too low an osmolality (Bohman, 1974).

2.3.2. Henle's Loop

The descending and ascending thin limbs of Henle's loop from the juxtamedullary (long) nephrons are found in the inner zone. They form hairpin turns at different levels and this progressive reduction in the number of loops contributes to the tapering off of the papilla. Although the descending thin limb of long nephrons has slightly higher and more complex epithelial cells in the outer zone and in the outermost levels of the inner zone, both limbs have a very flat and relatively simple epithelium in the inner zone (Osvaldo and Latta, 1966a). The total cell height is in most places 0.5–1.0 μm and the cytoplasm contains only a few small, rounded mitochondria, occasional small cisternae of rough endoplasmic reticulum, some free ribosomes, and few other organelles (Fig. 6).

The question of whether or not a significant active sodium transport could occur over the epithelium of the thin ascending limb has been much discussed. It was suggested that such an active transport constituted the so-called "single effect," which then was reinforced by the countercurrent multiplication system in the medulla, but the ultrastructural appearance of the epithelium of the thin limbs was not in agreement with this concept (Osvaldo and Latta, 1966a). More recent models of the countercurrent multiplication, however (Kokko and Rector, 1972) seem to be able to explain this mechanism without postulating an active transport in the thin limbs. Instead, emphasis is placed on the different passive permeability characteristics of the descending and ascending thin limbs.

Recently, an elegant ultrastructural correlate to the differences in permeability of the various parts of the thin limbs was described by Schwartz and Venkatachalam (1974). They found that the descending thin limb has in its first part (in the inner stripe of the outer zone) epithelial cells with extensive and complex lateral interdigitations with each other and very shallow tight junctions (Type I). Somewhere in the outer level of the inner zone the epithelium changes into cells with few lateral interdigitations and with deep tight junctions (Type II). The latter type constitutes most of the ascending thin limb. The epithelium of the thin descending segment of the the loop, the epithelium again changes to one with complex interdigitations and shallow tight junctions (Type I), which makes up the whole of the ascending thin limb. The epithelium of the thin descending segment of the short nephrons is of Type II only.

2.3.3. *Blood Vessels*

The blood vessels supplying the renal medulla are derived from the efferent arterioles of the juxtamedullary glomeruli. The arterioles break up into the descending vasa recta, which run down parallel to each other in the vascular bundles. As the vascular bundles traverse the medulla a large part of the descending vasa recta leaves the bundles to form a dense capillary network in the inner stripe. The rich blood supply gives the inner stripe a dark red color in a freshly cut kidney while the inner zone is whitish. Because of the successive loss of vasa recta from the vascular bundles the latter taper off considerably as they pass through the inner stripe and outer part of the inner zone. In the depth of the inner zone this architectural element becomes rather inconspicuous.

In the inner zone all vessels are of capillary structure and form a relatively sparse, elongated plexus. Two types of medullary capillaries, fenestrated and nonfenestrated (continuous) were described in early electron microscopic investigations (Sakaguchi and Suzuki, 1958). Recent studies (Schwartz *et al.*, 1976) have proven that the descending vessels are those with continuous endothelium and that the ascending vessels all have a fenestrated endothelium.

The continuous endothelium of the descending vessels, which has a thickness of 0.1–0.5 μm, is characterized by a multitude of micropinocytotic vesicles in the cytoplasm. These are about 700 Å in diameter and are most abundant close to the basal (outer) surface of the endothelial cells where numerous small invaginations of the plasma membrane are also seen.

The fenestrated endothelium is in most places very thin (Fig. 6) and has numerous round fenestrations 500–800 Å in diameter, which are bridged by a thin (about 40 Å) diaphragm. In the fenestrated regions, the endothelial thickness is about 600–1000 Å, while in intervening nonfenestrated regions it may be 0.1–0.5 μm. In the region containing the nucleus it is several micrometers thick.

2.3.4. *Interstitium*

The volume of the interstitium (here defined as the tissue compartment outside the tubules and vessels) increases from 10–20% of the tissue volume in the outer zone, through the inner zone, to over 40% at the papilla tip (Bohman and Jensen, 1976, Knepper *et al.*, 1977).

The interstitium contains interstitial cells and an extracellular space. The latter is filled with a rather evenly distributed loose flocculent material (Fig. 6). This represents the extracellular matrix substances, i.e., sulfated and nonsulfated glucosaminoglycans (Furusato, 1977), which are abundant in the renal medulla. The rate of production of sulfated glucosaminoglycans seems to be influenced by changes in the osmotic gradient in the tissue (Farber *et al.*, 1971) but the theory that changes in the composition of the extracellular material are of major importance for the regulation of water excretion (Ginetzinsky, 1958) has not been generally accepted. The thin basal laminae of collecting ducts, thin limbs, and vessels outline the borders of the interstitial space. Numerous wisps of basement-membrane-like material are also found scattered in the interstitium and around the interstitial cells (Fig. 6). In many species small bundles of collagen fibrils are also present.

The interstitial cells of the rat (Bohman, 1974) and rabbit (Bulger and Nagle, 1973) renal medulla are of three types. Type 1 is the lipid-containing type which is present in the inner stripe of the outer zone and throughout the inner zone. This type will be described and discussed in further detail in the succeeding sections. Interstitial cell Type 2 is a lymphocytelike cell that is found in the cortex, outer zone, and outer levels of the inner zone (Bohman, 1974). Type 3 is a pericyte that is found in the outer zone (Moffat, 1967a) and in the outer levels of the inner zone. It is always closely related to the descending vasa recta where it is embedded between two layers of the basal lamina (Bohman, 1974). Thus, in the major part of the inner zone all interstitial cells are of Type 1.

3. THE INTERSTITIAL CELLS

3.1. Occurrence and Distribution

As indicated previously, only the lipid-containing or Type 1 interstitial cells (Bohman, 1974) will be discussed here, since this is the cell type that has been suggested to be a new endocrine cell type (Muirhead *et al.*, 1975).

The ultrastructure of the Type 1 interstitial cells has been studied primarily in the rat (Novikoff, 1960; Gloor and Neiditsch-Halff, 1965; Osvaldo and Latta, 1966*b*; Bulger and Trump, 1966; Abrahams and Pirani, 1966) but ultrastructurally very similar cells have also been described in the rabbit (Johnson and Darnton, 1967; Bulger and Nagle, 1973; Bohman and Jensen, 1978), the gerbil (Bohman and Jensen, 1978), the dog (Bulger *et al.*, 1979), and man (Bulger *et al.*, 1967; Mandal *et al.*, 1979). Light microscopic studies have suggested that similar cells are present in the renal medulla of a number of other species, such as the guinea pig (Renaut and Dubreuil, 1907), the kangaroo rat (Vimtrup and Schmidt-Nielsen, 1952), and other species (Sternberg *et al.*, 1956). Experimental studies indicating endocrine antihypertensive functions of these cells have been performed only in rats, rabbits, and dogs (Muirhead *et al.*, 1975).

The abundance of interstitial cells may vary somewhat among species. They seem to be somewhat less prominent in humans than· in rodents (Bulger *et al.*, 1967). The concept that they are particularly abundant in the kidneys of desert rodents (Vimtrup and Schmidt-Nielsen, 1952; Sternberg *et al.*, 1956; Gloor and Neiditsch-Halff, 1965) could not be confirmed in a recent comparative study (Bohman and Jensen, 1978).

The distribution of different types of interstitial cells in the kidney has been studied in only a few species. In the rat (Bohman, 1974) the Type 1 interstitial cells are predominant in the inner stripe of the outer zone as well as in the inner zone. In the apical half of the inner zone of rats, rabbits, and gerbils it is the only type of interstitial cell. In the gerbil the interstitial cells increase considerably in number toward the papilla tip, whereas this increase is less pronounced in the rat and the rabbit (Bohman and Jensen, 1978).

3.2. The Ultrastructure of Type 1 Interstitial Cells

3.2.1. *Cell Shape and Topographical Relations*

As mentioned above, the interstitial cells are located in the medullary interstitium between the collecting ducts, loops of Henle, and capillaries. The cell shape is very varied. It may be rounded, fusiform, or, most commonly, irregularly star-shaped with long cytoplasmic projections (Figs. 4 and 6). In the outer zone the Type 1 cells often have a very irregular shape with large invaginations, which are enclosed by thin cytoplasmic walls (Fig. 10). In longitudinal sections, cut parallel to the tubules and vessels of the medulla, it can be seen that the interstitial cells in many places are rather evenly distributed (Renaut and Dubreuil, 1907). They are extended between the thin limbs and vessels at relatively regular distances and many but not all interstitial cells have a somewhat flattened appearance when viewed from this aspect (Fig. 7). Close to the tip of the papilla, where the interstitial space becomes very wide, the interstitial cells to a large extent lose this characteristic orientation and most of them have a round shape.

At the ultrastructural level it can be seen that the cytoplasmic projections or the bodies of the interstitial cells often have a very close and regular relation to the basal laminae of loops of Henle and capillaries. One interstitial cell may have several projections that are in contact with a number of capillaries and thin limbs (Fig. 6). Apart from the close and regular apposition to the outer surface of the basal lamina, no specialized contact regions or structures are found. Very rarely an interstitial cell projection is seen to penetrate the basal lamina, of a blood vessel (Fig. 8).

In contrast to the striking relationship between interstitial cells, thin limbs and vessels, a close contact between interstitial cells and collecting ducts is practically never seen.

3.2.2. *Plasma Membrane and Surface Specializations*

The plasma membrane of the interstitial cells has an ordinary triple-layered appearance with a thickness of 80–90 Å in routine preparations. The surface coat is not prominent. No gaps in the plasma membrane are seen in well-fixed preparations.

Specialized cell junctions occur between projections from two interstitial cells or between two apposed surfaces of the same cell (Osvaldo and Latta, 1966*b*, Bulger and Trump, 1966) (Fig. 9). They have been described as an obliteration of the intercellular space over a rather large area, creating a five-layered structure, which thus resembles a very large tight junction (Osvaldo and Latta, 1966*b*). However, it appears unlikely that they represent true tight junctions. Rather, they resemble gap junctions, as observed between other types of interstitial and endocrine cells (Larsen, 1977; Burghardt and Anderson, 1979). Recently, Schiller and Taugner (1979) have presented freeze-fracture data indicating both tight and gap junction structures in these areas.

Occasional cilia may be seen extending from the surface of interstitial cells (Bulger and Trump, 1966) (Figs. 10 and 11).

3.2.3. *Nucleus*

The nucleus may have different shapes according to the general shape of the cell. In some species, such as rabbits (Bohman and Jensen, 1978) it often has several deep invaginations, giving it a lobulated shape. A moderate amount of heterochromatin is present, mainly as a peripheral rim inside the nuclear membrane. Nucleoli are not prominent.

As in many other cell types, continuity between the outer layer of the nuclear membrane and the endoplasmic reticulum may be seen in some places, but dilation of the perinuclear cisternae is not prominent in well-fixed cells (Bohman, 1974).

3.2.4. *Rough Endoplasmic Reticulum*

Cisternae of rough endoplasmic reticulum are a constant finding in the cytoplasm of the interstitial cells, although the amount is variable. The rough endoplasmic reticulum is especially abundant in the outer levels of the inner zone and in the outer zone of the medulla.

In some interstitial cells cisternae of the rough endoplasmic reticulum are expanded and filled with a flocculent material of moderate electron density that probably represents newly synthesized protein (Novikoff, 1960; Osvaldo and Latta, 1966*b*; Bulger and Trump, 1966; Bohman, 1974) (Figs. 12 and 13). These "filled" cisternae should be distinguished from the widely dilated, empty-looking cisternae of rough or smooth endoplasmic reticulum that have been repeatedly described as characteristic for the interstitial cells. In well-fixed tissue such highly dilated cisternae, as well as dilated perinuclear cisternae (Fig. 14), are virtually absent and probably represent fixation artifacts (Bohman, 1974). Certain other features described in the literature, such as lipid droplets bulging into a widely dilated empty-looking cisterna or lipid droplets lying seemingly within cisternae, may also arise from swelling of the endoplasmic reticulum during fixation.

In addition to the rough-sufaced endoplasmic reticulum the cytoplasm of the interstitial cells contains a moderate number of free ribosomes in the form of polysomes.

3.2.5. *Smooth Cytoplasmic Membranes*

The interstitial cells do not contain a well-developed tubular smooth endoplasmic reticulum comparable to that of hepatocytes, adrenocortical cells, or small intestine epithelial cells. However, smooth cytoplasmic membranes with a thickness of 60–70 Å are often seen in the interstitial cells either in the form of relatively large cisternae or as small vesicles. The smooth cisternal elements are often continuous with the rough-surfaced endoplasmic reticulum (Figs. 13 and 15).

The smooth cytomembranes are often seen in close relation to the cytoplasmic lipid droplets. They may form concentric "whorls" around one or a group of lipid droplets (Bulger and Trump, 1966) (Fig. 15) and the innermost membranes may be very closely apposed to part of the lipid droplet surface (Fig. 15, inset). Single smooth-surfaced cisternae and smooth-surfaced vesicles may have the same close relation to lipid droplets (Bohman and Jensen, 1978) (Fig. 13).

3.2.6. *Mitochondria*

Mitochondria are moderate in number in the interstitial cells. They show no preferential orientation, neither towards the plasma membrane nor towards the lipid droplets. The mitochondria are usually enlongated and have no striking ultrastructural features (Figs. 6 and 12). Dense matrix granules are very few. Occasionally, crystalloid inclusions are found (Osvaldo and Latta, 1966b).

Peroxisomes have not been described in the interstitial cells.

3.2.7. *Lysosomes and Vacuoles*

A small number of lysosomelike bodies are seen in the interstitial cells (Fig. 13). These probably give rise to the acid phosphatase activity seen by light microscope histochemistry (Bulger and Trump, 1966; Nissen and Andersen, 1971). These lysosomes are 0.2–0.8 μm in diameter, are limited by a 90-Å-thick, triple-layered membrane, and may have a variable content (Bohman and Maunsbach, 1972). Some have a homogeneously granular content while others contain membraneous material or areas of low electron density, suggesting the presence of a lipid material.

Endocytic vacuoles or invaginations of the plasma membrane are rather sparse in the interstitial cells. This finding indicates that endocytosis is not a very active process in the interstitial cells under normal conditions. However, when challenged with foreign proteins such as horseradish peroxidase (Straus, 1971; Bohman, unpublished observations) or with particulate material (Bohman, 1980) the interstitial cells of both the inner and outer zone show endocytotic capacity. The reason why ferritin, given intravenously to normal and potassium-deficient rats (Morrison and Schneeberger-Keeley, 1969), accumulates exclusively in the interstitial cells of the outer zone is not clear.

3.2.8. *Filaments and Microtubules*

Bundles of 60-Å-thick filaments are in most interstitial cells seen immediately inside and parallel to the plasma membrane (Fig. 12). They are particularly abundant in those regions where the plasma membrane is closely related to a thin limb or capillary and are oriented mainly in a horizontal plane, perpendicular to the long axis of the medulla. It is possible that these filaments contain actin although this has not been directly demonstrated. Microtubules are also present (Fig. 15). These show no obvious specific localization or orientation.

3.2.9. *Cylindrical Bodies*

A peculiar type of cytoplasmic cylindrical bodies was first described by Bulger *et al.* (1966) in the interstitial cells of dehydrated rats. Further information was provided by Moffat (1967*b*), Osvaldo-Decima and Latta (1970), Osvaldo-Decima (1973), and Ledingham and Simpson (1973). The latter study showed that the occurrence of this organelle is not a response to dehydration. It was found sporadically without striking quantitative differences in a variety of experimental conditions.

The bodies, which are relatively rarely observed (Fig. 16), occur in bundles of up to 50 parallel cylinders. Each cylinder is 1300–1800 Å in diameter and may be over 11 μm in length (Ledingham and Simpson, 1973). The wall of the cylindrical tube is about 130–140 Å thick and in oblique sections a line pattern with a 170 Å periodicity appears (Bulger *et al.*, 1966).

Further information about the substructure of the cylindrical bodies can be obtained in high-magnification micrographs (Fig. 17). In cross sections of the wall two layers can be resolved, each about 50–60 Å thick. The intervening electron-lucent layer is thus about 20 Å thick. Each of the two 50- to 60-Å layers is resolved as a triple-layered structure with two electron-dense layers and a middle electron-lucent layer.

Bulger *et al.* (1966) suggested that the cylindrical bodies are derivatives of the endoplasmic reticulum since the walls of the cylinders seemed to be continuous in some places with the endoplasmic reticulum membranes. The lumen of the cylinder, filled with a flocculent material, was not, however, continuous with the cisterna of the endoplasmic reticulum, but separated from it by a thin membrane (Bulger *et al.*, 1966). These observations were confirmed by Ledingham and Simpson (1973) and are also in good agreement with the present demonstration that the wall of the cylinders in high magnification can be resolved as two parallel triple-layered membranes, each with a thickness of about 60 Å. The latter correspond very closely to the ultrastructure of the endoplasmic reticulum membranes (without ribosomes). In fact, this structure could be explained on the basis of the hypothetical model for the connection between cylindrical bodies and endoplasmic reticulum drawn by Bulger *et al.* (1966, Fig. 2) if it is assumed that the membrane separating the cylinder lumen is of the same structure as the membrane of the rest of the endoplasmic reticulum cisterna and that both these membranes are reflected off to form the double wall of the cylinder.

The functional significance of this endoplasmic reticulum derivative remains obscure. It should be pointed out that very similar, although not identical, structures continuous with the endoplasmic reticulum have also been described in other cell types (King and Tibbits, 1977), indicating that this is not a specific reaction pattern of the interstitial cells.

3.2.10. *Lipid Inclusions (Lipid Droplets)*

The cytoplasmic lipid inclusions or lipid droplets are the hallmark of the Type 1 interstitial cells. In contrast to the cylindrical bodies, the lipid droplets are present in all Type 1 interstitial cells although in varying numbers (Fig. 7). The lipid droplets have a smooth round shape in perfusion-fixed material (Figs. 6, 13, and 15). They usually have a completely homogeneous, rather electron-lucent content as observed after glutaraldehyde fixation, postosmication, embedding in Vestopal or Epon, thin sectioning, and double staining. However, the electron density may vary somewhat with variations in fixation methods, section thickness, staining procedures, and possibly also with physiological variations of the composition of the lipid material.

The size of the lipid droplets varies within each cell and the size distribution as well as the number of lipid droplets varies from species to species. In the rat, the lipid droplets make up 2–4% of the interstitial cell volume depending, on, for example, diuresis (Bohman and Jensen, 1976). The mean diameter of the rat lipid droplets has been estimated at about 0.4–0.5 μm (Bohman and Jensen, 1976) and lipid droplet profiles with a diameter of up to 1 μm are frequently observed in the sections. In both rabbits and gerbils the lipid droplets are smaller than in the rat. Profiles with a diameter of more than 0.5 μm are rare in these species (Bohman and Jensen, 1978).

The lipid droplets of the interstitial cells have been isolated in relatively pure form from homogenates of rat (Nissen and Bojesen, 1969; Bohman and Maunsbach, 1969, 1972) and rabbit (Änggård *et al.*, 1972) renal medulla and were found to consist mainly of triglycerides and small but variable amounts of cholesterol esters and phospholipids (see Chapter 6 of this volume). The lipid droplets do not have a surrounding (triple-layered) membrane (Osvaldo and Latta, 1966b) but are often seen to be limited by a 20- to 50-Å-thick, electron-dense outer zone (Bohman and Maunsbach, 1972) (Fig. 13). This thin rim is not clearly discerned in sections away from the center of the droplet. In some places, a coarsely granular electron-dense material (Fig. 15, inset) or a lamellar material with a 40 Å periodicity (Fig. 18, inset) can be seen associated with the outer zone of the lipid droplets (Bohman and Jensen, 1978). The thin electron-dense outer border is similar in ultrastructure to that surrounding chylomicrons, which contains a monolayer of phospholipids in addition to some cholesterol and protein (Salpeter and Zilversmit, 1968; Blanchette-Mackie and Scow, 1973).

Both the granular and the lamellar electron-dense material is often located in parts of the droplet periphery that are close to smooth 60- to 70-Å cytoplasmic membranes (Bohman and Jensen, 1978) (Fig. 15). The chemical composition of the different types of electron-dense material has not been determined. However, since the electron-dense outer zone of chylomicrons is known to be composed *inter alia* of a phospholipid monolayer, and since a lamellar structure with a 40 Å periodicity closely resembles the structure of phospholipid "myelin figures" (Stoeckenius, 1962), it is possible that the material seen at the lipid droplet periphery also contains polar lipids. This is interesting in view of the fact that a specific functional role for the interstitial cell lipid droplets in the turnover of membrane phsopholipids has been suggested (Comai *et al.*, 1975; Bojesen, Chapter 6 of this volume). However, it should be pointed out that a thin electron-dense outer border as well as electron-dense granular and lamellar material is seen associated with other types of lipid droplets that are not believed to have the same function (Palade, 1959; Thoenes, 1962; Schoefl, 1968).

In addition to the ordinary lipid droplets described above, which are present in virtually all of the interstitial cells, occasional cells contain a few very large or "giant" lipid droplets that may have a diameter of up to 5 μm (Bohman and Jensen, 1978). Such droplets are more frequently seen in the gerbil than in the rat or rabbit medulla. They seem to take up a very large part of the cytoplasm and are often surrounded by large amounts of concentrically arranged lamellar material with a 40 Å periodicity (Bohman and Jensen, 1978) (Fig. 18).

3.3. Experimental Alterations of the Interstitial Cell Lipid Droplets

Since the first studies showing that the number of lipid droplets was altered in different physiological or pathophysiological conditions (Mandal *et al.*, 1967; Nissen, 1968a,b) a number of studies of experimentally induced alterations in the lipid droplets have been presented. The main results obtained in a number of such studies have been summarized in Table 1, where the investigations have been grouped according to the general type of experimental situation studied. Potentially, such studies should be valuable in elucidating the function of the interstitial cells. However, so far results have often been difficult to interpret. This is largely the result of the complex and partially unknown mechanisms involved in many of the experimental models, but also of the fact that contradictory results have sometimes been obtained and that considerable species differences seem to exist.

Furthermore, methodological problems in the estimation of the amount of stored lipid may be of some significance (Bohman and Jensen, 1976). Since many of the lipid droplets have a diameter close to the resolution of the light microscope (0.25 μm) underestimations may be obtained in light microscopic studies. In most of the cited studies (Table 1) the *number* of lipid droplets per cell or per unit area was determined by light or electron microscopy. However, in order to estimate the amount of stored lipid, both the *number and size* of droplets must be taken into account. This can be done by using stereological methods for the determination of the relative volume (volume density) of lipid droplets. The major methodological problem, however, may be the fact that a possible osmotic swelling of the medullary tissue and the interstitial cells without a concomitant swelling of the lipid droplets will create a false decrease both in the number of lipid droplets per cell profile or unit area and in the relative volume of lipid droplets. The papilla with its high tissue osmolality has a considerable tendency to swell during fixation (see Section 2.2). It is possible that the degree of swelling can differ under different physiological or experimental circumstances where the tissue electrolyte and urea concentrations have been altered to various degrees. Therefore, rigorous control of possible volume changes of the tissue is desirable in this type of study. Since this may be difficult to attain in practice, small or moderate changes in the amount of stored lipid in the interstitial cells may be difficult to detect.

Bojesen (Chapter 6 in this volume) has advocated biochemical determination of triglyceride glycerol as a better way to assess the amount of lipid stored in the interstitial cells. Such biochemical data have been in good agreement with electron microscope stereological determinations of the volume density of lipid droplets in water-loaded animals (Bojesen, chapter 6 of this volume; Bohman and Jensen, 1976). However, the biochemical method rests upon the assumption that all the extractable triglycerides are derived from the interstitial cells. This condition may not be completely fulfilled since the collecting duct cells also contain cytoplasmic inclusions that ultrastructurally suggest the presence of neutral lipids, albeit in relatively small amounts (Bohman and Jensen, 1976).

3.4. Theories about the Possible Functions of the Interstitial Cells

A number of functions have been suggested for the interstitial cells with more or less experimental support. Some of these suggested functions will be mentioned and briefly commented on below. It should be noted that several of the functions discussed are not mutually exclusive. On the contrary, the interstitial cells may have more than one function and some of the functions discussed below may theoretically be interconnected and form

TABLE 1

Studies of Alterations in the Lipid Droplets of the Interstitial Cells in the Renal Medulla under Different Experimental Conditions

Experimental model or treatment	Species	Alteration of lipid droplet	Method[a]	Other comments	Reference
Hypertension (unilateral nephrectomy + DOCA + salt)	Rat	↓	EM, no.		Mandal et al. (1967)
	Rat	↓	LM + EM, no.	Severe vascular lesions observed in the kidneys	Muehrcke et al. (1969)
Hypertension ("postsalt")	Rat	↓	LM, no.	No alteration by unilateral nephrectomy only. Hypertensive rats also had low papillary sodium concentration	Tobian et al. (1969)
Hypertension (renal artery clipping)	Rat	↓	LM, no.	Both in clipped and untouched kidney. Good correlation between granule count and papillary sodium concentration	Ishii and Tobian (1969)
Hypertension ("post-Goldblatt")	Rat	↓	LM, no.	Hypertensive animals had low sodium concentration in the papilla	Tobian and Ishii (1969)
Hypertension (66% renal ablation)	Rat	↑	LM, no.		Muirhead et al. (1977)
Hypertension (renal artery clipping)	Rabbit	↓	EM, no.	Transient decrease	Nekrasova et al. (1973)
	Rat	↓	LM, no.	Both in right and left kidneys, not well correlated with degree of hypertension, decrease also in animals with clipping but having no hypertension	Latta et al. (1975)
	Rat	↓	LM, no.	Nonclipped kidney studied after 20–30 days. Decrease only in malignant course of hypertension, prevented by positive sodium balance	Szokol et al. (1979)

Condition	Species		Method	Comment	Reference
	Rat	0	EM, vol.	The nonclamped kidneys studied in hypertensive and resistant rats at intervals between 3 weeks and 1 year	Perov and Postnov (1976b)
Hypertension (malignant)	Man	→	EM. no.		Muehrcke et al. (1970)
Hypertension (spontaneous)	Rat	→	EM, no.		Mandal et al. (1974, 1975)
	Rat	0	LM, subj.		Simpson (1970)
	Rat	↑	EM, vol.	Rats 1 year old, no difference from control at 1.5 months' age	Perov and Postnov (1976a)
	Rat	↑	LM, no.		Nissen (1968b)
Salt repletion of salt-depleted animals	Rat	↑	LM, no.		Nissen (1968a)
Acute hydration of dehydrated animals	Rat	↑	EM, vol.	Both size and number of lipid droplets increased	Bohman and Jensen (1976, 1978)
Water load (5 hr)	Rat	↑	EM, vol.		Bohman and Jensen (1978)
	Rabbit	→	LM + EM, subj.		Bohman and Jensen (1978)
	Gerbil	→	LM + EM, subj.		Bohman and Jensen (1978)
Water diuresis (2 weeks)	Rat	→	LM, no.	Returned to control values after 3 months of water diuresis. Strong correlation between lipid counts and papillary sodium concentration	Azar et al. (1970)
	Rat	→	LM, no.	Decrease in rats on butter fat diet, not in rats fed safflower oil (polyunsaturated lipids)	Tobian and Azar (1971)

(Continued)

TABLE 1 (Continued)

Experimental model or treatment	Species	Alteration of lipid droplet	Method[a]	Other comments	Reference
Water diuresis (24 hr)	Rat	↓	Biochem.	Good correlation between degree of diuresis and amount of triglycerides	Bojesen (Chapter 6)
Saline diuresis (48 hr)	Rat	↑	Biochem.		Bojesen (Chapter 6)
Water deprivation (24 hr)	Rat	↓	Biochem.		Bojesen (Chapter 6)
	Rat	↓	EM, subj.		Osvaldo and Latta (1970)
(36 hr)	Rat	↓	LM, subj.		Simpson (1970)
Indomethacin	Rabbit	↑	EM, no.	In vivo experiments, dose-dependent effect	Comai et al. (1974, 1975)
	Rat	↓	LM, no.	In vivo experiments	Limas et al. (1976)
	Rat	↑	EM, vol.	In vitro experiments on cultured interstitial cells from rat	Muirhead et al. (1975), Pitcock et al. (1976)
Hydronephrosis	Rabbit	↑	EM, no.	48 or 72 hr of ureter ligation, slight or no change in contralateral kidney	Comai et al. (1974, 1975), Bohman (unpublished)
	Rat	↑	LM, subj.		Bohman (unpublished)
Furosemide	Rat	↓	LM, subj.		Simpson (1970)
Mercuric chloride-induced acute tubular necrosis	Rat	↓	EM, subj.	Dose-dependent	Bulger and Siegel (1975)

[a] LM, light microscopic investigation; EM, electron microscopic investigation; subj., subjective evaluation of number and size of lipid droplets; no., number of lipid droplets counted per cell or unit area; vol., volume density (volume fraction) of lipid droplets estimated by stereological techniques; biochem., based on biochemical determination of triglyceride in whole papilla extract.

part of some physiologically or pathophysiologically important systemic mechanism.

3.4.1. Mechanical Function

A supporting function for the interstitial cells has been considered since the 19th century (Bowman, 1842). The special arrangement of these cells perpendicular to the tubules and vessels, as well as their close relationship to the basal laminae of the loop of Henle and vessels, is consistent with this hypothesis.

The abundant filaments inside the plasma membrane suggest that the interstitial cells may be motile, a characteristic which would be consistent with a more active mechanical role—e.g., changing the form or size of the interstitial space—but there is at present no experimental evidence to support this theory. The hypothesis that the interstitial cells could constrict the blood vessels (Novikoff, 1960) appears unlikely since, although the cytoplasmic processes of the interstitial cells are found in close apposition to the vessels, they rarely enclose more than a small part of the vessel circumference.

3.4.2. Monitoring Function

The very close and regular relationship between the interstitial cell suface and the basal surface of thin limbs and capillaries suggests some kind of interaction between these structures. Although this is not ultrastructurally evident in the interstitial cell cytoplasm, one may speculate that the interstitial cells could have a polarity, with the side facing the thin limb being the "receptor" side and that facing a capillary being the "effector" side, or vice versa. The interstitial cells could in such a case monitor the composition of the fluid in the loop of Henle and react accordingly, e.g., by secreting some substance into the blood.

3.4.3. Metabolic Function

The possibility that the lipid droplets of the interstitial cells represent metabolic energy stores appears unlikely since: (1) the lipid droplets have a special fatty acid composition that is quite different from that of, for example, adipose tissue and plasma lipids (Nissen and Bojesen, 1969); (2) fatty acid oxidation is not a major pathway in the renal medulla (Lee et al., 1962); and (3) the close relation between mitochondria and lipid inclusions seen in some other cell types such as hepatocytes (Palade, 1959) and cardiac-muscle cells (Maunsbach and Wirsén, 1966) is rarely observed in the interstitial cells (Bohman and Jensen, 1978).

Alternative theories hold that fatty acids from the lipid droplet triglycerides are specifically transesterified into membrane phospholipids (Bojesen,
1974, Bojesen *et al.*, 1976). This theory will be presented in detail in
Chapter 6 of this volume.

3.4.4. *Secretory Function*

A secretory function has been suggested for the interstitial cells by
many investigators. This suggestion is based on the observation of a well-
developed rough endoplasmic reticulum (Novikoff, 1960; Bulger and
Trump, 1966) and the lipid droplets which have been regarded as some kind
of secretory granules (Muehrcke, *et al.*, 1965; Nissen, 1968b; Fourman and
Moffat, 1971; Mandal *et al.*, 1975).

It can at present not be determined with certainty whether the
abundant rough endoplasmic reticulum and the lipid droplets are functionally directly related or reflect different functional aspects of the interstitial cells. However, it seems clear that the lipid droplets are not secretory
granules in the usual sense. Although it has been suggested that the lipid
droplets are secreted as such either through gaps in the plasma membrane
(Fourman and Moffat, 1971) or by exocytosis (Mandal *et al.*, 1975) this
appears unlikely. Gaps in the plasma membrane as well as extracellular
lipid droplets are extremely rare in successfully fixed medullary· tissue
(Bohman, 1974; Schifferli, 1975). Exocytosis has not been clearly documented and seems difficult to explain in the absence of a well-defined
membrane around the droplet that could fuse with the plasma membrane
during this process. It seems more likely that the deposition and removal of
the lipid material is mediated by the activity of enzymes within the cell.
Some of these enzymes may be located in the smooth cytoplasmic
membranes sometimes seen in close apposition to the lipid droplet surface
(Bohman, 1974; Bohman and Jensen, 1976, 1978). It has not been directly
established whether the material thus released within the cell is directly
secreted, utilized as a precursor in the synthesis of some secretory product,
or utilized in some other metabolic pathway.

3.4.4a. Interstitial Substances. The interstitial cells have repeatedly
been suggested to be the site of synthesis of the extracellular matrix that is
abundant in the medulla, especially in the apical part (Novikoff, 1960;
Gloor and Neiditsch-Halff, 1965; Osvaldo and Latta, 1966b; Bulger and
Trump, 1966). The observation of expanded cisternae of rough endoplasmic
reticulum, which contain a flocculent material with a certain ultrastructural
resemblance to the extracellular material, supports this theory (Novikoff,
1960). However, it is puzzling that the rough endoplasmic reticulum is more
prominent in the interstitial cells in the outer zone where the interstitium is
relatively narrow and the extracellular material less abundant.

3.4.4b. Prostaglandins. During the last 10 years many investigators have tended to regard the interstitial cells of the renal medulla as a specialized prostaglandin-producing cell type and the lipid droplets as a store of prostaglandin precursor (Lee, 1973; Comai *et al.*, 1975; Limas *et al.*, 1976; Verberckmoes *et al.*, 1976). However, this theory (Mandal *et al.*, 1967; Nissen and Andersen, 1968), which emanated from the observation of a lipid-containing cell type in the renal medulla that had just been found to have a high prostaglandin content (Lee *et al.*, 1967), has generally been based on rather indirect evidence (for discussion, see Bohman 1977, 1979).

Direct measurements of the prostaglandin-synthesizing capacity in isolated cell preparations have shown that close to 50% of the prostaglandin synthetase of the medulla is located in the collecting duct cells while the remaining 50% is present in other cell types of the medulla (including the interstitial cells) (Bohman, 1977; W. L. Smith, personal communication). Thus, although the interstitial cells have prostaglandin synthetase activity (Zusman, Chapter 9 of this volume), this is by no means a unique feature of the interstitial cells and there is little support for the theory that prostaglandin production is their main function. The fact that isolated lipid droplets contain a certain amount of arachidonic acid (Nissen and Bojesen, 1969; Änggård *et al.*, 1972) does not necessarily mean that they are directly involved in prostaglandin synthesis. The same or higher relative concentrations of arachidonic acid are present in the microsomal and mitochondrial phospholipids in the medulla (Änggård *et al.*, 1972) and there is some evidence that these fatty acids are the main precursor pool for prostaglandin synthesis (Kunze and Vogt, 1971; Nishikawa *et al.*, 1977).

3.4.4c. Antihypertensive Substances. The most exciting theory about the functional role of the interstitial cells is that they may be endocrine cells involved in the regulation of blood pressure. This theory will be treated in detail in other chapters of this volume and only some aspects will be briefly discussed here.

The first suggestion that the interstitial cells reacted to changes in blood pressure was presented by Mandal *et al.* (1967), who found a reduction of the number of interstitial cell lipid droplets in experimentally hypertensive rats. However, the same group of investigators (Muehrcke *et al.*, 1969) also noted that significant alterations in the number of lipid droplets occurred only in those experimental groups where arteriolosclerosis and glomerulosclerosis were prominent, suggesting that the direct cause of the decrease in lipid droplets was not the elevated blood pressure *per se* but secondary derangements in the medullary circulation. The latter possibility has found strong support in studies by Tobian *et al.* (see Table 1), which have shown that in different types of experimental hypertension the number of lipid droplets is strongly correlated with the medullary sodium and urea content. The latter is reduced in many forms of hypertension and this reduction may be due to reversible or irreversible hemodynamic alterations (Muehrcke *et al.*, 1969; Ganguli, Chapter 8 in this volume).

New support for a role of the interstitial cells in blood pressure regulation was obtained when Muirhead *et al.* found that renomedullary tissue transplants, which have a blood-pressure-lowering effect in different types of experimental hypertension, consisted mainly of one proliferating cell type that was characterized by numerous cytoplasmic lipid droplets. On the basis of their morphology, these cells were identified by Muirhead *et al.* (1972) as interstitial cells. Initially, there was some uncertainty about the identification of the cells and the cytoplasmic lipid droplets were referred to as "vesicles" or "membrane-limited vesicles" (Muirhead *et al.*, 1970, 1972). Furthermore, cytoplasmic accumulation of neutral lipids appears to be a common reaction pattern for different cell types, especially when removed from their natural environment (Paul, 1965; Cohn *et al.*, 1966; Zucker-Franklin *et al.*, 1978), and is not in itself pathognomonic for the interstitial cells. However, altogether it seems highly likely that the identification of the cells in the transplants as interstitial cells was correct and many studies have since been carried out by Muirhead's group and by others to further elucidate the antihypertensive properties of the interstitial cells. The mediator of the antihypertensive effect appears to be a lipid but its molecular structure is not known. It is generally assumed that the cytoplasmic lipid droplets of the interstitial cells represent some kind of precursor depot, but their precise relation to the antihypertensive lipid has not been clarified. The nature of the "signal" that stimulates the activity of the interstitial cells is likewise not known. It may be alterations in the medullary blood flow, as suggested by Tobian and Ishii (1969), but there are also other possibilities, such as hormone stimulation (Florendo *et al.*, 1978; Zusman, Chapter 9 in this volume) or changes in the electrolyte composition. It seems clear that the function of the cells is in some way related to the sodium content of the papilla (Table 1). It is hoped that parallel studies of interstitial cells *in situ* in the medulla and transplanted or cultured interstitial cells will resolve these questions.

REFERENCES

Abrahams, C., and Pirani, C. L., 1966, The renal papilla of the rat: Electronmicroscopic and histochemical studies, *S. Afr. J. Med. Sci.* **31**:107.

Änggård, E., Bohman, S.-O., Griffin, J. E. III, Larsson, C., and Maunsbach, A. B., 1972, Subcellular localization of the prostaglandin system in the rabbit renal papilla, *Acta Physiol. Scand.* **84**:231.

Azar, S., Tobian, L., and Ishii, M., 1970, Prolonged water diuresis affecting solutes and interstitial cells of renal papilla, *Am. J. Physiol.* **221**:75.

Blanchette-Mackie, E. J., and Scow, R. O., 1973, Effects of lipoprotein lipase on the structure of chylomicrons, *J. Cell Biol.* **58**:689.

Bohman, S.-O., 1974, The ultrastructure of the rat renal medulla as observed after improved fixation methods, *J. Ultrastruct. Res.* **47**:329.

Bohman, S.-O., 1977, Demonstration of prostaglandin synthesis in collecting duct cells and other cell types of the rabbit renal medulla, *Prostaglandins* **14**:729.

Bohman, S.-O., 1979, The interstitial cells of the renal medulla. Ultrastructure and relation to prostaglandin formation, Ph.D. thesis, University of Aarhus, Denmark.

Bohman, S.-O., 1980, The ultrastructure and function of the interstitial cells of the renal medulla with special regard to prostaglandin synthesis, in: *Functional Ultrastructure of the Kidney* (A. B. Maunsbach, T. Steen Olsen, and E. I. Christensen, eds.), Academic Press, London, in press.

Bohman, S.-O., and Jensen, P. K. A., 1976, Morphometric studies on the lipid droplets of the interstitial cells of the renal medulla in different states of diuresis, *J. Ultrastruct. Res.* **55**:182.

Bohman, S.-O., and Jensen, P. K. A., 1978, The interstitial cells in the renal medulla of rat, rabbit and gerbil in different states of diuresis, *Cell Tissue Res.* **189**:1.

Bohman, S.-O., and Maunsbach, A. B., 1969, Isolation of the lipid droplets from the interstitial cells of the renal medulla, *J. Ultrastruct. Res.* **29**:569.

Bohman, S.-O., and Maunsbach, A. B., 1972, Ultrastructure and biochemical properties of subcellular fractions from rat renal medulla, *J. Ultrastruct. Res.* **38**:225.

Bojesen, I., 1974, Quantitative and qualitative analyses of isolated lipid droplets from interstitial cells in renal papillae from various species, *Lipids* **9**:835.

Bojesen, I., Bojesen, E., and Capito, K., 1976, In vitro and in vivo synthesis of long chain fatty acids from [1-¹⁴C]acetate in the renal papillae of rats, *Biochim. Biophys. Acta* **424**:8.

Bowman, W., 1842, On the structure and use of the malpighian bodies of the kidney, with observations on the circulation through that gland, *Philos. Trans. R. Soc. London* **B132**:57.

Bulger, R. E., and Nagle, R. B., 1973, Ultrastructure of the interstitium in the rabbit kidney, *Am. J. Anat.* **136**:183.

Bulger, R. E., and Siegel, F. L., 1975, Alterations of the renal papilla during mercuric chloride-induced acute tubular necrosis, *Lab. Invest.* **33**:712.

Bulger, R. E., and Trump, B. F., 1966, Fine structure of the rat renal papilla, *Am. J. Anat.* **118**:685.

Bulger, R. E., Griffith, L. D., and Trump, B. F., 1966, Endoplasmic reticulum in rat renal interstitial cells: Molecular rearrangement after water deprivation, *Science* **151**:83.

Bulger, R. E., Tisher, C. C., Myers, C. H., and Trump, B. F., 1967, Human renal ultrastructure. II. The thin limb of Henle's loop and the interstitium in healthy individuals, *Lab. Invest.* **16**:124.

Bulger, R. E., Cronin, R. E., and Dobyan, D. C., 1979, Survey of the morphology of the dog kidney, *Anat. Rec.* **194**:41.

Burghardt, R. C., and Andersen, E., 1979, Hormonal modulation of ovarian interstitial cells with particular reference to gap junctions, *J. Cell Biol.* **81**:104.

Cohn, Z. A., Hirsch, J. G., and Fedorko, M. E., 1966, The in vitro differentiation of mononuclear phagocytes. IV. The ultrastructure of macrophage differentiation in the peritoneal cavity and in culture, *J. Exp. Med.* **123**:747.

Comai, K., Prose, P., Farber, S. J., and Paulsrud, J. R., 1974, Correlation of renal medullary prostaglandin content and renal interstitial cell lipid droplets, *Prostaglandins* **6**:375.

Comai, K., Farber, S. J., and Paulsrud, J. R., 1975, Analyses of renal medullary lipid droplets from normal, hydronephrotic and indomethacin treated rabbits, *Lipids* **10**:555.

Dieterich, H. J., 1968, Die Ultrastruktur der Gefässbündel im Mark der Rattenniere, *Z. Zellforsch.* **84**:350.

Dousa, T. P., and Barnes, L. D., 1974, Effects of colchicine and vinblastine on the cellular action of vasopressin in mammaliam kidney. A possible role of microtubules, *J. Clin. Invest.* **54**:252.

Farber, S. J., Walat, R. J., Benjamin, R., and van Praag, D., 1971, Effect of increased osmo-lality on glycosaminoglycan metabolism of rabbit renal papilla, *Am. J. Physiol.* **220**:880.

Florendo, N. T., Pitcock, J. A., and Muirhead, E. E., 1978, Cyclic 3′,5′-nucleotide phos-phodiesterase; cytochemical localization in rat renomedullary interstitial cells, *J. His-tochem. Cytochem.* **26**:441.

Fourman, J., and Moffat, D. B., 1971, *The Blood Vessels of the Kidney*, Blackwell, Oxford.

Furusato, M., 1977, Ultrastructure and histochemistry of the medullary interstitial matrix of rat kidney, *Acta Pathol. Jpn.* **27**:331.

Ginetzinsky, A. G., 1958, Role of hyaluronidase in the reabsorption of water in renal tubules: The mechanism of action of the antidiuretic hormone, *Nature* **182**:1218.

Gloor, F., and Neiditsch-Halff, L. A., 1965, Die interstitiellen Zellen des Nierenmarkes der Ratte, *Z. Zellforsch.* **66**:488.

Ishii, M., and Tobian, L., 1969, Interstitial cell granules in renal papilla and the solute com-position of renal tissue in rats with Goldblatt hypertension, *J. Lab. Clin. Med.* **74**:47.

Johnson, F. R., and Darnton, S. J., 1967, Ultrastructural observations on the renal papilla of the rabbit, *Z. Zellforsch.* **81**:390.

Kaissling, B., and Kriz, W., 1979, *Structural analysis of the rabbit kidney*, Advances in Anatomy, Embryology, and Cell Biology, Vol. 56, Springer Verlag, Berlin, 123 pp.

King, B. F., and Tibbits, F. D., 1977, Ultrastructural observations on cytoplasmic lamellar inclusions in oocytes of the rodent *Thomomys*, *Anat. Rec.* **189**:263.

Knepper, M. A., Danielson, R. A., Saidel, G. M., and Post, R. S., 1977, Quantitative analysis of renal medullary anatomy in rats and rabbits, *Kidney Int.* **12**:313.

Kokko, J. P., and Rector, F. C., 1972, Countercurrent multiplication system without active transport in inner medulla, *Kidney Int.* **2**:214.

Kunze, H., and Vodgt, W., 1971, Significance of phospholipase A for prostaglandin formation, *Ann. N. Y. Acad. Sci.* **180**:123.

Larsen, W. J., 1977, Gap junctions and hormone action, in: *Transport of Ions and Water in Animals* (B. L. Gupta, R. B. Moreton, J. L. Oschman, and B. J. Wall, eds.), Academic Press, London, pp. 333–361.

Latta, H., White, F. N., Osvaldo, L., and Johnston, W. H., 1975, Unilateral renovascular hypertension in rats. Measurements of medullary granules, juxtaglomerular granularity and cellularity and area of adrenal zones, *Lab. Invest.* **33**:379.

Ledingham, J. M., and Simpson, F. O., 1973, Bundles of intracellular tubles in renal medullary interstitial cells, *J. Cell Biol.* **57**:594.

Lee, J. B., 1973, Renal homeostasis and the hypertensive state: A unifying hypothesis, in: *Prostaglandins*, Vol. 1 (P. W. Ramwell, ed.), Plenum Press, New York, pp. 133–160.

Lee, J. B., Vance, V. K., and Cahill, G. F., Jr., 1962, Metabolism of C^{14}-labeled substrates by rabbit kidney cortex and medulla, *Am. J. Physiol.* **203**:27.

Lee, J. B., Crowshaw, K., Takman, B. H., Attrep, K. A., and Gougoutas, J. Z., 1967, The identification of prostaglandins E_2, $F_{2\alpha}$ and A_2 from rabbit kidney medulla, *Biochem. J.* **105**:1251.

Limas, C., Limas, C. J., and Gesell, M. S., 1976, Effects of indomethacin on renomedullary interstitial cells, *Lab. Invest.* **34**:522.

Mandal, A. K., Muehrcke, R. C., Epstein, M., and Volini, F. I., 1967, Relationship of the renomedullary interstitial cells to experimental hypertension, *J. Lab. Clin. Med.* **70**:872.

Mandal, A. K., Frohlich, E. D., Chrysant, K., Pfeffer, M. A., Yunice, A, and Nordquist, J. A.,

1974, Ultrastructural analysis of renal papillary interstitial cell of spontaneously hypertensive rats, *J. Lab. Clin. Med.* **83**:256.

Mandal, A. K., Frohlich, E. D., Chrysant, K., Nordquist, J., Pfeffer, M. A., and Clifford, M., 1975, A morphological study of the renal papillary granule: Analysis in the interstitial cell and in the interstitium, *J. Lab. Clin. Med.* **85**:120.

Mandal, A. K., Nordquist, J. A., Thigpen, M. W., and James, T. M., 1979, Electron microscopy studies of papillary interstitial granules in normal human kidneys, *Ann. Clin. Lab. Sci.* **9**:37.

Maunsbach, A. B., and Wirsén, C., 1966, Ultrastructural changes in kidney, myocardium and skeletal muscle of the dog during excessive mobilization of free fatty acids, *J. Ultrastruct. Res.* **16**:35.

Moffat, D. B., 1967*a*, The fine structure of the blood vessels of the renal medulla with particular reference to the control of the medullary circulation, *J. Ultrastruct. Res.* **19**:532.

Moffat, D. B., 1967*b*, A new type of cell inclusion in the interstitial cells of the medulla of the rat kidney, *J. Microsc. (Paris)* **6**:1073.

Morrison, A. B., and Schneeberger-Keeley, E. E., 1969, The phagocytic role of renal medullary interstitial cells and the effect of potassium deficiency on this function, *Nephron* **6**:584.

Muehrcke, R. C., Rosen, S., and Volini, F. I., 1965, The interstitial cells of the renal papilla: Light and electron microscopic studies, in: *Progress in Pyelonephritis* (E. H. Kass, ed.), F. A. Davis, Philadelphia, pp. 422–433.

Muehrcke, R. C., Mandal, A. K., Epstein, M., and Volini, F. I., 1969, Cytoplasmic granularity of the renal medullary interstitial cells in experimental hypertension, *J. Lab. Clin. Med.* **73**:299.

Muehrcke, R. C., Mandal, A. K., and Volini, F. I., 1970, A pathophysiological review of the renal medullary interstitial cells and their relationship to hypertension, *Circ. Res.* **26,27**:I-109.

Muirhead, E. E., Stirman, J. A., and Jones, F., 1960, Renal autoexplantation and protection against renoprival hypertensive cardiovascular disease and hemolysis, *J. Clin. Invest.* **39**:266.

Muirhead, E. E., Leach, B. E., Daniels, E. D., and Hinman, J. W., 1968, Lapine renomedullary lipid in murine hypertension, *Arch. Pathol.* **85**:72.

Muirhead, E. E., Brown, G. B., Germain, G. S., and Leach, B. S., 1970, The renal medulla as an antihypertensive organ, *J. Lab. Clin. Med.* **76**:641.

Muirhead, E. E., Brooks, B., Pitcock, J. A., Stephenson, P., and Brosius, W. L., 1972, Role of the renal medulla in the sodium-sensitive component of renoprival hypertension, *Lab. Invest.* **27**:192.

Muirhead, E. E., Germain, G. S., Armstrong, F. B., Brooks, B., Leach, B. E., Byers, L. W., Pitcock, J. A., and Brown, P., 1975, Endocrine-type antihypertensive function of renomedullary interstitial cells, *Kidney Int.* **8**:271.

Muirhead, E. E., Clapp, W. L., Pitcock, J. A., Brown, P., Brooks, B., and Brosius, W. L., 1977, Renomedullary interstitial cell (RIC) damage and the evolution of salt-dependent hypertension, *Kidney Int.* **12**:505.

Nekrasova, A. A., Sokolova, R. I., and Lantsberg, L. A., 1973, Prostaglandinlike renal vasodepressor lipids and electrolyte exchange in the kidney, in: *Advances in the Biosciences*, Vol. 9, International Conference on Prostaglandins (S. Bergström, ed.), Pergamon Press–Vieweg, Oxford, pp. 307–312.

Nishikawa, K., Morrison, A., and Needleman, P., 1977, Exaggerated prostaglandin biosynthesis and its influence on renal resistance in the isolated hydronephrotic rabbit kidney, *J. Clin. Invest.* **59**:1143.

Nissen, H. M., 1968a, On lipid droplets in renal interstitial cells. II. A histological study on the number of droplets in salt depletion and acute salt repletion, *Z. Zellforsch.* **85**:483.

Nissen, H. M., 1968b, On lipid droplets in renal interstitial cells. III. A histological study on the number of droplets during hydration and dehydration, *Z. Zellforsch.* **92**:52.

Nissen, H. M., and Andersen, H., 1968, On the localization of a prostaglandin-dehydrogenase activity in the kidney, *Histochemie* **14**:189.

Nissen, H. M., and Andersen, H., 1971, On the enzyme histochemistry of the renal interstitial cells, *Histochemie* **27**:109.

Nissen, H. M., and Bojesen, I., 1969, On lipid droplets in renal interstitial cells. IV. Isolation and identification, *Z. Zellforsch.* **97**:274.

Novikoff, A. B., 1960, The rat kidney: Cytochemical and electron microscopic studies, in: *Biology of Pyelonephritis* (E. L. Quinn and E. H. Kass, eds.), Little, Brown, Boston, pp. 113–144.

Osvaldo, L., and Latta, H., 1966a, The thin limbs of the loop of Henle, *J. Ultrastruct. Res.* **15**:144.

Osvaldo, L., and Latta, H., 1966b, Interstitial cells of the renal medulla, *J. Ultrastruct. Res.* **15**:589.

Osvaldo-Decima, L., 1973, Ultrastructure of the lower nephron, in: *Handbook of Physiology*, Section 8: *Renal physiology* (J. Orloff and R. W. Berliner, eds.), American Physiological Society, Washington, D.C., pp. 81–102.

Osvaldo-Decima, L., and Latta, H., 1970, The renal medulla of diuretic and antidiuretic rats studied by electron microscopy, in: *Proceedings of the 4th International Congress of Nephrology*, Vol. I (N. Alwall, F. Berglund, and B. Josephson, eds.), Karger, Basel, pp. 116–123.

Palade, G. E., 1959, Functional changes in the structure of cell components, in: *Subcellular Particles* (T. Hayashi, ed.), Ronald Press, New York, pp. 64–83.

Paul, J., 1965, Carbohydrate and energy metabolism, in: *Cells and Tissues in Culture. Methods, Biology and Physiology*, Vol. 1 (E. N. Willmer, ed.), Academic Press, London, pp. 239–276.

Pease, D. C., 1964, *Histological Techniques for Electron Microscopy*, 2nd ed., Academic Press, New York.

Perov, Y. L., and Postnov, Y. V., 1976a, Interstitial cells of the renal medulla in rats with genetic spontaneous hypertension, *Bull. Exp. Biol. Med. (USSR)* **82**:938.

Perov, Y. L., and Postnov, Y. V., 1976b, Lipid droplets of interstitial medullary cells of intact rat kidney with two-kidney Goldblatt hypertension, *Virchows Arch. B* **22**:163.

Pitcock, J. A., Rightsel, W. A., Brown, P., Brooks, B., and Muirhead, E. E., 1976, Functional–morphological correlates of renomedullary interstitial cells, *Clin. Sci. Mol. Med.* **51**:291s.

Renaut, J., and Dubreuil, G., 1907, Note sur l'histologie, la cytologie des tubes de Bellini et le tissu conjonctif de la pyramide du rein, *C. R. Assoc. Anat.* **9**:94.

Sakaguchi, H., and Suzuki, Y., 1958, Fine structure of renal tubule cells, *Keizyo J. Med.* **7**:17.

Salpeter, M. M., and Zilversmit, D. B., 1968, The surface coat of chylomicrons: Electron microscopy, *J. Lipid Res.* **9**:187.

Schifferli, J., Grandchamp, A., and Chatelanat, F., 1975, Ultrastructure of the interstitial cells of the rat renal papilla, *Kidney Int.* **7**:366.

Schiller, A., and Taugner, R., 1979, Junctions between interstitial cells of the renal medulla: A freeze-fracture study, *Cell Tissue Res.* **203**:231.

Schoefl, G. I., 1968, The ultrastructure of chylomicra and of the particles in an artificial fat emulsion, *Proc. R. Soc. Ser. B* **169**:147.

Schwartz, M. M., and Venkatachalam, M. A., 1974, Structural differences in thin limbs of Henle: Physiological implications, *Kidney Int.* **6**:193.

Schwartz, M. M., Karnovsky, M. J., and Venkatachalam, M. A., 1976, Ultrastructural differences between rat inner medullary descending and ascending vasa recta, *Lab. Invest.* **35**:161.

Schweigger-Seidel, F., 1865, Die Nieren des Menschen und der Säugethiere in ihrem feineren Baue, Thesis, University of Halle, Halle.

Simpson, F. O., 1970, Renal vasculature and hypertensive mechanisms, *Circ. Res.* **26,27**:II-235.

Sternberg, W. H., Farber, E., and Dunlap, C. E., 1956, Histochemical localization of specific oxidative enzymes: II. Localization of diphosphopyridine nucleotide and triphosphopyridine nucleotide diaphorases and the succindehydrogenase system in the kidney, *J. Histochem. Cytochem.* **4**:266.

Stoeckenius, W., 1962, Some electron microscopical observations on liquid crystalline phases in lipid–water systems, *J. Cell. Biol.* **12**:221.

Straus, W., 1971, Comparative analysis of the concentration of injected horseradish peroxidase in cytoplasmic granules of the kidney cortex, in the blood, urine and liver, *J. Cell. Biol.* **48**:620.

Szokol, M., Schömig, A., Thomázy, V., and Kovács, Z., 1979, On the lipid granularity of renomedullary interstitial cells in benign and malignant courses of renal hypertension, *Exp. Pathol.* **17**:143.

Thoenes, W., 1962, Fine structure of lipid granules in proximal tubule cells of mouse kidney, *J. Cell Biol.* **12**:433.

Tisher, C. C., 1976, Anatomy of the kidney, in: *The Kidney*, Vol. I (B. M. Brenner and F. C. Rector Jr., eds.), W. B. Saunders, Philadelphia, pp. 3-64.

Tobian, L., and Azar, S., 1971, Antihypertensive and other functions of the renal papilla, *Trans. Assoc. Am. Phys.* **84**:281.

Tobian, L,. and Ishii, M., 1969, Interstitial cell granules and solutes in renal papilla in post-Goldblatt hypertension, *Am. J. Physiol.* **217**:1699.

Tobian, L., Ishii, M., and Duke, M., 1969, Relationship of cytoplasmic granules in renal papillary interstitial cells to "postsalt" hypertension, *J. Lab. Clin. Med.* **73**:309.

Vimtrup, B. J., and Schmidt-Nielsen, B., 1952, The histology of the kidney of kangaroo rats, *Anat. Rec.* **114**:515.

Verberckmoes, R., van Damme, B., Clement, J., Amery, A., and Michielsen, P., 1976, Bartter's syndrome with hyperplasia of renomedullary cells: Successful treatment with indomethacin, *Kidney Int.* **9**:302.

Wade, J. B., O'Neil, R. G., Pryor, J. L., and Boulpaep, E. L., 1979, Modulations of cell membrane area in renal collecting tubules by corticosteroid hormones, *J. Cell Biol.* **81**:439.

Zucker-Franklin, D., Grunsky, G., and Marcus, A., 1978, Transformation of monocytes into "fat" cells, *Lab. Invest.* **38**:620.

CHAPTER 2

Evidence for an Involvement of the Renal Papilla in Hypertension

E. E. MUIRHEAD and J. A. PITCOCK

1. INTRODUCTION

Several classic experiments support the view that the kidney exerts a nonexcretory antihypertensive function. Bilateral nephrectomy plus a sodium–volume load causes hypertension (Braun–Menendez and Von Euler, 1947; Grollman et al., 1949), while ureterovenous anastomosis (Grollman et al., 1949; Floyer, 1955; Muirhead, 1962) under similar circumstances prevents hypertension. Destruction of the renal papilla is attended by hypertension induced by sodium and volume (Muirhead et al., 1950, 1960a) on the one hand, and by aggravation of existing hypertension, on the other (Heptinstall et al., 1975). Unclipping of a one-kidney, one-clip hypertensive rat is followed by normalization of the arterial pressure within 24 hr or less (Byrom and Dodson, 1949; Floyer, 1955; Muirhead et al., 1976). Ureterovenous anastomosis plus unclipping is also attended by normalization of the arterial pressure (Floyer, 1955; Muirhead et al., 1976), even though a longer time interval may be required. Indeed, ureterovenous anastomosis plus a saline load given intravenously (1.25–2.5% of the body weight) followed by unclipping is also attened by normalization of the arterial pressure, but additional time is needed (Muirhead and Brooks, 1980). Unclipping while an intravenous saline infusion equal to or greater than the urine loss is maintained is also attended by a normal pressure within 20 hr (Muirhead et al., 1976; Neubig and Hoobler, 1975). Thus, the recession of the arterial pressure in the ureterovenous experiment is not caused by substances entering the circulation via the ureter. Paired sham-operated controls for these manipulations had no change of the arterial pressure over the same time

E. E. MUIRHEAD and J. A. PITCOCK • University of Tennessee Center for the Health Sciences and Baptist Memorial Hospital, Memphis, Tennessee 38146.

period. There is no loss of sodium and volume to the outside of the body when ureterovenous anastomosis is imposed. The interpretation given, under these conditions, is that the kidney performs an internal function that allows the pressure to be either maintained when sodium–volume is added to the normotensive animal or lowered after its elevation due to the previous arterial constriction.

It is especially noteworthy that either whole kidney transplantation or whole kidney perfusion lowers the arterial pressure of hypertensive animals even though a positive sodium–volume load is maintained (Kolff and Page, 1954; Muirhead et al., 1956; Gomez et al., 1960).

It has been suggested that the nonexcretory antihypertensive function of the kidney is performed to a great extent by renomedullary tissue (Muirhead, 1974). The main candidate for such function in this area is the unique group of cells known as the renomedullary interstitial cells (RIC). It is the purpose of this chapter to examine the evidence supporting this position.

2. ANTIHYPERTENSIVE ACTION OF TRANSPLANTS OF FRAGMENTED RENAL PAPILLA

We have modified our procedure for transplantation of fragmented renal papilla as follows: The kidney is removed under pentobarbital anesthesia (30 mg/kg ip). After delivery, the kidney is sectioned across the convex surface of the cortex slightly to the left of center with a 5.5-cm straight razor blade. This opens the pelvis and exposes the papilla in an intact state. With a small pair of curved scissors, the papilla is cut across its base and removed. The papilla(ae) is placed in a Petri dish containing 0.1 ml of Hank's balanced salt solution. With the same razor blade the renal tissue is minced for 1½ min, using right-angle up and down strokes. A curved spatula is used to maintain the minced papilla(ae) in one spot on the Petri dish. After the mincing procedure the tissue is placed in a 25-ml conical centrifuge tube along with 5 ml of Hank's solution. The particles are suspended and centrifuged for 1 min in a table model centrifuge. The supernatant is decanted and the particles of tissue are taken up in a tuberculin syringe containing 0.2 ml of Hank's solution plus 500 units of penicillin and 100 μg gentamicin. Operating-room-type sterile procedures are used throughout. The recipient's skin is prepared by shaving, scrubbing with PHisoHex,® washing with 70% alcohol, and then treating with tincture of iodine for 1 min. The iodine is removed with alcohol. With a 21 gauge, ~4 cm needle, the particles of papilla are injected. The needle is driven subcutaneously to the hilt and slowly removed as the injection occurs, thereby making a thin long track of tissue. The entire procedure takes 10–15 min.

Three points are crucial: (1) the mincing procedure must not be over-

TABLE 1
Hypertensive States Affected by Tr Pap

Animal	Hypertensive state	Reference
Dog	Renoprival	Muirhead et al. (1960a)
Rabbit	Renoprival	Muirhead et al. (1972b)
		Muirhead et al. (1973b)
	Malignant	Muirhead et al. (1972a)
Rat	One kidney, one clip	Muirhead et al. (1970)
	Two kidneys, one clip	Manthorpe, (1973)
		Manthorpe (1975)
	Postsalt	Tobian and Azar (1971)
	Genetic hydronephrosis–salt	Sušić et al. (1976)
		Sušić et al. (1978)
	Angiotensin–salt	Muirhead et al. (1975)
	SHR	Sušić et al. (1977)
	SHR and hydronephrosis	Solez et al. (1976)
	Partial nephrectomy–salt	Muirhead, unpublished
	DOCA–salt	Muirhead, unpublished

done lest the tissue not take (particles of 1 mm or less are preferable); (2) there must be a track and not a bolus, lest necrosis of much of the transplant occur; and (3) a palpable nodule that appears to expand must develop by the next day or so.

Such transplants of renal papilla (Tr Pap) are incapable of performing an excretory function and yet they exerted a powerful antihypertensive action in a variety of settings (Table 1). After 10–21 days, these transplants consisted almost entirely of RIC and capillaries. The other structures (vasa recta, Henle's loop, and collecting duct) underwent atrophy and disappeared (Muirhead et al., 1972a,b). A clustering effect of the RIC within the transplant suggested proliferation of these cells. A close relationship between the RIC and the capillaries developed (termed positive tropism). The appearance was reminiscent of an endocrine gland (Figs. 1 and 2*).

Of the twelve types of hypertensive states listed in Table 1, in which Tr Pap were shown to be effective in either preventing or reversing the hypertension, at least nine are currently considered to have a salt component in their pathogenesis. Thus, the RIC of the Tr Pap appeared to mitigate, in a major way, the influence of salt and volume on the arterial pressure. In renoprival hypertension this effect could not be due to an influence on the degree of sodium and water retention.

This relationship between the RIC and salt–volume may be formulated in more specific terms. It would seem that salt–volume excess alone is not prohypertensive (witness various edematous states bordering on anasarca

* Figures 1, 2, 4, 5, 8–11, 13, 19, and 22 appear on an insert following page 40.

and various polycythemias attended by little or no hypertension). By the same token, the diminution or absence of the antihypertensive function of the RIC alone may not be prohypertensive (witness bilateral nephrectomy alone and no hypertension, at least for a few days). Rather, the combination of salt–volume excess and the absence of the antihypertensive function of the RIC is prohypertensive (as in early renoprival hypertension following a sodium–volume load). Stated differently, the absence (or depression) of the antihypertensive function of the RIC is not necessarily prohypertensive, but the absence of this function seems to allow prohypertensive mechanisms to operate out of control, salt–volume excess apparently being one of the prohypertensive mechanisms so implicated. In this framework, Floyer (1957) discussed the existence of an extrarenal prohypertensive mechanism that is set in motion when the antihypertensive function of the kidney seemingly is compromised, as in renoprival and late renal hypertension. Although the nature of this mechanism remained unknown, one major possibility entertained, based on work by Ledingham (1957), was that of increased electrolytes in the vascular smooth muscle causing increased vascular resistance.

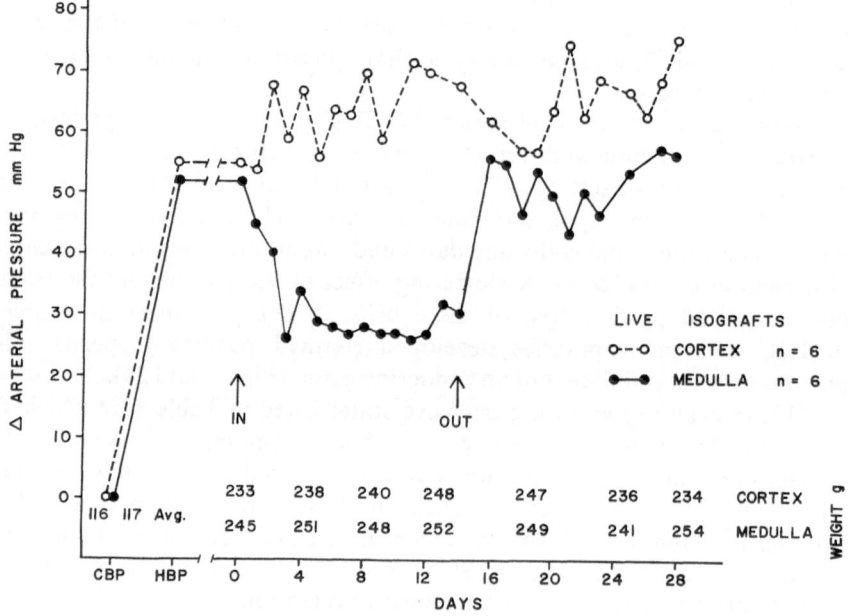

FIGURE 3. The antihypertensive effect of Tr Pap in one-kidney, one-clip hypertension of the rat is demonstrated by the solid line and solid circles. The Tr Pap was introduced at the arrow IN and removed at the arrow OUT. Note the "make" and "break" effects. The broken line and open circles represent the lack of antihypertensive action of renocortical transplants in paired controls. [From Muirhead et al. (1970).]

The antihypertensive action of Tr Pap and their RIC must be mediated by a substance(s) that is secreted into the blood and carried elsewhere for its action, i.e., a hormone. The positive tropism RIC to capillaries is in keeping with this contention. Moreover, removal of the Tr Pap after its antihypertensive action reaches maximum is followed by return of the hypertensive state (Muirhead et al., 1970; Muirhead, 1974), a "make" and "break" effect characteristic of endocrine organs (Fig. 3).

3. MONOLAYER TISSUE CULTURE OF RIC

The concentration of RIC within the Tr Pap made possible the derivation of monolayer cultures of RIC (Muirhead et al., 1972c). These were shown to be potent secretors of prostaglandins (PG), mainly PGE_2.* The first cell line was derived from lapine tissue following the demonstration of the antihypertensive action of Tr Pap in renoprival and malignant hypertension of the rabbit (Fig. 4) (Muirhead et al., 1972a,b). The second cell line was a syngeneic one derived following the demonstration of the antihypertensive action in angiotensin–salt hypertension within our syngeneic rat line (Wistar/GM) (Muirhead et al., 1973a) (Fig. 5). It was possible to use this culture for retransplantation into hypertensive recipients.

4. ANTIHYPERTENSIVE ACTION OF CULTURED RIC

Transplantation of cultured RIC (Tr TCric) into syngeneic hypertensive recipients was followed by a sharp decline of the arterial pressure (Muirhead et al., 1975; Muirhead, 1974). This type of experiment netted several interesting results. Three major patterns of antihypertensive activity were noted: In one, the arterial pressure began to recede shortly after the transplant and reached a maximal effect in 12–24 hr (Figs. 6 and 7). In another, the arterial pressure receded slowly over a few days (2–5 days) to its minimal level. In a third pattern, the antihypertensive action was transient, reaching maximum in 12–24 hr but returning to prior hypertensive levels in 24–48 hr. Even in the syngeneic recipient the antihypertensive action of the transplant was not permanent, being dissipated after an interval of two or more weeks. The loss of antihypertensive action was invariably associated with the disappearance of the transplanted cells (Muirhead et al., 1975). This dissipation of antihypertensive function and of the

---

* The prostaglandin synthetase system appears to be associated with the microsomal membranes (Bohman and Larsson, 1975). The lipid granules are biologically inactive (Änggård et al., 1972; Muirhead, unpublished observations; Bohman and Larsson, 1975).

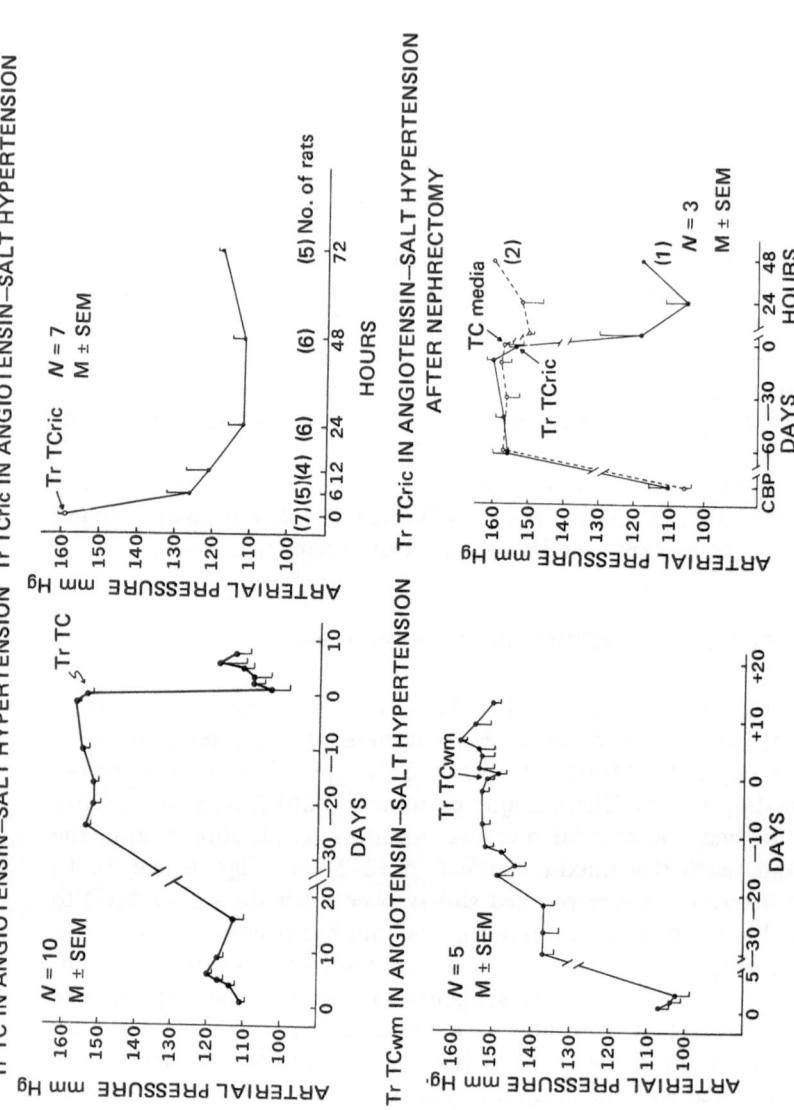

FIGURE 6. The antihypertensive action of Tr TCric. In the upper left panel, the control blood pressure 150–160 mm Hg for 30 days before the transplant. The transplant (16–30 million cells, 85% viable) caused the blood pressure to recede to control levels within 24 hr. The pressure remained so depressed for the 8 days of observation. The upper right panel shows the drop in blood pressure at 6, 12, 24, 48, and 72 hr. Note a major recession at 6 hr and maximal recession by 12–24 hr. In the lower left panel are results when a tissue culture devoid of RIC was transplanted (Tr TCwm). There was no change in blood pressure. The lower right panel demonstrates that Tr TCric exert their antihypertensive action in the absence of normal renal tissue, i.e., in the renoprival state. [From Muirhead et al. (1975).]

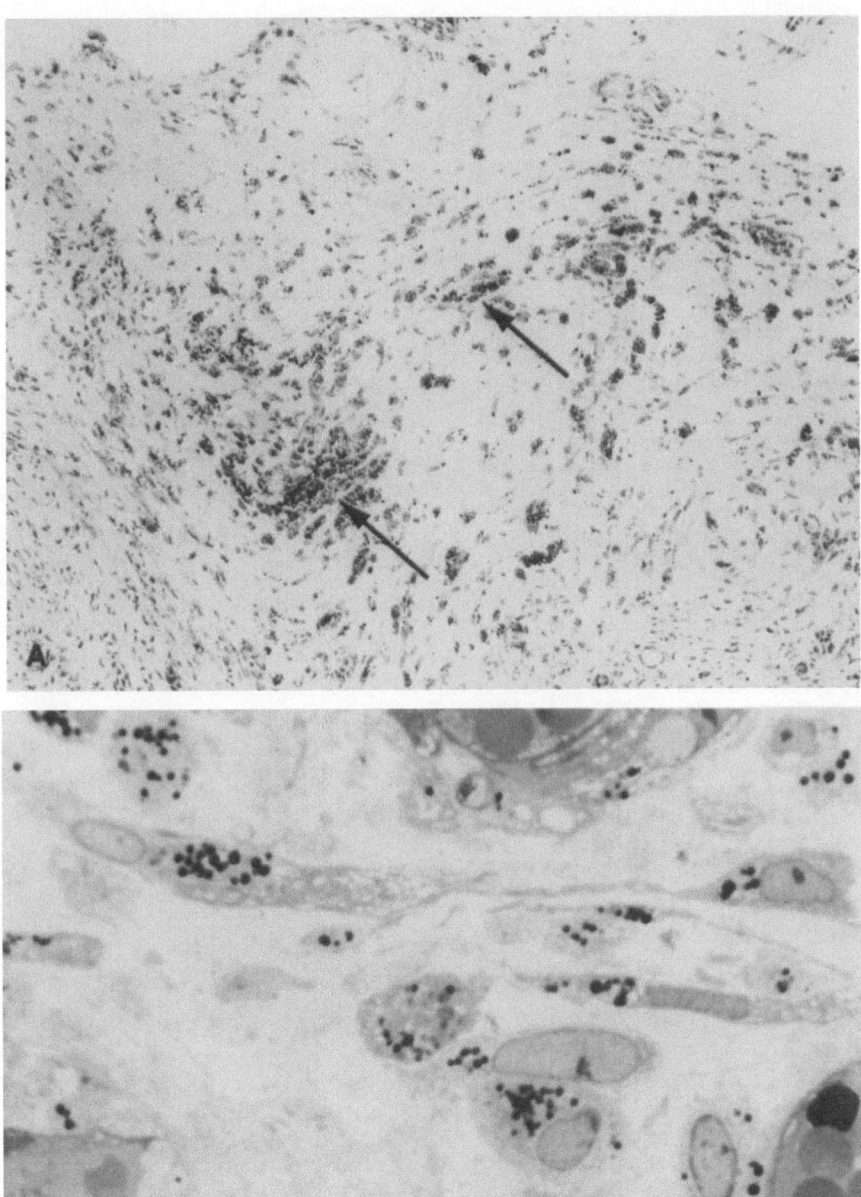

FIGURE 1. (A) Oil Red O stain, 5-μm frozen section of Tr Pap. This Tr Pap exerted an antihypertensive action in renoprival hypertension of the rabbit. Note the clustering of oil Red O-positive (lipid-containing) cells at arrows. [From Muirhead *et al.* (1972*b*).] (B) Toluidine blue stain of a 0.5-μm section. These RIC are from a Tr Pap that prevented malignant hypertension of the rabbit. The granules and cisternae are evident. In the micrograph a cell is

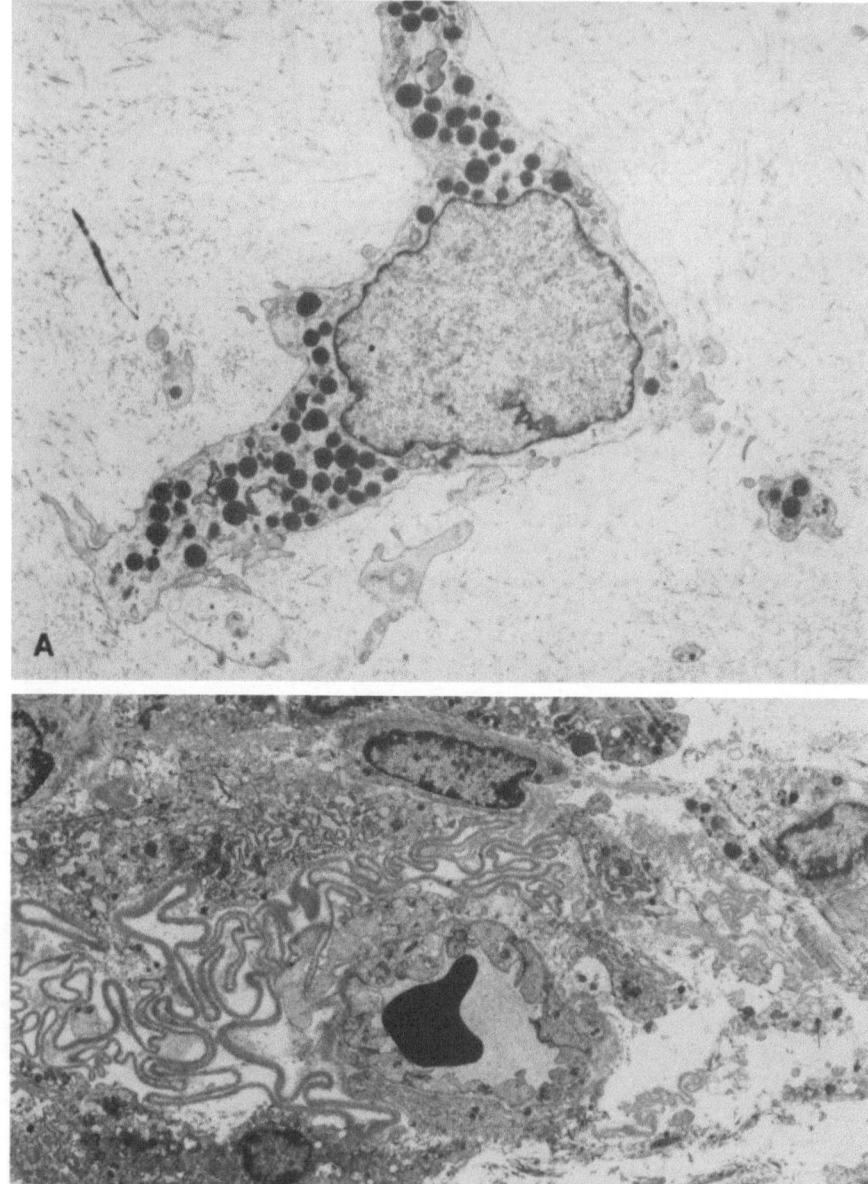

FIGURE 2. (A) Transmission electron microscopy (TEM). An RIC from the Tr Pap of 1A. Note the cytoplasmic processes and numerous dense (osmiophilic) granules characteristic of RIC in an active Tr Pap. [From Muirhead *et al.* (1972*b*).] (B) TEM. A Tr Pap similar to that of 1B. RIC and their processes, granules and cisternae are shown. In the center is a capillary surrounded by nearby RIC and processes of RIC (interpreted as positive tropism). The

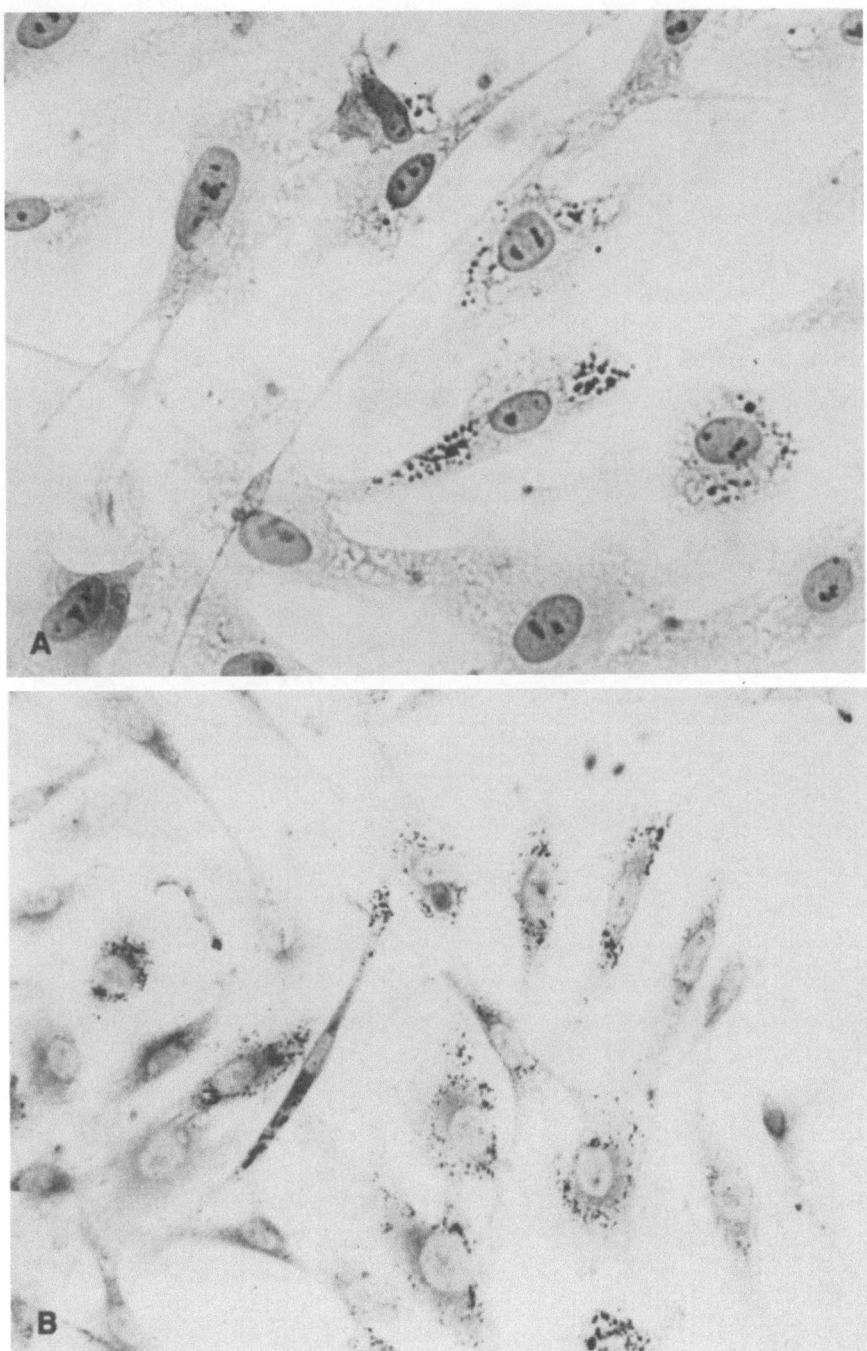

FIGURE 4. (A) Oil Red O stain of a cover-slip culture of RIC. Two features of the cytoplasm are prominent, the oil Red O-positive granules and the cisternae. (B) Sudan black B stain of a cover-slip culture of RIC. The Sudan black B-positive granules are evident.

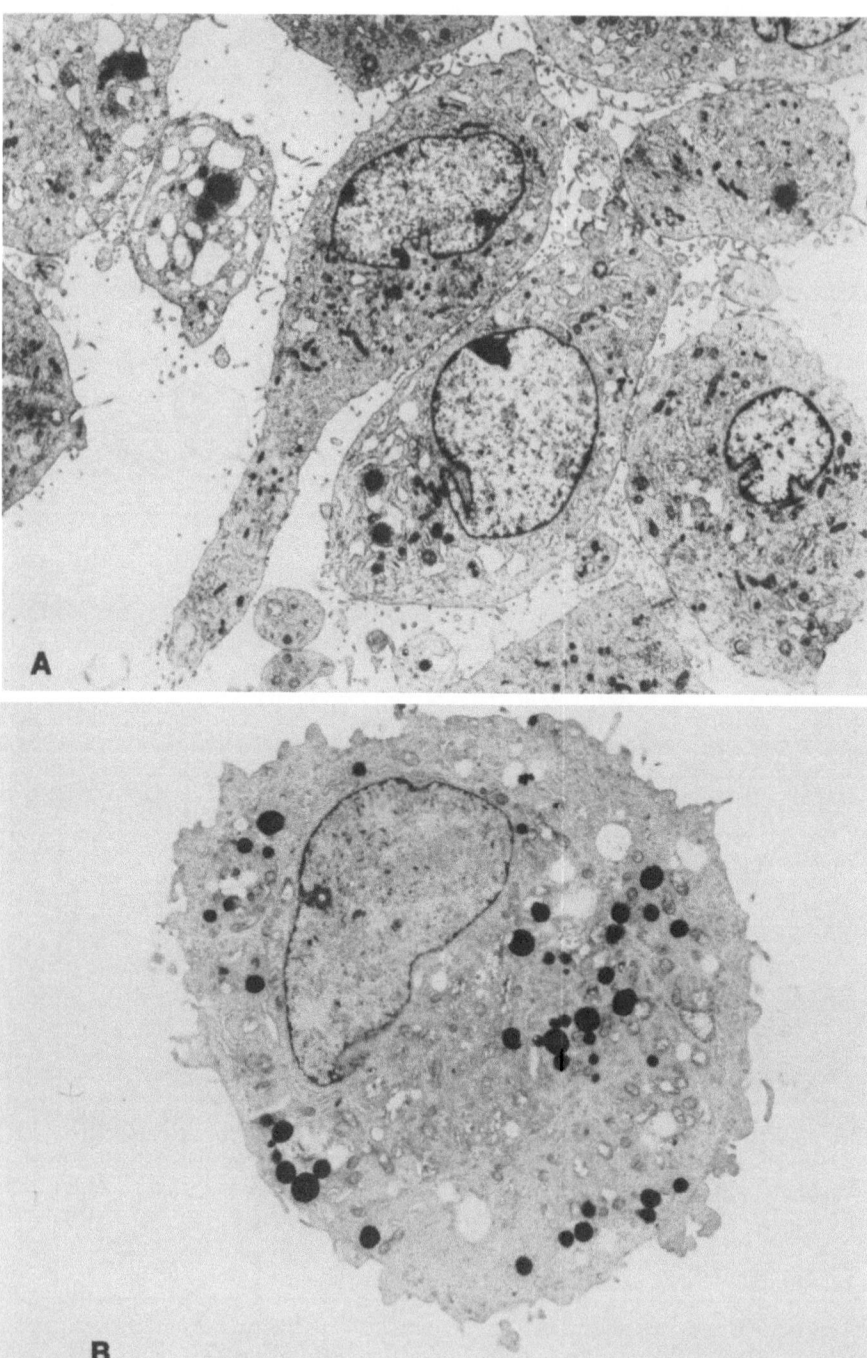

FIGURE 5. (A) TEM. RIC from a syngeneic rat line (Wistar/GM) in tissue culture. The cells
reveal processes and the lipid granule–cistern relationship. [From Muirhead *et al*. (1974*d*).]
(B) TEM. A cell from a monolayer tissue culture of rabbit RIC. The dense granules, cisternae
and Golgi apparatus are depicted. On occasions the cells become round in tissue culture. [From
Muirhead *et al*. (1972*c*).]

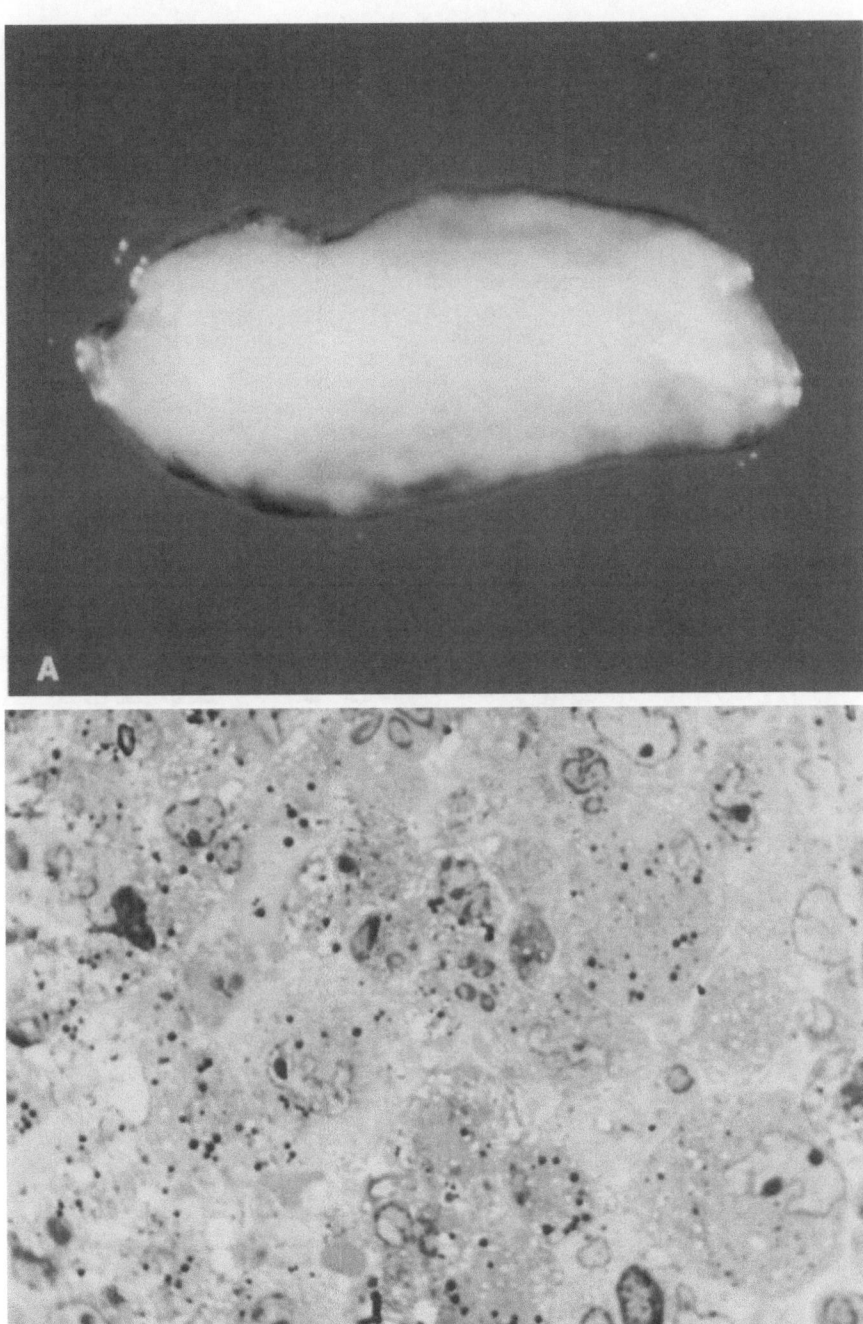

FIGURE 8. (A) This Tr TCric was removed 6 hr after its introduction into the subcutaneous tissue. At that time, the arterial pressure of the hypertensive recipient (angiotensin–salt hypertension) had decreased significantly. This compact nodule, which could be shelled out, was presumably the result of the aggregating properties of the cells. (B) Toluidine blue stain of a 0.5-μm section from the nodule shown in A. The RIC apparently are aggregated. A polymorphonuclear granulocyte is present in the center of the figure. [A and B from Muirhead *et al.* (1974a).]

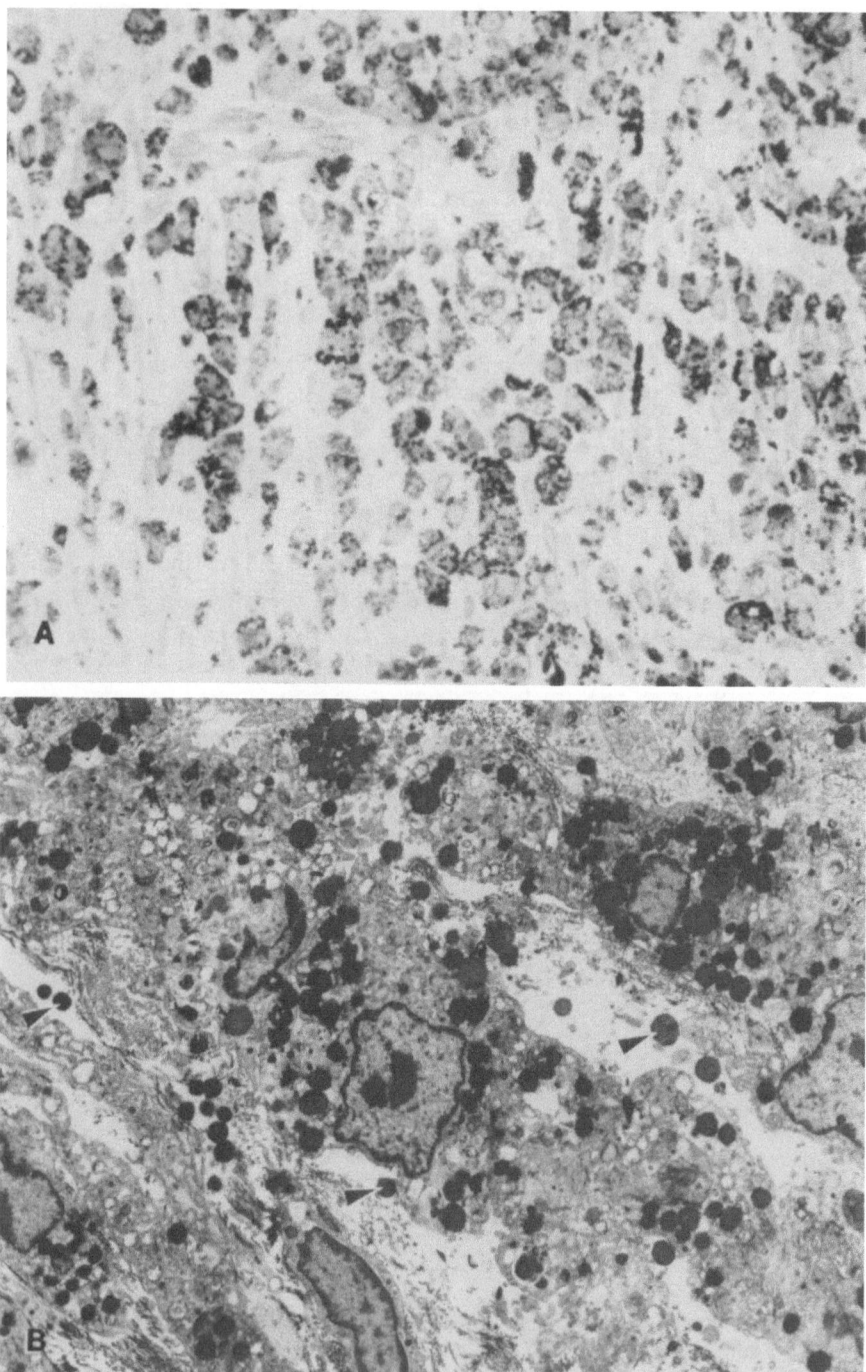

FIGURE 9. (A) This is an example of Tr TCric that lowered the arterial pressure of a rat having angiotensin–salt hypertension. Note the numerous granules in the cytoplasm (Toluidine blue stain, 0.5-μm section). (B) TEM. These cells are from the same Tr TCric as in A. The lipid granule–cisternal relationship is evident. Some granules appear free in the stroma (arrows). Whether this represents an artifact or extrusion is not known. [A and B from Muirhead (1974).]

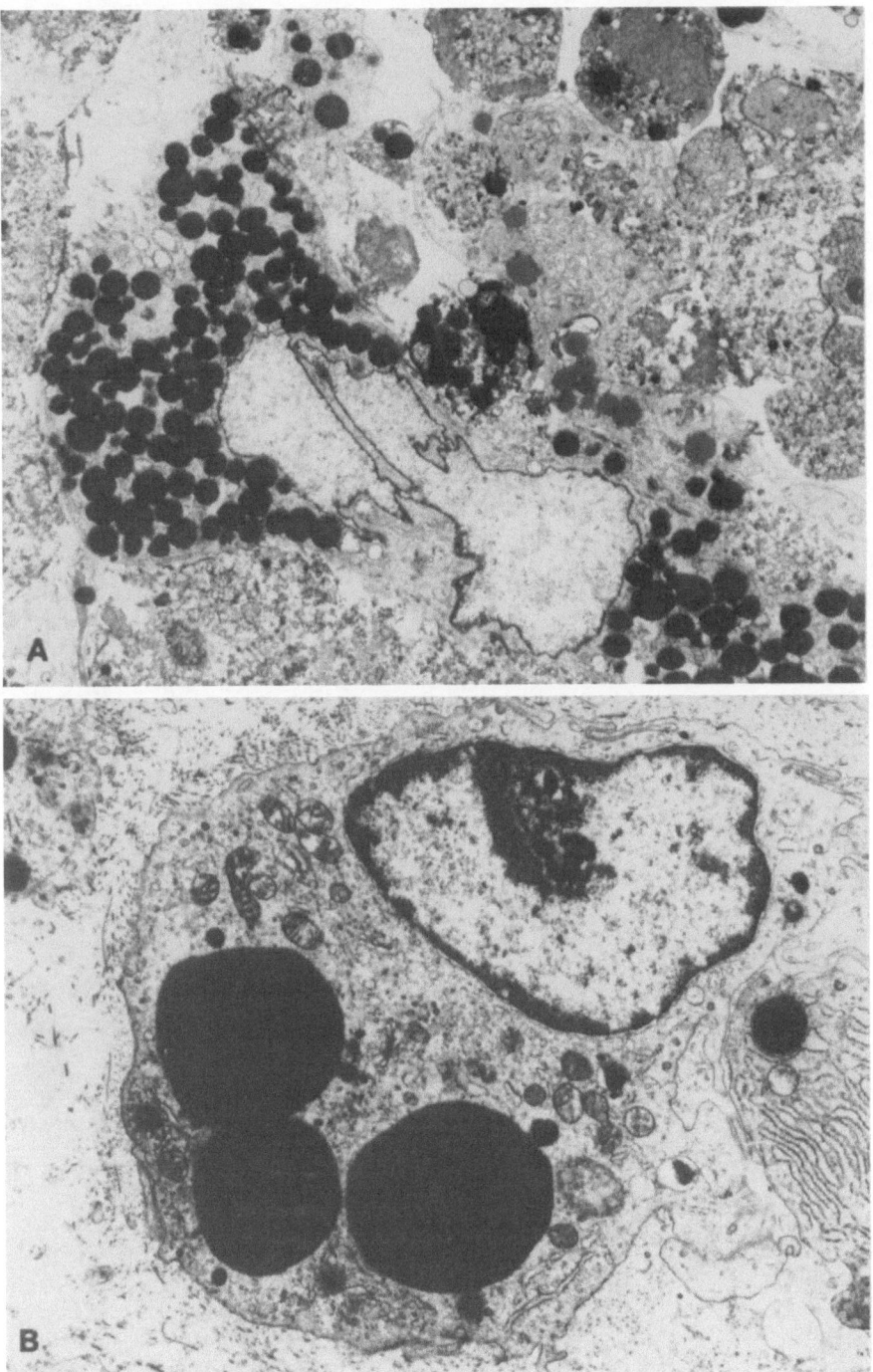

FIGURE 10. (A) TEM. The treatment of cultured RIC with indomethacin (4 μg/ml of culture media) caused enlargement of the cells and the presence of numerous dense granules. The many granules made the cisterns appear obscure. (B) TEM. Indomethacin also gave rise to very large dense granules in the cultured RIC. [From Muirhead *et al.* (1975).]

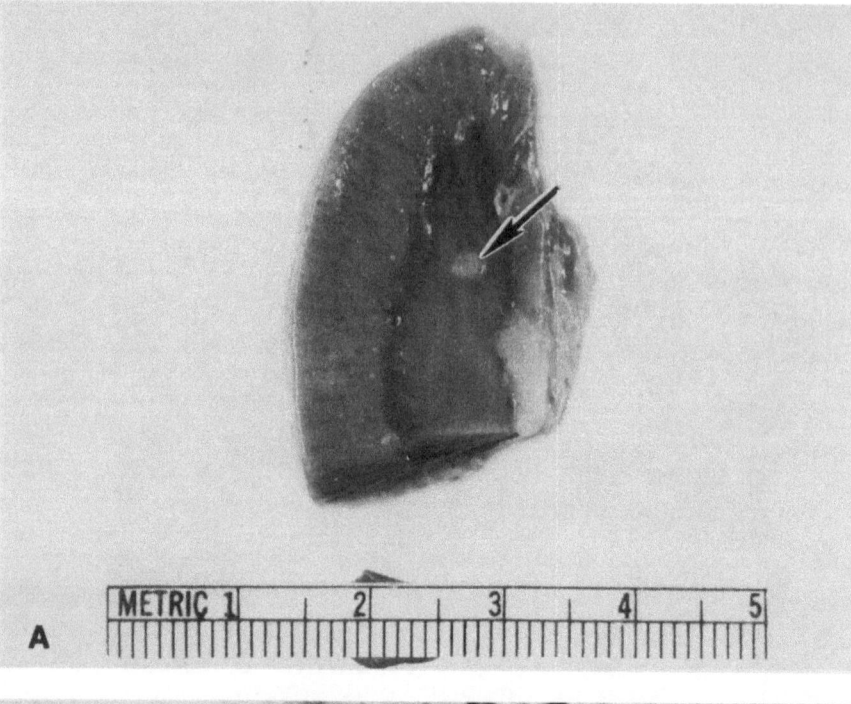

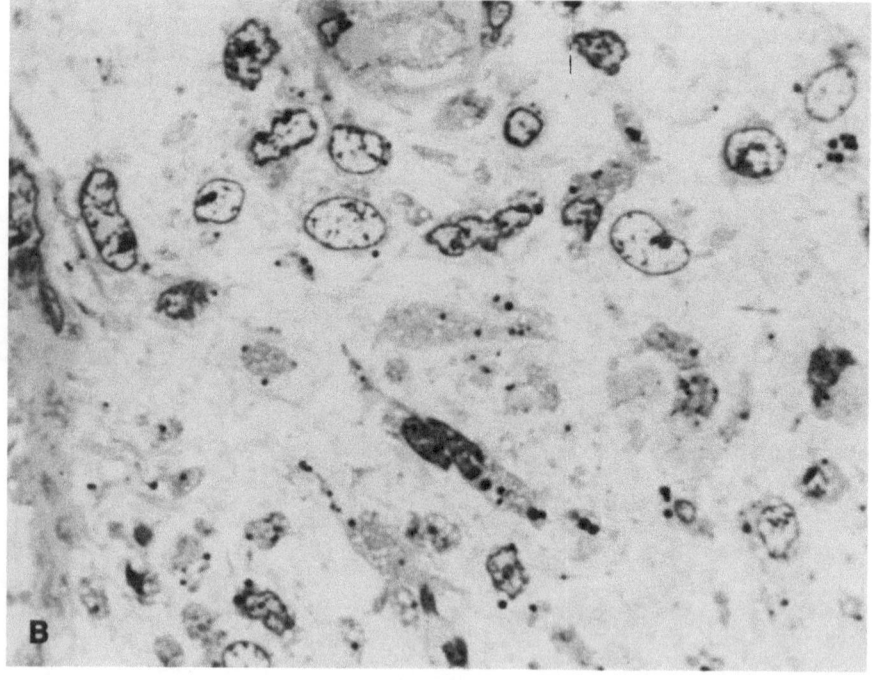

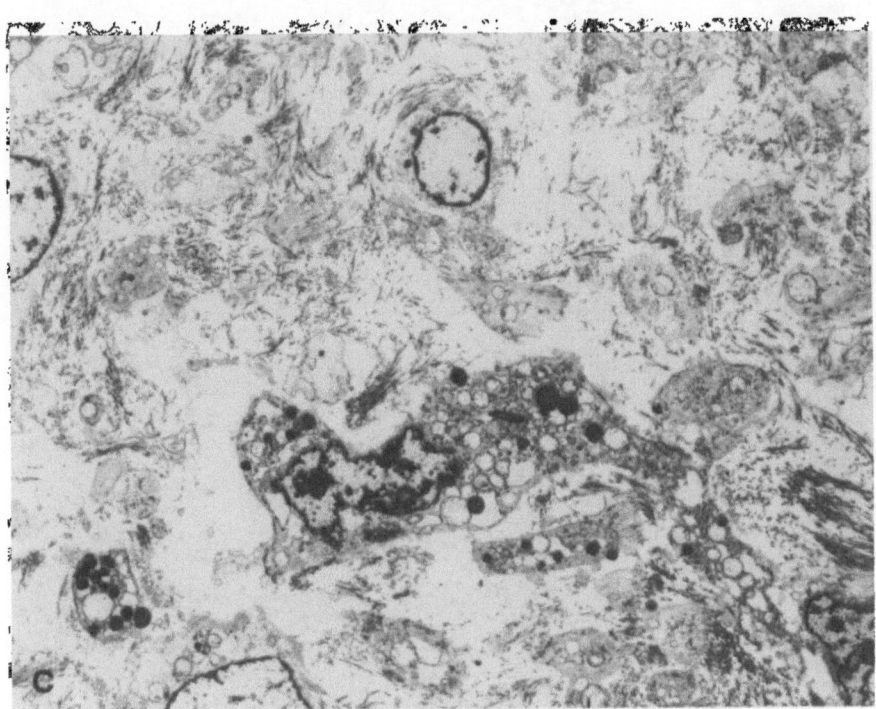

FIGURE 13. (A) The gross appearance of the RICT as seen in the human kidney. The nodule is in the middle level of the papilla (arrow). (B) Cells of the RICT displaying cytoplasmic processes, granules, and cisterns (Toluidine blue stain, 0.5-μm section). (C) TEM. Cell from RICT showing the processes and typical dense granule–cisternal relationship. (The poor quality of B and C results from the postmortem source.) [A, B, and C from Lerman *et al.* (1972).]

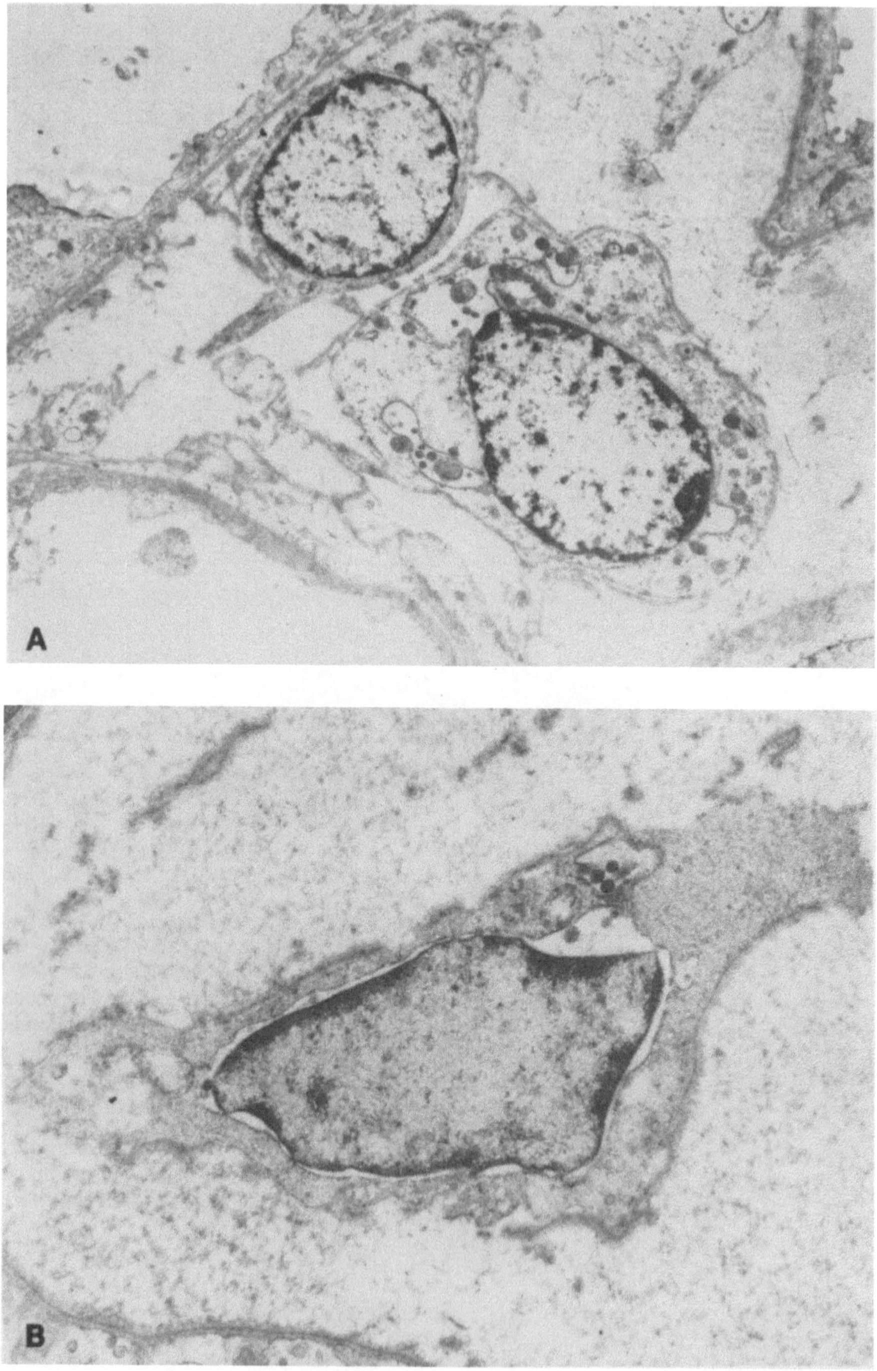

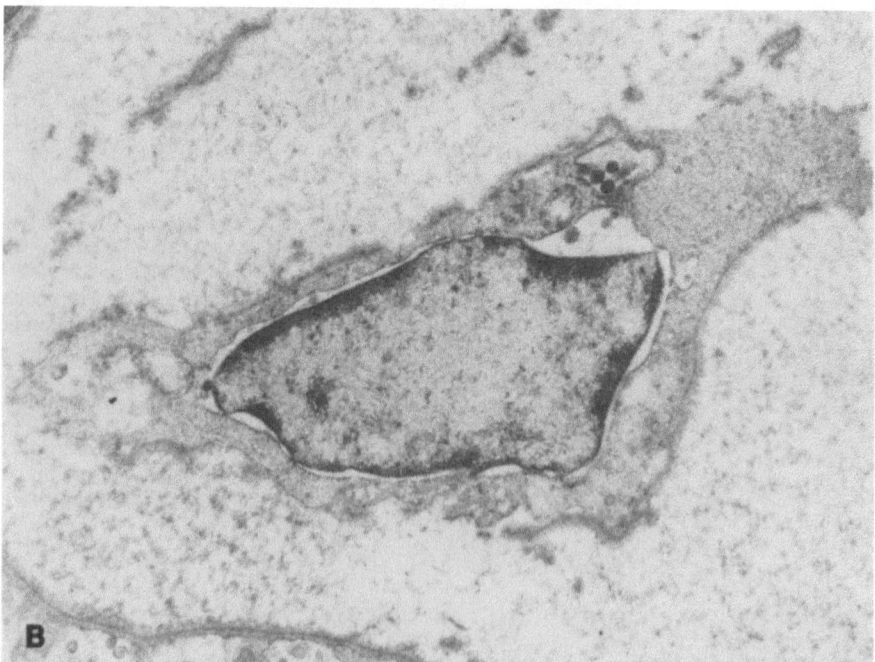

FIGURE 11. (A) TEM. The RIC in PN-SH. These cells became rounded and displayed a paucity of granules and cisterns. (B) This RIC from PN-SH of 30 days' duration reveals loss of cytoplasmic processes, granules and cisterns. The cytoplasm is finely granular. [A and B from Pitcock *et al.* (1980).]

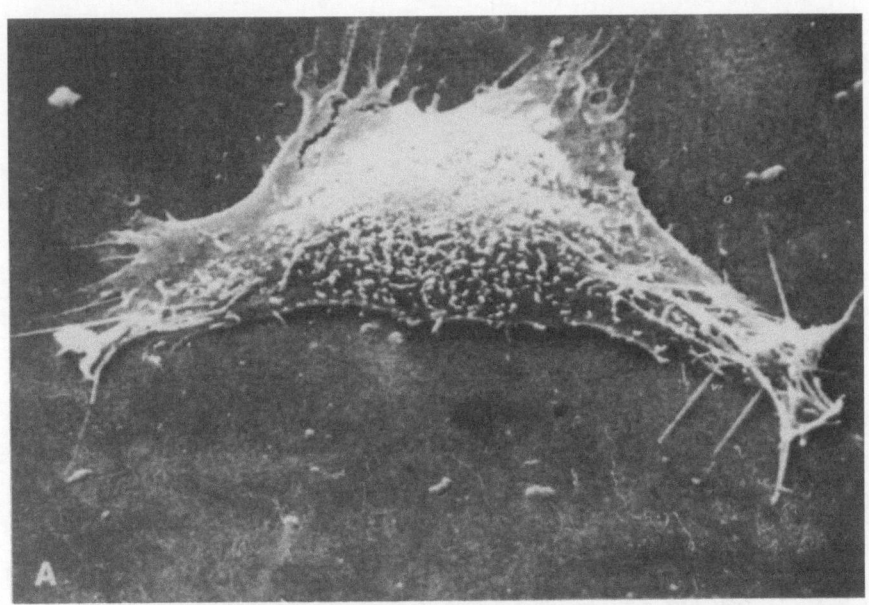

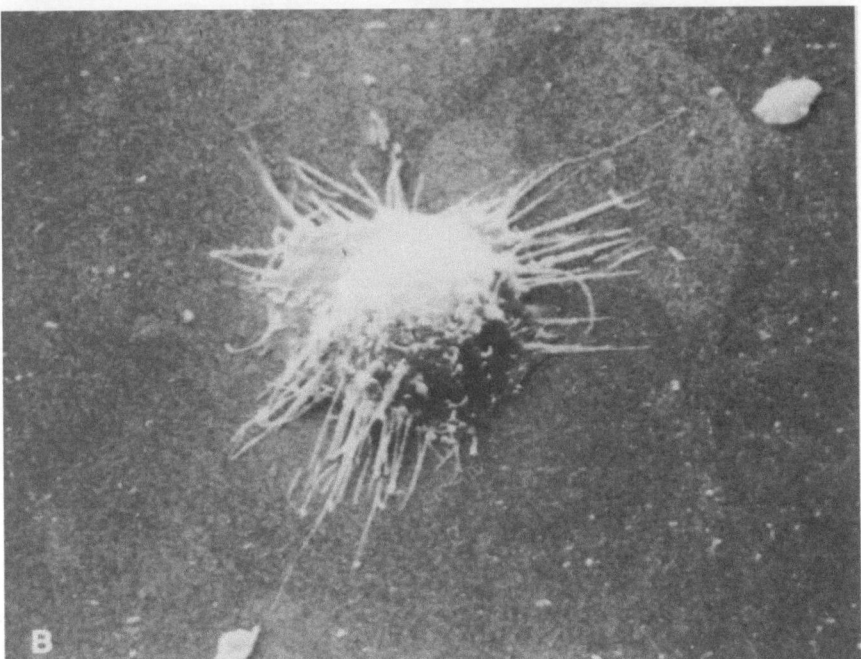

FIGURE 19. Scanning electron microscopy (SEM). A photomicrograph of RIC in tissue culture. The cytoplasmic processes are evident. (B) This cell, also from tissue culture of RIC, displays numerous surface projections, typical of a highly mobile cell. [These pictures were made available through the courtesy of Dr. D. W. DuCharme and Ms. Marcia McCandlis of The Upjohn Company, Kalamazoo, Michigan.]

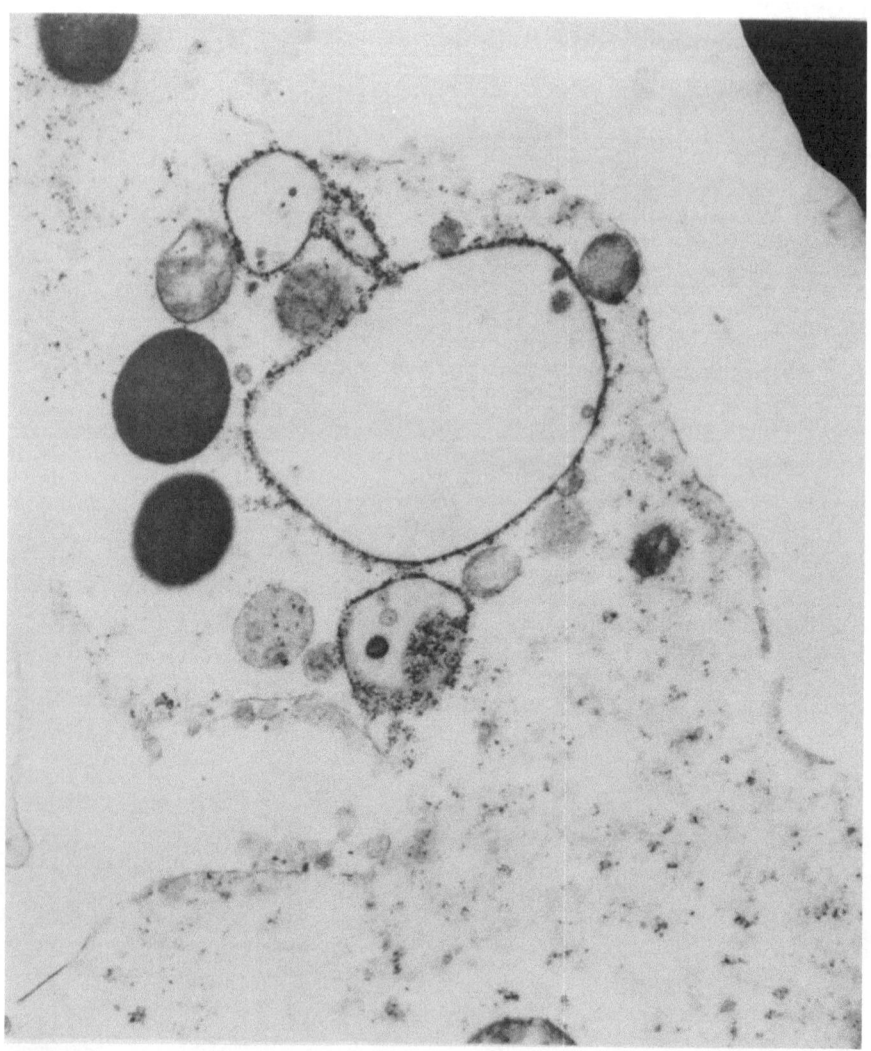

FIGURE 22. A lipid granule–cisternal complex convincingly illustrating the presence of reaction product indicative of phosphodiesterase activity on the cytoplasmic border of the membrane of the dilated cistern. The plasma membrane does not contain electron opacities. There are scattered opaque granules in the area of the cytosol.

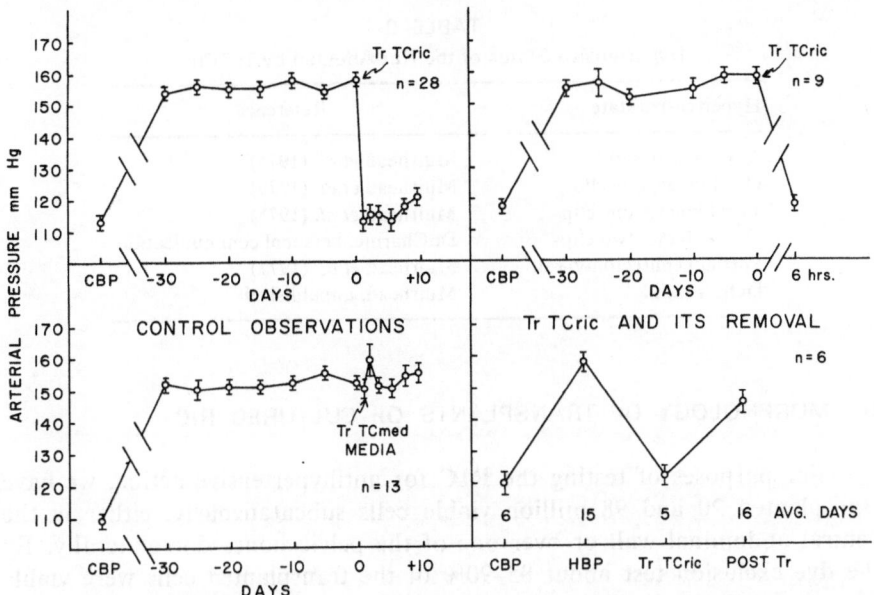

FIGURE 7. A summary of the antihypertensive effect of Tr TCric in recipients having angio-tensin–salt hypertension. Preculture tissue culture media were injected into the control animals. In the 28 examples of the upper left panel, the arterial pressure was lowered to normal within 24 hr and remained depressed for the 10 days of observation. No change in pressure occurred in the 13 control animals (lower left). The upper right panel demonstrates the lowering of the pressure over 6 hr in nine examples. The lower right panel demonstrates the return of the pressure toward the hypertensive levels after removal of the transplant. CBP, control blood pressure. HBP, hypertensive blood pressure. [From Muirhead et al. (1974b).]

cells themselves suggests either that the RIC are unstable in an extrarenal environment or that forces are at play in the hypertensive state that are constraining and injurious to these cells. The latter suggestion is invoked as part of the hypothesis explaining failure of RIC within the kidney to prevent hypertension in various hypertensive states.

Other results indicated that the antihypertensive action of the Tr TCric was not mediated by diuresis–natriuresis–kaliuresis (Muirhead et al., 1975). Indeed, this action occurred when regular renal tissue was removed, i.e., in the renoprival state (Fig. 6). This interpretation was further supported by the lack of weight loss as the arterial pressure receded.

Tr TCric have been effective against a variety of hypertensive states of the rat (Table 2). The antihypertensive action of these transplants made up of pure (or near-pure) RIC resembled closely that of the Tr Pap. This is another reason to consider the results of both transplants as the result of the actions of a single cell type, namely the RIC.

TABLE 2

Hypertensive States of the Rat Affected by Tr TCric

Hypertensive state	Reference
Angiotensin–salt	Muirhead *et al.* (1975)
One kidney, one clip	Muirhead *et al.* (1975)
Two kidneys, one clip	Muirhead *et al.* (1975)
Two kidneys, two clips	DuCharme, personal communication
Partial nephrectomy–salt	Muirhead *et al.* (1977)
DOCA–salt	Muirhead, unpublished

5. MORPHOLOGY OF TRANSPLANTS OF CULTURED RIC

For purposes of testing the RIC for antihypertensive action, we have transplanted 20 and 98 million viable cells subcutaneously, either in the ventral abdominal wall or over one of the pelvic bones dorsolaterally. By the dye exclusion test about 85–90% of the transplanted cells were viable after separation from the culture bottle, washing and suspending for injection. It is preferable to consider the morphology of Tr TCric during two phases of their existence: (1) early phase, i.e., within 24 hr, and (2) later phase, i.e., after 1–2 weeks or longer.

5.1. Early Phase of the Transplant

Within 24 hr the transplanted cells underwent aggregation that made it possible to shell out a mass (Fig. 8A) (Muirhead *et al.*, 1974*a*). This mass, naturally, was without an intrinsic vasculature. The small blood vessels about the mass were dilated, there being a regional hyperemia. Overwhelmingly, the cells of the transplant appeared viable (Fig. 8B). The cells retained the characteristics of RIC, such as the typical lipid granules of Bohman's Type 1 cell, the cisterns and the cytoplasmic processes (Muirhead *et al.*, 1974*a*). However, there were foci of degeneration and necrosis involving small groups of cells. Here polymorphonuclear neutrophils and macrophages infiltrated. We suggest that these inflammatory cells likely were derived as an aftermath of disintegration of the 10–15% of nonviable cells injected during the transplantation.

It is important to remember that a transplant of this type is capable of exerting a prominent antihypertensive action. In other words, some of these transplants lower the arterial pressure either significantly or to near-normal levels within the first 24 hr of their existence. Since there is no intrinsic vasculature of the transplant and, therefore, no blood flow, it appears most unlikely that the cells exert their antihypertensive action by neutralizing circulating vasopressor agents in situ. Rather, the antihypertensive action clearly results from the seeping out of an antihypertensive substance(s) from the cells that is picked up by nearby capillaries or lymphatics and is circulated in the manner of a hormone.

5.2. Later Phase of the Transplant

Within one to two weeks, the active transplant formed a nodule that expanded and was readily palpable in its subcutaneous location. Removal of the transplant at that time was followed by return of the arterial pressure to prior hypertensive levels (Fig. 7) (Muirhead et al., 1974b; Muirhead, 1974).

The cells retained the characteristics of RIC. At this stage, they formed a compact nodule in which there was a rich network of capillaries. The close association of the RIC to the capillaries was evident (positive tropism). The structure indeed resembled an endocrine gland (Fig. 9) (Muirhead, 1974).

The RIC of the transplant at this stage had a very high concentration of granules and the relationship of the lipid laden granules to the cisterns was evident (see Section 6). Staining the transplant with Alcian blue and colloidal iron indicated the presence of positive material within and about the cells. This suggested the production of acid mucopolysaccharide by the transplanted RIC.

6. THE LIPID GRANULE–CISTERNAL ORGANELLE RELATIONSHIP OF RIC

The two most unique intracellular structures of the RIC are the lipid granules and cisternal system [dilated rough endoplasmic reticulum (RER)]. In the normal cell, either, either in situ in the kidney, in tissue culture, or in transplants of either papillae or cultured RIC, a close relationship is commonly observed between the granule and cistern such that the granule appears to bulge into the cistern (Osvaldo and Latta, 1966). At times, the granule is seen inside the cistern but this could be an artifact.

A functional–morphological correlation seems to exist between the lipid granule and the cisternal organelle (Pitcock et al., 1976). We studied this possibility by comparing cultured RIC under three different circumstances: ordinary or normal circumstances, under the influence of indomethacin, and after numerous passages (>35) in tissue culture. The antihypertensive action of these cultures was tested in the syngeneic rat system while the transplanted cells were studied morphologically by a point-counting technique (Principle of Delesse) with which a true measure of various organelles could be determined and volume densities calculated by Weibel's approach (Weibel, 1970). The organelles singled out included the

TABLE 3
Organelle Volume Density[a]

	Nucleus	Droplets	Golgi apparatus	Dilated cisterns	Gray lipid
Functionally active RIC	0.2521	0.0424	0.0260	0.1466	0
	(0.1077)	(0.0374)	(0.0224)	(0.0877)	
Indomethacin-treated functionally active RIC	0.2182	0.3183	0.0404	0.0518	0
	(0.0663)	(0.0911)	(0.0265)	(0.0469)	
Late-passage non-functionally active RIC	0.2649	0	0.0236	0.0155	0.0142
	(0.1049)		(0.0332)	(0.0173)	(0.0100)

[a] Mean values with SD in parentheses are shown.

nucleus, dense lipid granules, Golgi apparatus, cisternal sacs, and less dense granules. The volume density measurements are depicted in Table 3.

Indomethacin (4 μg/ml culture medium) produced a tremendous increase in the number of dense lipid granules, at times almost obscuring the normal cytoplasmic structures (Fig. 10). Many very large granules were present (Muirhead et al., 1975). The cisternal system appeared smaller, apparently being compressed by the granules. The Golgi apparatus was larger. The chromatin pattern of the nucleus became more dispersed. In short-term experiments, the antihypertensive action was not altered by these changes.

The cultured RIC, after many passages, lost their antihypertensive action. This was attended by major morphological changes. The normal dense lipid granules disappeared or became very rare. A smaller number of less osmiophilic (gray) granules were present. The dilated cisternal pattern gave way to a flattened RER resembling that of the fibroblast.

It appears that the dense lipid granule–cisternal organelle relationship is essential for the antihypertensive action of the RIC to be maintained.

7. RENOMEDULLARY (RIC) DEFICIENCY IN HYPERTENSION

The absence of RIC appears to allow certain prohypertensive mechanisms to operate out of control (see Section 2). Sodium and volume excess is one such mechanism. Accordingly, renomedullary or RIC deficiency seems to be a state permissive toward hypertension (Muirhead et al., 1973b). This deficiency also seems to make possible the acute cardiovascular lesions of renoprival hypertension of the dog (Muirhead et al., 1951). Extracts of renal medulla protect against both renoprival hypertension and its cardiovascular damage, even when exaggerated by the vasopressor action of renin (Muirhead and Kosinski, 1962; Muirhead, 1963).

The relationship of renomedullary (RIC) deficiency to the hypertensive state has been evaluated in partial nephrectomy–salt hypertension (PN-SH) (the Chanutin–Ferris model). Two approaches were used: a morphometric study of the RIC with emphasis on the number of cells and granules within the cells (Pitcock *et al.*, 1977, 1978), and transplantation of the renal papilla into hypertensive recipients.

7.1. Morphometric Study of the Renal Papilla in Partial Nephrectomy–Salt Hypertension

PN-SH of the rat was induced by ablating 70–75% of the renal tissue (removal of one kidney and the poles of the opposite kidney) and by giving the animals 1% NaCl to drink. Under these conditions the papilla remained in the renal nubbin. The arterial pressure elevated sharply within 3–4 days and remained elevated as long as the salt intake was maintained (blood pressure ~150–180 mm Hg, control 110–120 mm Hg).

The morphometric study was conducted according to the principles proposed by Weibel (Weibel, 1970) and as described by Bohman and Jensen (1976). After 25–30 days of hypertension there was a marked reduction in the number of RIC and in the number of dense granules in their cytoplasm (for normal controls number of cells/grid: 11.04 ± 1.5, number of granules/cell: 4.48 ± 0.4; for hypertensive animals: 3.7 ± 0.1 and 1.1 ± 0.1, respectively; $N = 10$, $p < 0.001$). The RIC not only were depleted in numbers and granules but also became degenerated. Degeneration was indicated by loss of cytoplasmic processes and organelles, and by the cytoplasm becoming granular (Fig. 11).

7.2. Transplantation of Renal Papilla from Animals Having Partial Nephrectomy–Salt Hypertension

The renal papilla derived from the remaining renal remant of two rats having PN-SH of 30 days' duration failed to lower the mean arterial pressure (MAP) of one kidney, one clip hypertensive recipients when transplanted as Tr Pap. Transplants of two papillae from normal kidneys did lower the MAP significantly ($+13 \pm 4$ vs. -23 ± 3 mm Hg, $N = 10$, $p < 0.001$) (Fig. 12).

The morphological component of this study indicated considerable degeneration of RIC in terms of numbers and lipid granule–cisternal relationship. The functional component of the study suggests a deficiency in the antihypertensive function of the RIC. The maintenance of PN-SH of the rat, like renoprival hypertension of the dog and rabbit, appears to depend on a sodium–volume load in the absence of the controlling influence of the RIC. The specific cause of the damage to the RIC was not determined, but

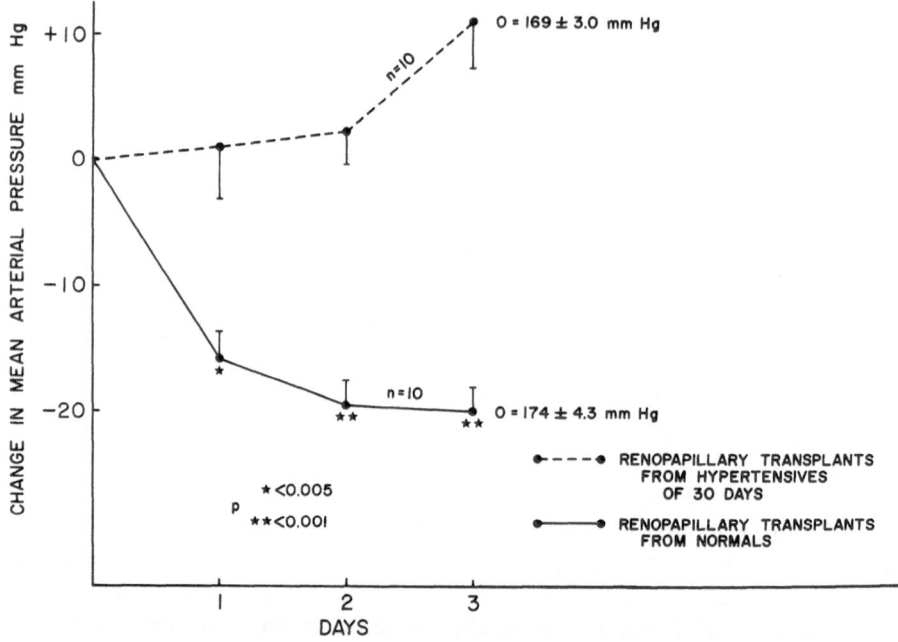

FIGURE 12. The transplantation of minced and washed renal papillae from two normal rat kidneys (solid line) caused a significant lowering of the MAP of hypertensive recipients having one kidney, one clip hypertension by 24 hr; this reduced pressure was maintained at 48 and 72 hr. By way of contrast, the transplantation of minced and washed papillae from two kidneys of rats having partial nephrectomy–salt hypertension of 30 days' duration failed to change the MAP.

it related to the high salt load since partial nephrectomy alone did not disturb the appearance of the RIC.

8. RENOMEDULLARY INTERSTITIAL CELL TUMOR

We reasoned that if the RIC represent an endocrine organ then, in keeping with most endocrine structures, they should, under certain circumstances, undergo either a hyperplastic or an adenomatous change. It turned out that the so-called fibroma of the renal medulla of the human kidney represented a collection of RIC surrounded by acid mucopolysaccharide, collagen, and PAS-positive material (Fig. 13). We renamed this structure the renomedullary interstitial cell tumor (RICT) (Lerman et al., 1972).

This small tumor is usually situated in the middle of the renal papilla where RIC are most numerous. In a human autopsy service having a high rate of deaths due to cardiovascular disease, this tumor is encountered in about 30% of cases, if carefully searched for (Lerman *et al.*, 1972). However, Stuart *et al.* (1976) did not find a correlation between the existence of this structure at autopsy and evidence of hypertension during life.

9. INHIBITION OF THE CONVERTING ENZYME (KININASE II) AND THE ACTION OF RIC

Tr Pap and their RIC prevented malignant hypertension (MH) of the rabbit.* Under the conditions of this experimental model, the early elevation of the MAP was not prevented by the RIC but the lethal rise of the third week was prevented (Fig. 14). After three weeks, removal of the Tr Pap, which by then consisted almost entirely of RIC, was followed by a sharp elevation of the MAP and a lethal outcome.

The inhibition of kininase II by teprotide or SQ 20,881 also prevented MH of the rabbit and in the same manner as did the RIC (Muirhead *et al.*, 1974c). Discontinuance of the drug after 3 weeks was followed by a sharp elevation of the MAP and death, similar to the effect of removal of the Tr Pap and its RIC.

Teprotide failed to prevent MH if initiation of therapy was delayed for 6–8 days. Thus, teprotide prevented a fairly early event in the pathogenesis of MH.

Combining Tr Pap and teprotide delayed the early rise in MAP but did not prevent it. This combination also prevented MH in the same manner as either approach alone. Since Tr Pap and teprotide do not potentiate each other beyond 1 week, there is the suggestion that each operates through a similar mechanism.

The similarities in the antihypertensive actions of RIC and teprotide could be fortuitous. On the other hand, they could indicate a relationship between the antihypertensive action of RIC and either the prevention of generation of angiotensin II or the potentiation of the action of bradykinin, the two known developments following the inhibition of kininase II. An attractive hypothesis considers that either angiotensin II within the kidney

---

* By malignant hypertension (Muirhead *et al.*, 1972a) is meant the development of severe hypertension (mean aortic pressure of 130 mm Hg or higher) associated with diffuse fibrinoid necrosis of the viscera, uremia, encephalopathy, and death. This syndrome was produced in the rabbit by placing a narrow clip on the left renal artery and removing the right kidney. The mean aortic pressure elevated sharply during the first 24–36 hr (from 60–70 to 90–100 mm Hg), leveled off for 10–14 days, and elevated rapidly to lethal levels during the third week. By standardizing the experimental approaches (use of male rabbits aged 14–16 weeks and weighing 3 kg, and use of a rigid clip having a fixed gap), all animals died within three weeks, giving a sharp end point.

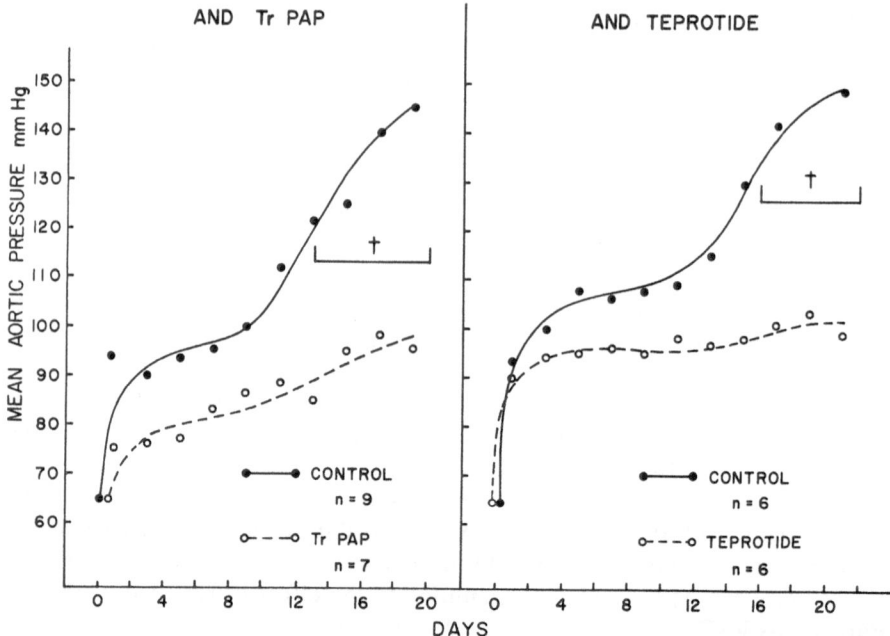

FIGURE 14. A comparison of the antihypertensive action of Tr Pap and teprotide in MH of the rabbit. The solid lines and closed circles represent the sequence of MAP change in control rabbits subjected to the MH procedure. The broken lines and open circles demonstrate protection against the lethal rise of MAP in MH by Tr Pap and teprotide. The similarity in results is apparent. All control animals died by 16–22 days. All animals receiving either Tr Pap or teprotide survived beyond 22 days. [Modified from Muirhead *et al.* (1972*a*, 1974*c*).]

effects a constraining influence on the antihypertensive action of the RIC, or bradykinin has a stimulating influence on these cells.

10. ANTIHYPERTENSIVE LIPIDS DERIVABLE FROM FRESH RENAL MEDULLA

Soon after it was demonstrated that transplants of renal medulla (Tr Pap) were protective toward the hypertensive state (Muirhead *et al.*, 1960*b*), extracts of fresh renal medulla were prepared and were shown to exert a similar action (Muirhead *et al.*, 1960*c*). These extracts were refined by at least eight separate techniques and were demonstrated to be lipid in nature (Muirhead *et al.*, 1963, 1965, 1966). About this time, the prostaglandins entered this picture by the work of Lee *et al.* (1963). It soon became apparent that there were at least two classes of lipids extractable from fresh renal medulla (Muirhead *et al.*, 1965). One was determined to be a neutral lipid by chromatographic and solubility characteristics, and the other was acidic and, in time, was identified as prostaglandin (Daniels *et al.*, 1967; Lee *et al.*, 1967), mainly PGE_2.

Currently there are two nonprostanoic lipid entities, derived from renal medulla, under scrutiny. One is a highly polar lipid, termed antihypertensive polar renomedullary lipid (APRL), and the other is neutral, termed antihypertensive neutral renomedullary lipid (ANRL) (Prewitt *et al.*, 1979).

ANRL is a native substance obtained by total lipid extraction followed by column and thin-layer chromatography (Muirhead *et al.*, 1977). It has not been characterized.

APRL is obtained by total lipid extraction followed by a reduction step using Vitride [$NaAlH_2(OCH_2CH_2OCH_3)_2$], acetylation, silicic acid column chromatography, two thin-layer chromatographic steps, and high-pressure liquid chromatography. In view of the Vitride step it has been considered semisynthetic.

Intravenous injection of ANRL as a bolus dose into the hypertensive rat is followed by a lag period lasting 2 min or more, after which the MAP slowly declines to a minimum over 15 to >60 min, depending on the potency of the extract (Fig. 15). Administration of APRL as a bolus iv dose

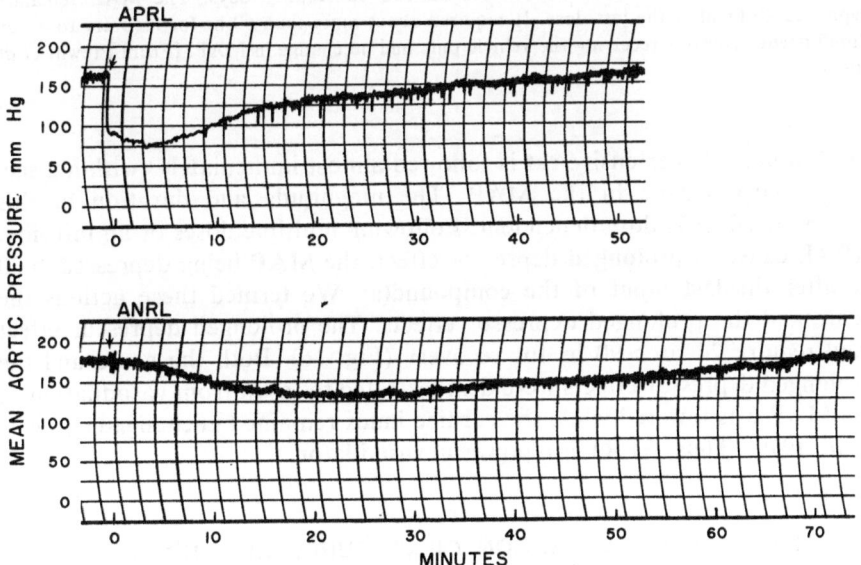

FIGURE 15. The contrasting effects of APRL and ANRL when injected intravenously as a bolus dose into a one kidney, one clip hypertensive rat. APRL caused an almost immediate acute depressor effect requiring over 60 min for complete recovery, while injection of ANRL was followed by a lag period of 3 min, then a slow decline in the MAP to a minimum in 20–30 min. Recovery after ANRL also required over 60 min. [From Prewitt *et al.* (1979).]

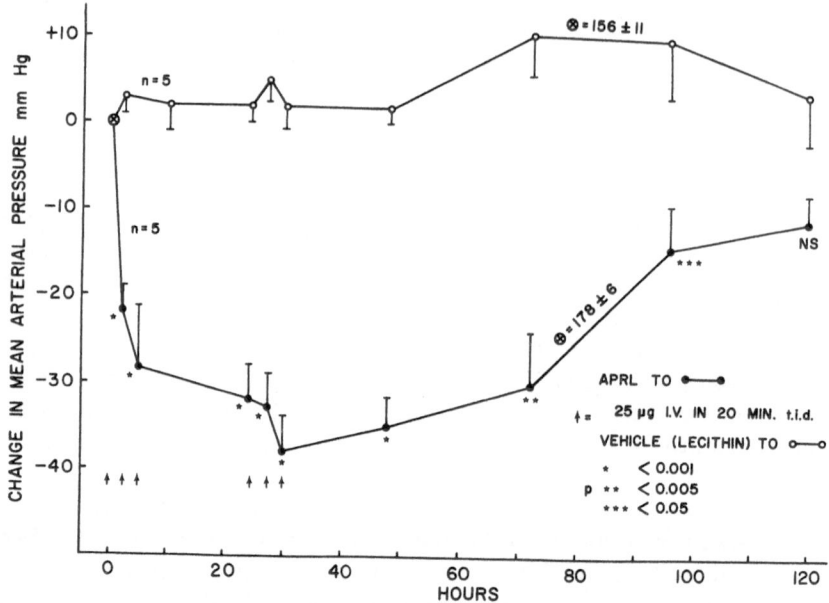

FIGURE 16. Prolonged depressor effect of APRL in one-kidney Goldblatt hypertensive rats. Three doses of APRL were administered on two consecutive days. The MAP remained depressed 20 hr after the last dose. It required about more than 60 hr for recovery to occur. Simultaneous controls receiving the vehicle only had no change in MAP. [From Prewitt *et al.* (1979).]

to a similarly hypertensive rat is followed almost immediately (within 2 sec) by a sharp decline in the MAP. The magnitude and duration of this depressor effect is dose dependent. Following multiple doses or an infusion, APRL causes a prolonged depressor effect, the MAP being depressed >20 hr after the last input of the compound(s). We termed these actions the acute and the prolonged depressor effects. The prolonged depressor effect may require 24 to >90 hr for recovery (Fig. 16). Both the acute and the prolonged depressor effects were demonstrated to result from vasodilation as the MAP was lowered while the cardiac index remained unchanged (Prewitt *et al.*, 1979). Thus, APRL is a powerful vasodilator.

11. ANTIHYPERTENSIVE ACTION OF CULTURED RIC AND OF LIPIDS DERIVED FROM THE SAME TISSUE CULTURE

RIC grown in tissue culture (TCric) were subjected to two procedures at about the same time (Muirhead *et al.*, 1977). (1) TCric was transplanted into hypertensive recipients (20–30 million viable cells). (2) The RIC tissue cultures were extracted for lipids according to the sequence described in Section 12 (Muirhead *et al.*, 1977) and injected iv into the same types of hypertensive recipients. The results indicated that both the intact cells and the lipids extracted from the cells exerted a similar antihypertensive action (Fig. 17). Thus, these lipids are the major candidates for the mediation of the antihypertensive action of the RIC. Moreover, it is of interest that similar antihypertensive lipids can be derived from fresh renal medulla (Fig. 18) (Muirhead *et al.*, 1977).

12. THREE ADDITIONAL SPECIAL FEATURES OF RIC

12.1. Surface Mobility in Tissue Culture

One of the major features of the RIC, termed Type I cell by Bohman (1974), is the projection of cytoplasmic processes. This, in itself, is indicative of the mobile nature of the cell. In ordinary preparations of the renal papilla these processes appear irregularly distributed, touching all three major nearby structures, but especially the vasa recta and Henle's loop (Bohman, 1974). In tissue culture, this mobility is also indicated by scanning electron microscopy (D. W. DuCharme, M. R. McCandlis, and J. Mathews, unpublished observations). The surface of the cell displays prominent cytoplasmic projections (Fig. 19A), at times being porcupinelike (Fig. 19B), similar to other highly mobile cells. The functional implications of this mobility within the papilla of the kidney are unknown at present.

12.2. Milieu of the RIC

Within the papilla the main substance holding the structures together consists of proteoglycans (acid mucopolysaccharide) (Farber *et al.*, 1970). The RIC are in a ladderlike arrangement within the gel-like milieu. The indications are that the RIC secrete the proteoglycans (Fig. 20) (Pitcock *et al.*, 1978), thus creating their own environment as well as the environment for the other related local structures (vasa recta, Henle's loop, collecting ducts).

12.3. Phosphodiesterase and Its Localization within RIC

The RIC are rich in phosphodiesterase (Fig. 21) (Florendo *et al.*, 1978). This, in itself, suggests that cyclic AMP (cAMP) is an active messenger within the cells. The message conveyed by cAMP within these cells is unknown. It could be related to any of their known synthetic activities,

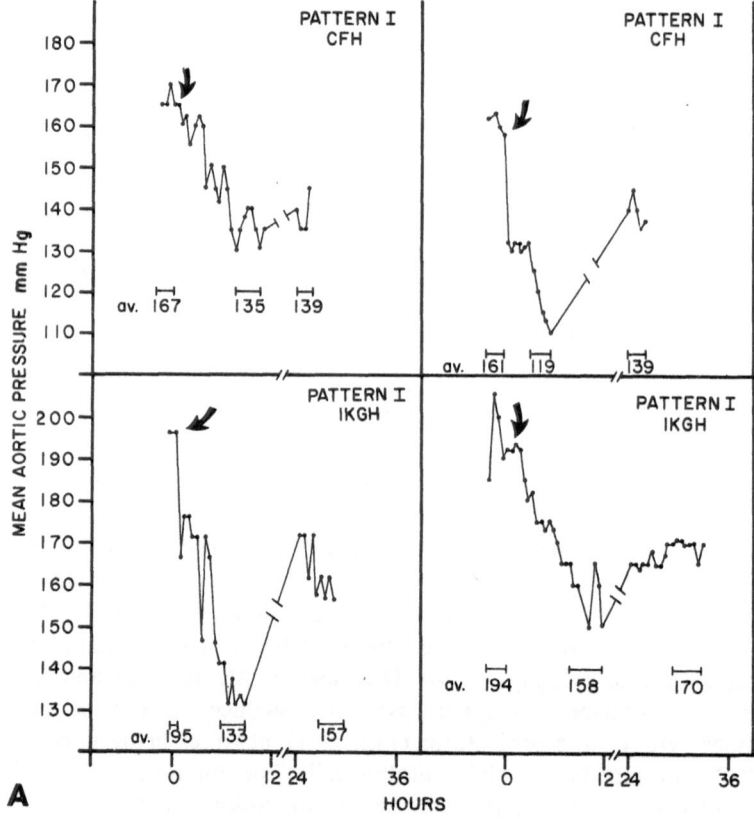

FIGURE 17. The antihypertensive action of transplants of cultured RIC (Tr TCric) and lipid extracted from the same cell line. (A) At the arrows, 20–30 million viable RIC were injected subcutaneously. The MAP was recorded every 30 min in an automated assembly. Two hypertensive models were used: partial nephrectomy–salt (PN-SH) and one kidney, one clip

namely the synthesis of prostaglandin (mainly PGE_2), proteoglycans, and an antihypertensive hormone.

The phosphodiesterase is concentrated on the cytoplasmic side of the cisternal membranes but is also appears to be diffusely scattered over the cytosol. It is absent in the cell membrane, nuclear membrane, and membrane of the mitochondria and granules (Fig. 22).

13. DISCUSSION

As indicated by other chapters in this volume, the RIC are considered to perform various functions. Indeed, it seems evident that differentiation of

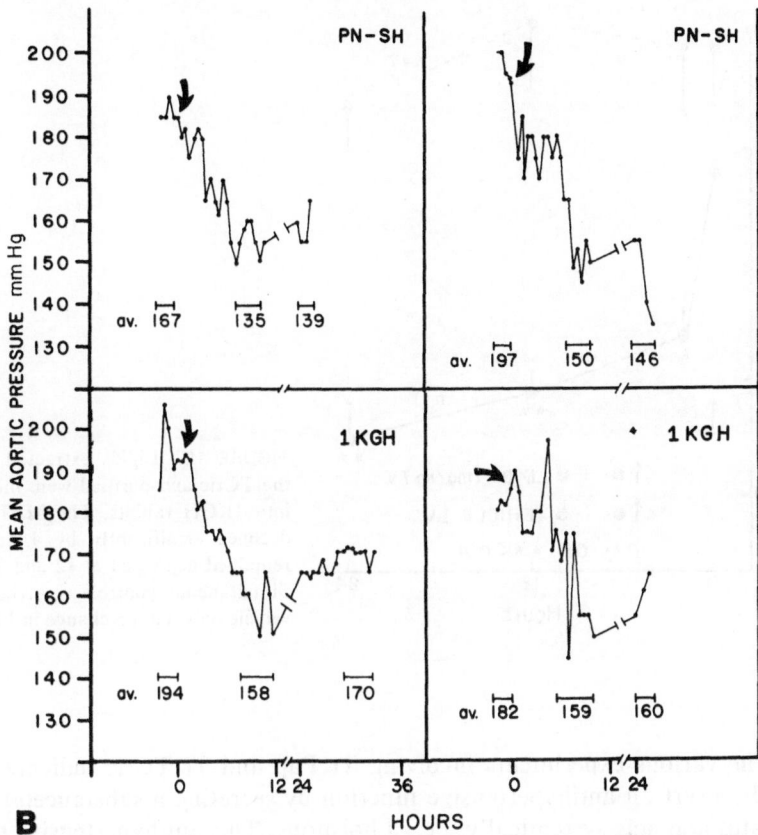

B

HOURS

(1KGH). The MAP declined to a maximum within 6–12 hr and remained depressed the following day. (B) Lipids extracted from the TCric were injected iv into hypertensive recipient rats. The MAP receded in a manner comparable to that noted when the RIC themselves were transplanted. [From Muirhead *et al.* (1977).]

these cells in their special location resulted from demands for special functions. These functions could be localized or they could be generalized, through the secretion of messengers into the bloodstream to act elsewhere. Our studies are consistent with both types of functions.

The indications are that the RIC synthesize and secrete proteoglycans. They may be the cells that produce the main interstitial substances (interstitial gel) of the papilla. This raises questions as to whether there are local modulators of gel secretion and gel compliance within the papilla.

These cells also synthesize prostaglandins, mainly PGE_2, most likely for local purposes.*

* It is now established that cells of the papilla other than RIC synthesize prostaglandin. The

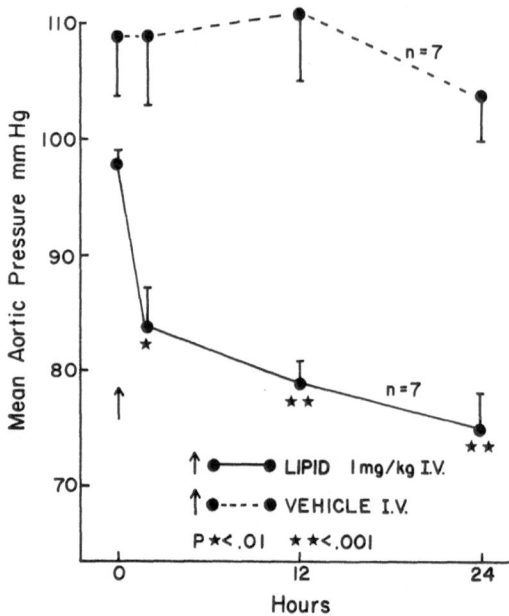

FIGURE 18. Lipids extracted from the TCric and purified were injected into 1KGH rabbits. The MAP had declined significantly by 4 hr and remained depressed at 12 and 24 hr. Simultaneous controls receiving the vehicle only had no change in MAP.

The various experiments involving Tr Pap and Tr TCric indicate that the RIC exert an antihypertensive function by secreting a substance(s) that circulates and acts systemically, i.e., a hormone. This antihypertensive function has been demonstrated by both the prevention and the reversal of the hypertensive state by the RIC. The two organelles within the RIC that appear essential for this function are the lipid-laden granules and the cisternal system (dilated RER). Antihypertensive lipids can be derived from both the renal medulla and cultured RIC (Muirhead *et al.*, 1977), raising the question as to whether such lipids are the mediators of the antihypertensive function of the RIC.

Lucas and Floyer (1972, 1973) have approached the question of the renal function involved during the ureterovenous manipulation from the viewpoint of the interstitial gel compliance. According to this view, a factor from the kidney increases interstitial gel compliance in such way as to hold sodium and water in the gel, thereby protecting the circulating volume from overexpansion. Conversely, in the absence of kidneys the compliance of the gel, according to these workers, is decreased, allowing more intravascular

original suggestion of Janszen and Nugteren (1971), using a histochemical method, that the collecting duct synthesizes prostaglandin had been confirmed by Bohman (1977) by a direct method.

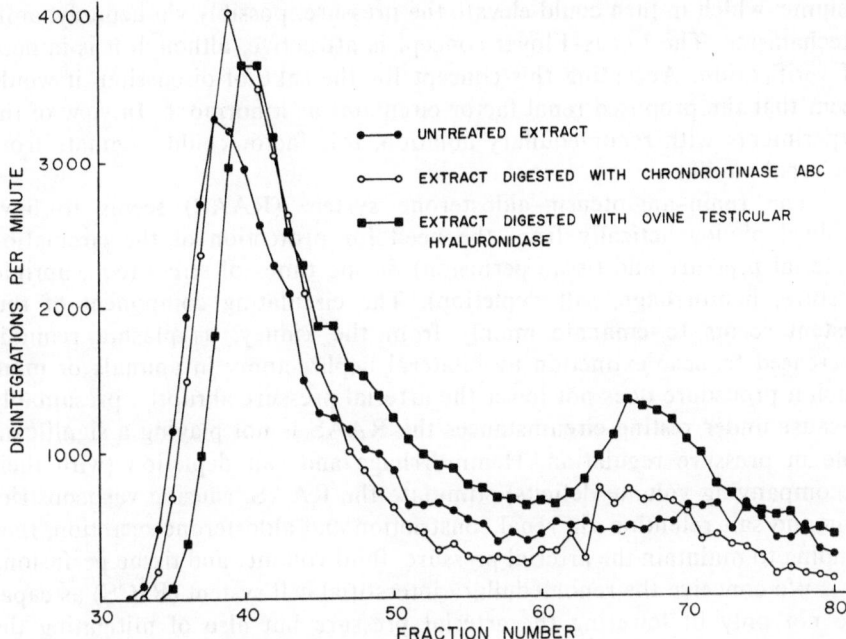

FIGURE 20. Chromatography of an extract of RIC tissue culture medium. A tissue culture of RIC was labeled with tritiated glucosamine and the medium was collected 24 hr later. The medium was precipitated with trichloracetic acid (TCA) and the soluble portion was dialyzed. The nondialyzable fraction contained about 10% of the initial radioactivity. This fraction was chromatographed (Sephadex G-25 column) before and after digestion with glycosaminoglycan-degrading enzymes. The chromatography indicates partial digestion of the TCA-soluble, non-dialyzable fraction of RIC tissue culture medium by ovine testicular hyaluronidase, a further indication of production of glycosaminoglycans by the RIC.

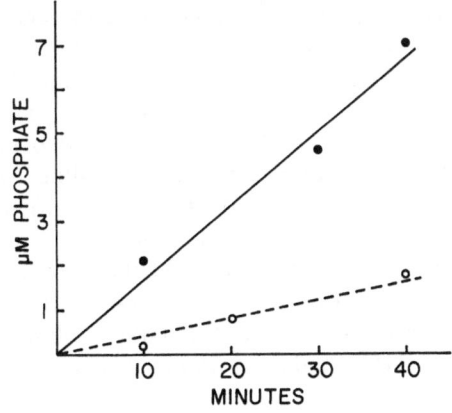

FIGURE 21. Phosphodiesterase activity in renal medulla (procedure of Butcher and Sutherland, 1962). The addition of theophylline (dashed line) decreased inorganic phosphate release by 75%. The solid line depicts the activity without theophylline. [From Florendo *et al.* (1978).]

volume, which in turn could elevate the pressure, possibly via hemodynamic mechanisms. The Lucas–Floyer concept is attractive, although it is in need of verification. Accepting this concept for the sake of discussion, it would seem that the proposed renal factor circulates as a hormone. In view of the experiments with renomedullary ablation, this factor could originate from the renal papilla.

The renin–angiotensin–aldosterone system (RAAS) seems to have evolved phylogenetically from the need for protection of the circulation (arterial pressure and tissue perfusion) during times of stress (e.g., upright posture, hemorrhage, salt depletion). The circulating component of this system seems to emanate mainly from the kidney, as plasma renin is decreased to near extinction by bilateral nephrectomy in animals or man. Such a procedure does not lower the arterial pressure abruptly, presumably because under resting circumstances the RAAS is not playing a significant role in pressure regulation. Hemmorrhage and salt depletion (with their accompanying volume deficits) stimulate the RAAS, causing vasoconstriction and salt retention via renal constriction and aldosterone secretion, thus tending to maintain the arterial pressure, fluid volume, and tissue perfusion.

We conceive the renomedullary interstitial cell system (RICS) as capable not only of lowering the arterial pressure but also of mitigating the prohypertensive effect of sodium and volume. The antihypertensive internal secretion of the RIC does not seem to be called into play under ordinary resting conditions, much like the juxtaglomerular–cell secretion (renin-angiotensin). Therefore, one would not expect the arterial pressure to elevate abruptly because the RICS is removed (as by bilateral nephrectomy or renal papillary ablation). Rather, the arterial pressure remains unchanged.

As expressed previously, the absence or suppression of the RICS is considered to allow prohypertensive mechanisms to operate out of proper control. In this respect, the combination of an activated RAAS and the accompanying excessive vasoconstriction and sodium–volume load plus a markedly suppressed RICS should make for a pronounced elevation of the arterial pressure. We conceive the accelerated malignant hypertensive state to result from such a combination.

The two systems, RAAS and RICS, may be considered as stress responders within the framework of arterial pressure control. As such, a "push–pull" effect between the two systems has been proposed (Fig. 23) (Muirhead et al., 1977). According to this hypothesis, stimulation of the RAAS (hemorrhage, salt depletion) depresses the RICS and thus allows vasoconstriction to act unopposed, assisting in the maintenance of both pressure and perfusion. At the same time, sodium retention allows the activation of the blood-pressure-elevating actions of sodium. Conversely, suppression of the RAAS (sodium–volume expansion, hypervolemia) stimulates the RICS, inducing unopposed vasodilatation and suppression of the blood-

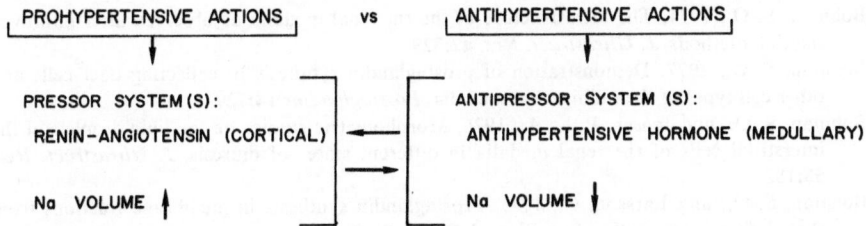

FIGURE 23. A schematic depiction of the proposed relationship between the prohypertensive and the antihypertensive actions of the kidney as related to renal hormones and the handling of sodium and volume by the kidney.

pressure-elevating actions of sodium. The "push–pull" view places emphasis on more or less angiotensin.*

Clearly, the RAAS and RICS were not developed, in the evolutionary sense, for the purpose of causing the hypertensive state. According to current views, the hypertensive state results when alterations occur in homeostatic mechanisms that control arterial pressure. Page's mosaic theory (Page, 1968) suggests that when one controlling system goes awry, other systems may follow, culminating in the state of sustained arterial pressure elevation. No matter how the elevated pressure is initiated, sooner or later, as emphasized by Guyton *et al.* (1972), the kidney plays a role in maintaining the heightened pressure. The questions at issue are how does the kidney enter into the maintenance of the elevated arterial pressure and how may the mechanisms involved be altered. The work of McGiff and associates (McGiff, 1975; Sullivan and McGiff, 1980) indicates that intrarenal vasoconstrictive mechanisms (such as the actions of angiotensin, norepinephrine, and an elevated adrenergic drive) are prohypertensive, while intrarenal vasodilator mechanisms (such as the actions of bradykinin and prostaglandins and the blockage of constrictor actions) are antihypertensive.

Our proposals add a dimension to those of the mosaic theory of Page and to the intrarenal mechanisms, such as those of Guyton and McGiff, by emphasizing the antihypertensive action of the RIC.

REFERENCES

Änggård, E., Bohman, S.-O., Griffin, J. E., III, Larsson, C., and Maunsbach, A. B., 1972, Subcellular localization of the prostaglandin system in the rabbit renal papilla, *Acta Physiol. Scand.* **84**:231.

---

* Angiotensin seems to be the agent most eligible for constraining RIC function. Is is conceivable that other renal vasoconstrictive agents may also constrain RIC function, either directly or via angiotensin generation within the kidney.

Bohman, S.-O., 1974, The ultrastructure of the rat renal medulla as observed after improved fixation methods, *J. Ultrastruct. Res.* **47**:329.

Bohman, S.-O., 1977, Demonstration of prostaglandin synthesis in collecting duct cells and other cell types of the rabbit renal medulla, *Prostaglandins* **14**:729.

Bohman, S.-O., and Jensen, P. K. A., 1976, Morphometric studies on the lipid droplets of the interstitial cells of the renal medulla in different states of diuresis, *J. Ultrastruct. Res.* **55**:182.

Bohman, S.-O., and Larsson, C., 1975, Prostaglandin synthesis in membrane fractions from the rabbit renal medulla, *Acta Physiol. Scand.* **94**:244.

Braun-Menendez, E., and Von Euler, U. S., 1947, Hypertension after bilateral nephrectomy in the rat, *Nature* **160**:905.

Butcher, R. W., and Sutherland, E. W., 1962, Adenosine 3',5'-phosphate in biological materials. 1. Purification and properties of cyclic 3',5'-nucleotide phosphodiesterase and use of this enzyme to characterize adenosine 3',5'-phosphate in human urine, *J. Biol. Chem.* **237**:1244.

Byrom F. B., and Dodson, L. F., 1949, The mechanism of the vicious circle in chronic hypertension, *Clin. Sci.* **8**:1.

Daniels, E. G., Hinman, J. W., Leach, B. E., and Muirhead, E. E., 1967, Identification of prostaglandin E$_2$ as the principal vasodepressor lipid of rabbit renal medulla, *Nature* **215**:1298.

Farber, S. J., Walat, R. J., Benjamin, R., and van Praag, D., 1970, Effect of increased osmolality on glucosaminoglycan metabolism of rabbit renal papilla, *Am. J. Physiol.* **220**:880.

Florendo, N. T., Pitcock, J. A., and Muirhead, E. E., 1978, Cyclic 3',5'-nucleotide phosphodiesterase: Cytochemical localization in rat renomedullary interstitial cells. Phosphodiesterase in rat renal medulla, *J. Histochem. Cytochem.* **26**:441.

Floyer, M. A., 1955, Further studies on the mechanism of experimental hypertension in the rat, *Clin. Sci.* **14**:163.

Floyer, M. A., 1957, Role of the kidney in experimental hypertension, *Br. Med. Bull.* **13**:29.

Gomez, A. H., Hoobler, S. W., and Blaquier, P., 1960, Effect of addition and removal of kidney transplant in renal and adrenocortical hypertensive rats, *Circ. Res.* **8**:464.

Grollman, A., Muirhead, E. E., and Vanatta, J., 1949, Role of the kidney in the pathogenesis of hypertension as determined by a study of the effects of bilateral nephrectomy and other experimental procedures on the blood pressure of the dog, *Am. J. Physiol.* **156**:21.

Guyton, A. C., Coleman, T. J., Cowley, A. W., Scheel, K. W., Manning, R. D., Jr., and Norman, R. A., Jr., 1972, Arterial pressure regulation: Overriding dominance of the kidneys in long-term regulation and in hypertension, *Am. J. Med.* **52**:584.

Heptinstall, R. H., Salyer, D. C., and Salyer, W. R., 1975, The effects of chemical ablation of the renal papilla on blood pressure of rats with and without silver-clip hypertension, *Am. J. Pathol.* **78**:297.

Janszen, F. H. A., and Nugteren, D. H., 1971, Histochemical localization of prostaglandin synthetase, *Histochemie* **27**:159.

Kolff, W. J., and Page, I. H., 1954, Blood pressure reducing function of the kidney: Reduction of renoprival hypertension by kidney perfusion, *Am. J. Physiol.* **178**:75.

Ledingham, J. M., 1957, Disturbances in water and electrolyte metabolism in experimental hypertension, *Br. Med. Bull.* **13**:33.

Lee, J. B., Hickler, R. B., Saravis, C. A., and Thorn, G. W., 1963, Sustained depressor effect of renal medullary extract in the normotensive rat, *Circ. Res.* **13**:359.

Lee, J. B., Crowshaw, K., Takman, B. H., Attrep, K. A., and Gougoutas, J. Z., 1967, The identification of prostaglandin E$_2$, F$_{2\alpha}$ and A$_2$ from rabbit kidney medulla *Biochem. J.* **105**:1251.

Lerman, R. I., Pitcock, J. A., Stephenson, P., and Muirhead, E. E., 1972, Renomedullary interstitial cell tumor, *Human Pathol.* **3**:559.

Lucas, J., and Floyer, M. A., 1972, Communications: 1. Body fluid distribution and pressure in experimental hypertension, *Clin. Sci.* **42**:2.

Lucas, J., and Floyer, M. A., 1973, Renal control of changes in the compliance of the interstitial space; a factor in the etiology of renoprival hypertension, *Clin. Sci.* **44**:397.

McGiff, J. C., 1975, Prostaglandins as regulators of blood pressure, *Hosp. Pract.* **10**:101.

Manthorpe, T., 1973, The effect on renal hypertension of subcutaneous isotransplantation of renal medulla from normal or hypertensive rats, *Acta Pathol. Microbiol. Scand.* **81**:725.

Manthorpe, T., 1975, Antihypertensive and hypertensive effects of the kidney, *Acta Pathol. Microbiol. Scand.* **83**:395.

Muirhead, E. E., 1962, Protection against sodium-overload hypertensive disease: Use of renal tissue and medullorenal extract, *Arch. Pathol.* **74**:214.

Muirhead E. E., 1963, Renal tissue and extracts vs cardiovascular injury, *Arch. Pathol.* **76**:613.

Muirhead, E. E., 1974, The role of the renal medulla in hypertension, in: *Advances in Internal Medicine*, Vol. 19 (G. H. Stollerman, ed.), Year Book Medical Publishers, Chicago, pp. 81–107.

Muirhead, E. E., and Brooks, B., 1980, Reversal of one-kidney, one clip hypertension by unclipping: The renal sodium–volume relationship reexamined, *Proc. Soc. Exp. Biol. Med.* **163**(4):540.

Muirhead, E. E., and Kosinski, M. 1962, Renal medulla and renoprival hypertension: Relationship between corticorenal (renin) and medullorenal extracts, *Circ. Res.* **11**:674.

Muirhead, E. E., Vanatta, J., and Grollman, A., 1950, Papillary necrosis of the kidney: A clinical and experimental correlation, *J. Am. Med. Assoc.* **142**:627.

Muirhead, E. E., Turner, L. B.,and Grollman, A., 1951, Hypertensive cardiovascular disease: Vascular lesions of dogs maintained for extended periods following bilateral nephrectomy or ureteral ligation, *Arch. Pathol.* **51**:575.

Muirhead, E. E., Stirman, J. A., Lesch, W., and Jones, F., 1956, The reduction of postnephrectomy hypertension by renal homotransplant, *Surg. Gynecol. Obstet.* **103**:673.

Muirhead, E. E., Jones, F., and Stirman, J. A., 1960a, Hypertensive cardiovascular disease of dog: Relation of sodium and dietary protein to ureterocaval anastomosis and ureteral ligation, *Arch. Pathol.* **70**:108.

Muirhead, E. E., Stirman, J. A., and Jones, F., 1960b, Renal autoexplantation and protection against renoprival hypertensive cardiovascular disease and hemolysis, *J. Clin. Invest.* **39**:266.

Muirhead, E. E., Jones, F., and Stirman, J. A., 1960c, Antihypertensive property in renoprival hypertension of extract from renal medulla, *J. Lab. Clin. Med.* **56**:167.

Muirhead, E. E., Hinman, J. W., and Daniels, E. G., 1963, Canine renoprival hypertension and the antihypertensive function of the kidney, in: *Proceedings of the Boerhaave Cursus Hypertension* (J. de Graeff, ed.), Boerhaave Kwartier Edition, Leiden, pp. 88–106.

Muirhead, E. E., Daniels, E. G., Booth, E., Freyburger, W. A., and Hinman, J. W., 1965, Renomedullary vasodepression and antihypertensive function, *Arch. Pathol.* **80**:43.

Muirhead, E. E., Brooks, B., Kosinski, M., Daniels, E. G., and Hinman, J. W., 1966, Renomedullary antihypertensive principle in renal hypertension, *J. Lab. Clin. Med.* **67**:778.

Muirhead, E. E., Brown, G. B., Germain, G. S., and Leach, B. E., 1970, The renal medulla as an antihypertensive organ, *J. Lab. Clin. Med.* **76**:641.

Muirhead, E. E., Brooks, B., Pitcock, J. A., and Stephenson, P., 1972a, Renomedullary antihypertensive function in accelerated (malignant) hypertension: Observations on renomedullary interstitial cells, *J. Clin. Invest.* **51**:181.

Muirhead, E. E., Brooks, B., Pitcock, J. A., Stephenson, P., and Brosius, W. L., 1972b, Role of the renal medulla in the sodium-sensitive component of renoprival hypertension, *Lab. Invest.* **27**:192.

Muirhead, E. E., Germain, G., Leach, B. E., Pitcock, J. A., Stephenson, P., Brooks, B., Brosius, W. L., Daniels, E. G., and Hinman, J. W., 1972c, Production of renomedullary prostaglandins by renomedullary interstitial cells grown in tissue culture, *Circ. Res.* **31**(Suppl. 2):161.

Muirhead, E. E., Germain, G. S., Leach, B. E., Brooks, B., and Stephenson P., 1973a, Renomedullary interstitial cells (RIC), prostaglandins (PG) and the antihypertensive function of the kidney, *Prostaglandins* **3**:581.

Muirhead, E. E., Brooks, B., and Brosius, W. L., 1973b, Renomedullary deficiency: A permissive factor in renoprival hypertension, *Arch. Pathol.* **95**:77.

Muirhead, E. E., Germain, G. S., Armstrong, F. B., Brooks, B., Leach, B. E., Byers, L. W., Pitcock, J. A., and Brown P., 1974a, Renomedullary endocrine system: Its antihypertensive action, *Trans. Assoc. Am. Physicians* **87**:288.

Muirhead, E. E., Leach, B. E., Pitcock, J. A., Germain, G. S., Byers, Ł. W., Armstrong, F. B., and Brown, P., 1974b, The antihypertensive action of renomedullary interstitial cells grown in tissue culture, *Acta Physiol. Lat. Am.* **24**:543.

Muirhead, E. E., Brooks, B., and Arora, K. K., 1974c, Prevention of malignant hypertension by the synthetic peptide SQ 20,881, *Lab. Invest.* **30**:129.

Muirhead, E. E., Germain, G. S., Pitcock, J. A., Brooks, B., and Leach, B. E., 1974d, The renal medulla and the hypertensive state, in: *Oral Contraceptives and Blood Pressure* (M. J. Fregley and M. S. Fregley, eds.), Dolphin Press, Gainesville, Florida, pp. 301–314.

Muirhead, E. E., Germain, G. S., Armstrong, F. B., Brooks, B., Leach, B. E., Byers, L. W., Pitcock, J. A., and Brown, P., 1975, Endocrine-type antihypertensive function of renomedullary interstitial cells, *Kidney Int.* **8**:S271.

Muirhead, E. E., Rightsel, W. A., Leach, B. E., Byers, L. W., Pitcock, J. A., and Brooks, B., 1976, The renomedullary antihypertensive function and its candidate antihypertensive hormone, *Ann. Acad. Med. (Singapore)* **5**:36s.

Muirhead, E. E., Rightsel, W. A., Leach, B. E., Byers, L. W., Pitcock, J. A., and Brooks, B., 1977, Reversal of hypertension by transplants and lipid extracts of cultured renomedullary interstitial cells, *Lab. Invest.* **36**:162.

Neubig, R., and Hoobler, S. W., 1975, Reversal of chronic renal hypertension. Role of salt water excretion, *Proc. Soc. Exp. Biol. Med.* **150**:254.

Osvaldo, L., and Latta, H., 1966, Interstitial cells of the renal medulla, *J. Ultrastruct. Res.* **15**:589.

Page, Irvine H., 1968, A unifying view of renal hypertension, in: *Renal Hypertension* (I. H. Page and J. W. McCubbin, eds.), Year Book Medical Publishers, Chicago, pp. 391–396.

Pitcock, J. A., Rightsel, W. A., Brown, P., Brooks, B., and Muirhead, E. E., 1976, Functional–morphologic correlates of renomedullary interstitial cells, *Clin. Sci. Mol. Med.* **51**:291s.

Pitcock, J. A., Brown, P., Brooks, B., Brosius, W. L., Clapp, W. L., and Muirhead, E. E., 1977, Partial nephrectomy–salt hypertension: Sodium balance and effect on renomedullary interstitial cells, *Fed. Proc. Fed. Am. Soc. Exp. Biol.* **36**:438.

Pitcock, J. A., Leach, B. E., Rightsel, W. A., and Muirhead, E. E., 1978, Proteoglycans of the rat renal papillary interstitium, ultrastructural observations and synthesis by renomedullary interstitial cells, *Fed. Proc. Fed. Am. Soc. Exp. Biol.* **37**:633 (abstr.).

Pitcock, J. A., Brown, P., Brooks, B., Clapp, W. L., Brosius, W. M., and Muirhead, E. E., 1980, Renomedullary deficiency in partial nephrectomy–salt hypertension, *Hypertension* **2**:281.

Prewitt, R. L., Leach, B. E., Byers, L. W., Brooks, B., Lands, W. E., and Muirhead, E. E.,

1979, Antihypertensive polar renomedullary lipid, a semisynthetic vasodilator, *Hypertension* **1**:299.

Solez, K., D'Agostini, R. J., Buono, R. A., Vernon, H., Wang, A. L., Finer, P. M., and Heptinstall, R. H., 1976, The renal medulla and mechanisms of hypertension in the spontaneously hypertensive rat, *Am. J. Pathol.* **85**:555.

Stuart, R., Salyer, W. R., Salyer, D. C., and Heptinstall, R. H., 1976, Renomedullary interstitial cell lesions and hypertension, *Hum. Pathol.* **7**:327.

Sullivan, J. M., and McGiff, J. C., 1980, Kallikrein–kinin and prostaglandin systems in hypertension, in: *Pathophysiology of Arterial Hypertension* (J. Rosenthal, ed.), Springer-Verlag, Heidelberg, in press.

Sušić, D., Sparks, J. C., and Machado, E. A., 1976, Salt-induced hypertension in rats with hereditary hydronephrosis: The effect of renomedullary transplantation, *J. Lab. Clin. Med.* **87**:232.

Sušić, D., Sparks, J. C., and Kentera, D., 1977, Suppressed antihypertensive function of the renal medulla in rats with spontaneous hypertension, *Pfleugers Arch.* **368**:173.

Sušić, D., Sparks, J. C., Machado, E. A., and Kentera, D., 1978, The mechanism of renomedullary antihypertensive action, haemodynamic studies in hydronephrotic rats with one-kidney renal-clip hypertension, *Clin. Sci. Mol. Med.* **54**:361.

Tobian, L., Jr., and Azar, S., 1971, Antihypertensive and other functions of the renal medulla, *Trans. Assoc. Am. Physicians* **84**:281.

Weibel, E. R., 1970, Serological technics for microscopic morphometry, in: *Principles and Technics of Electron Microscopy: Biological Applications*, Vol. III (M. A. Hayat, ed.), Van Nostrand Reinhold, New York, pp. 237–296.

CHAPTER **3**

Studies on the Mechanism
of the Renomedullary
Antihypertensive Action

DINKO SUŠIĆ

1. INTRODUCTION

The evidence gathered to date suggests that the renal medulla exerts a potent antihypertensive action and that the deficiency of renomedullary antihypertensive function is a contributory factor in the pathogenesis of various forms of hypertension. Yet, many questions concerning the role of the renal medulla in hypertension still remain to be answered. The most notable among them concerns the mechanism of the antihypertensive action. It is my objective to summarize the research dealing with this subject, although somewhat to my regret this chapter may not provide the reader with definite answers. The discussion on the mechanism of the renomedullary antihypertensive action will be restricted to endocrine-type mechanisms, although the medulla, as a part of the kidney, also participates in the regulation of blood pressure through its role in the regulation of sodium and water excretion and, therefore, in the regulation of body fluid volumes.

2. ENDOCRINE-TYPE ANTIHYPERTENSIVE ACTIVITY OF THE RENAL MEDULLA

Several lines of evidence clearly indicate that the renal medulla exerts an endocrinelike antihypertensive activity (for details see Chapter 2 by

DINKO SUŠIĆ • Institute for Medical Research, 11001 Belgrade, Yugoslavia.

Muirhead). Three main points are pertinent:

1. Subcutaneous transplantation of renomedullary tissue effectively lowers blood pressure in animals with various forms of hypertension (Muirhead et al., 1970; Tobian and Azar, 1971; Manthorpe, 1973; Manger et al., 1976; Solez et al., 1976; Sušić et al., 1976a). Of particular interest is the finding that renomedullary transplants prevent the rise in blood pressure in bilaterally nephrectomized animals subjected to saline loading (Muirhead et al., 1960b, 1972a, 1973).

2. Renomedullary transplants decrease the blood pressure in hypertensive animals even before vascularization of the transplant takes place (Muirhead, 1976), a finding which nullifies the hypothesis that the renal medulla exerts its antihypertensive activity by neutralizing circulating hypertensive substances.

3. Several substances capable of lowering blood pressure have been isolated from the renal medulla (Lee, 1972; Muirhead et al., 1971, 1977).

3. THE MEDIATOR OF RENOMEDULLARY ANTIHYPERTENSIVE FUNCTION

If we accept the fact that the antihypertensive function of the renal medulla is akin to the functions of endocrine organs, two questions immediately arise: what is the humoral mediator(s) and which of the renomedullary cells are involved?

The first question is a key issue in the discussion concerning the mechanism of renomedullary antihypertensive action. Although prostaglandins (PG) (Lee, 1972) and antihypertensive renomedullary lipids (ARL), both neutral (ANRL) and polar (APRL) (Muirhead et al., 1971, 1977; Prewitt et al., 1979), have been isolated from the medulla and implicated as mediators of antihypertensive function, their role in hypertension still remains to be determined. Since transplanted renomedullary tissue exerts antihypertensive activity even in the renoprival state (Muirhead et al., 1972a, 1973) the mediator is obviously a circulating substance, rather than a local hormone. In this context, ARL is a more likely possibility, since the action of renomedullary PG seems to be confined to the kidney (McGiff et al., 1974) and the renal medulla exerts its antihypertensive effect even after blockade of PG synthesis (Muirhead et al., 1975; Sušić et al., 1976a). Prostacyclin (PGI_2), the recently described member of the prostaglandin family, also fulfills the requirements of a circulating hormone (Moncada et al., 1978; Pace-Asciak et al., 1978) and has blood-pressure-reducing properties (Pace-Asciak et al., 1978). However, renocortical transplants do not exert antihypertensive activity even though renal cortex synthesizes PGI_2

(Whorton *et al.*, 1977). Furthermore, it does not seem likely that a substance, such as PGI_2, whose blood level neither solely nor predominantly depends on the medulla, could be a prime mediator of renomedullary antihypertensive action. It is possible that under certain conditions renomedullary PG, by an effect on renal blood flow and diuresis–natriuresis, operate in concert with ARL to prevent hypertension (Sušić and Sparks, 1975).

As for the site of production of the mediator(s), interstitial cells and collecting duct cells appear to be the main sources, at least in the case of PG (Muirhead *et al.*, 1972*b*; Bohman, 1977). It should also be noted that renomedullary interstitial cells synthesize both PG and ARL (Muirhead *et al.*, 1972*b*; 1975), and, probably, the same cellular organelles produce both compounds from common precursor(s) (Pitcock *et al.*, 1976). Since indomethacin blocks PG production in renomedullary interstitial cells grown in tissue culture but does not affect the synthesis of ARL (Muirhead *et al.*, 1975) the systems synthesizing the two compounds are probably different and may be under separate control. Detailed information on both substances is given elsewhere in this volume. Hereafter, the mediator of renomedullary antihypertensive function will be referred to as antihypertensive renomedullary substance (ARS).

4. WHAT SIGNALS THE MEDULLA TO RELEASE ANTIHYPERTENSIVE RENOMEDULLARY SUBSTANCE?

There is no evidence that renomedullary antihypertensive mechanisms are necessary for the maintenance of normotension under physiological conditions. Thus, blood pressure was found to be within physiological range in dogs following bilateral nephrectomy without volume loading (Leonards and Heisler, 1951), in rats with hereditary hydronephrosis (Lozzio *et al.*, 1972; Sušić *et al.*, 1975) in which the renal medulla was largely destroyed, and in Wistar rats in which the renal papilla was surgically removed (Sušić and Kentera, 1980). This does not necessarily indicate that the renal medulla is not involved in the regulation of blood pressure under physiological conditions; it could be that other factors may compensate for renomedullary deficiency. On the other hand, many reports indicate that the antihypertensive function of the medulla is essential for the preservation of normal blood pressure in animals exposed to hypertensive stimuli. For instance, hypertension developed rapidly in the above-mentioned animal models when the animals were consuming additional salt, while dogs and rats with a similar degree of renal excretory impairment but with either intact or transplanted medulla remained normotensive under the same conditions (Muirhead *et al.*, 1960*b*; Sušić *et al.*, 1976*a*; Sušić and Kentera, 1980).

   Some evidence points to salt overload as a possible stimulus for the production and/or release of ARS. In this respect, Dahl and Heine (1975) suggested that inherited differences in the antihypertensive capacity of the renal medulla may determine the ability of rats to withstand salt hypertension. A recent report from our laboratory supports this suggestion. Working on a salt-resistant substrain of Wistar rats (Sušić and Kentera, 1978, 1980 we have shown that animals in which a two-thirds nephrectomy (leaving the medulla intact) was performed do not develop hypertension when they were given excessive salt. In contrast, the rats in which unilateral nephrectomy was performed and the papilla of the remaining kidney was surgically removed became hypertensive, although the renal excretory function was similarly altered in both groups. Transplantation of renomedullary tissue prevented the rise in blood pressure in salt-loaded rats in which the renal papilla was dissected. Similarly, renomedullary transplants prevented the rise in blood pressure in salt-loaded rats with hereditary hydronephrosis, in which the renal medulla is largely destroyed (Sušić et al., 1976a). Thus, accepting the hypothesis that the antihypertensive activity of the renal medulla is necessary for the maintenance of normal blood pressure in salt-loaded animals, it is logical to assume that salt loading stimulates release of ARS. The finding that explantation of fragments of renal medulla from postsalt hypertensive rats lowered blood pressure in hypertensive animals more than did fragments of medullae from normotensive rats (Tobian and Azar, 1971) further supports this suggestion.

   It has also been reported that certain manipulations of the kidney, such as ureteral ligation (Muirhead et al., 1960a) or renal artery clipping (Sušić et al., 1976b), may induce a renomedullary deficiency that apparently contributes to the development of hypertension. Experiments performed in rats with unilateral hereditary hydronephrosis (Sušić et al., 1976b) may be used as an example. Unilateral nephrectomy was performed in all rats, so that one group of animals had a normal kidney (with intact medulla) remaining while the animals in the second group were left with a hydronephrotic kidney (with an almost completely atrophied medulla). After renal artery clipping (performed in all rats) the time course of blood pressure increase and the final level of blood pressure reached were similar in the two groups. In the same model, transplantation of renomedullary tissue outside the clipped kidney abolished the rise in blood pressure. These results clearly indicate that renal artery clipping interferes in some way with the antihypertensive function of the medulla. It has also been suggested that renomedullary deficiency contributes to the development of high blood pressure in spontaneously hypertensive (SH) rats (Sušić et al., 1977), since renomedullary transplants lower the blood pressure in SH rats with established hypertension (Solez et al., 1976; Manger et al., 1976) and abolish the spontaneous rise in blood pressure in young SH rats (Sušić et *al.*, 1977). Moreover, renal dysfunction of SH rats, which is thought to be induced either by an intrinsic kidney defect or by increased sympathetic activity, may be similar to the effects produced by clipping of the renal arteries (Coleman *et al.*, 1976). Thus, if the receptor sites involved in the control of the renomedullary antihypertensive function were located distal to the site of renal vascular abnormality, either a renal arterial clip or increased intrarenal resistance could result in a deceptively low blood pressure at the receptor site. If the mechanism that controls the renomedullary antihypertensive function operates as a negative feedback system it is possible that both arterial clipping (in Goldblatt hypertension) and the inherited renal defect of SH rats could cause the renal medulla to diminish or cease its antihypertensive function.

This is not to say that this hypothetical receptor is a mechano(baro)-receptor. It may be of interest to note that the electrolyte composition and osmolality of the interstitial fluid of the renal medulla are the variables affected by all of the procedures suggested above to influence the release of ARS. The osmolality of the interstitial fluid is obviously decreased in renomedullary transplants shown to exert an antihypertensive action. Similarly, saline overload decreases the tonicity of renomedullary interstitial fluid (Atherton, 1978). On the other hand, the osmolality of renomedullary interstitial fluid is most likely to be increased in states associated with a decrease in renomedullary antihypertensive activity, such as renal artery clipping and spontaneous hypertension. Renal blood flow and papillary plasma flow are decreased in SH rats (Albrecht, 1974; Ganguli *et al.*, 1976) and, obviously, in Goldblatt hypertensive rats, and since urinary concentrating ability is inversely proportional to renal blood flow (Thurau, 1964), medullary osmolality is in all likelihood increased under these two conditions. Thus, an inverse relationship between osmolality of interstitial fluid and the production of ARS may be proposed. It is worth noting that, in studies with rat renal papillae *in vitro*, hypertonic media were shown to increase the synthesis of PG (Danon *et al.*, 1978); however, experiments *in vivo* did not confirm this observation (Walker *et al.*, 1978). Perhaps the experiments on the renomedullary interstitial cells grown in tissue culture could give a better insight into the mechanism controlling the production of antihypertensive substance(s).

5. THE MECHANISM OF RENOMEDULLARY ANTIHYPERTENSIVE ACTION

5.1. Basic Considerations

The initial experiments that revealed the nonexcretory antihypertensive function of the kidney (Grollman *et al.*, 1949) and implied that the medulla was its source (Muirhead and Stirman, 1958; Muirhead *et al.*, 1960*a*) also pointed to a possible mechanism of renomedullary antihypertensive action. A review of these studies reveals that in the renoprival state the hypertensive stimulus of saline or saline–protein overload induced a significant increase of blood pressure in animals with either bilateral nephrectomy or bilateral ureteral ligation. In contrast, animals subjected to unilateral ureterocaval anastomosis and contralateral nephrectomy remained normotensive. Since the renal medulla underwent extensive destruction after ureteral ligation and remained intact following ureterocaval anastomosis, it was proposed that the medulla may be involved in the observed antihypertensive function of the kidney (Muirhead and Stirman, 1958). This idea is confirmed by studies that showed that renomedullary, but not renocortical, transplants prevented the development of hypertension in bilaterally nephrectomized animals subjected to volume overload (Muirhead *et al.*, 1960*b*, 1972*a*, 1973). From all the studies mentioned above it is reasonable to state that the renal medulla can prevent a rise in blood pressure in the presence of largely expanded plasma or extracellular fluid volume, and high sodium load. These findings suggested that the renal medulla exerts its antihypertensive activity by preventing hypertensive hemodynamic response to sodium–volume overload (Muirhead *et al.*, 1972*a*). This proposal is further supported by the reports showing the antihypertensive activity of the renal medulla in other hypertensive states associated with high sodium–volume loads, such as angiotensin–salt hypertension (Muirhead *et al.*, 1977), partial nephrectomy–salt hypertension (Muirhead *et al.*, 1977), salt hypertension in hydronephrotic rats (Sušić *et al.*, 1976*a*), and the early phase of one-kidney Goldblatt hypertension (Sušić *et al.*, 1978). It has been recently argued (Haddy and Overbeck, 1976) that the pathogenesis of sodium–volume expanded hypertension cannot be explained solely on the basis of classic autoregulation theory (Borst and Borst-DeGeus, 1963; Ledingham and Cohen, 1963; Guyton *et al.*, 1970). The same authors proposed that the altered concentration of some humoral agent(s), acting through a volume-independent mechanism, participates in the elevation of blood pressure in states associated with sodium–volume overload. In this context, the antihypertensive action of the renal medulla may be regarded volume independent.

There is evidence to indicate that the antihypertensive activity of the medulla is most pronounced in sodium–volume expanded hypertension (Muirhead *et al.*, 1975, 1977), yet renomedullary transplants exert a blood-pressure-lowering effect in hypertensive states not associated with an absolute increase in body sodium or fluid volumes, such as spontaneous hypertension in rats (Manger *et al.*, 1976; Solez *et al.*, 1976; Sušić *et al.*, 1977) and chronic one- (Muirhead *et al.*, 1970; Sušić *et al.*, 1976*b*, 1978) or two-kidney Goldblatt hypertension (Manthorpe, 1973). It should be noted according to Laragh (1974) that blood pressure is equivalent to volume $\times$

vasoconstriction, and according to Ulrych (1976) that blood pressure is equivalent to volume × vascular capacitance tone × vasoconstriction. *Circulatory filling* is the relation between the amount of fluid and the tone of capacitance vessels and this is the hemodynamic variable that actually determines the relation between volume and pressure, rather than volume itself. Therefore, in states where venous compliance is decreased, as it is in renovascular and spontaneous hypertension (Simon, 1976, 1978; Simon *et al.*, 1976), normal or even reduced blood volume may be considered as relative volume overload. Thus, in different states the renal medulla may exert its antihypertensive action by the same mechanism, regardless of the absolute volume load.

Theoretically, the ARS released from the renal medulla may prevent hypertension via a central nervous system mechanism, or it may somehow modulate the peripheral influence of sodium–volume loads on blood pressure (Muirhead, 1976). Although some of the circulatory effects of PG may be mediated via the central nervous system (Leach *et al.*, 1973; Laborit and Valette, 1973), there is no evidence whatsoever either to support or to refute the concept of central action of ARS. Thus, the discussion will be limited to the possible peripheral hemodynamic mechanisms.

5.2. The Effect of ARS on Peripheral Resistance

Generally speaking, the antihypertensive action of ARS may be accomplished via an effect on either peripheral resistance or cardiac output, or both. It is obvious that ARS, like any other blood-pressure-lowering agent, must evoke relaxation of resistance vessels in order to induce a permanent decrease in blood pressure. This notion is supported by the significantly lower blood pressure and peripheral resistance in chronic renal hypertensive rats with renomedullary transplants than in similarly hypertensive rats without renomedullary transplants (Sušić *et al.*, 1978). However, the question remains whether ARS primarily affects resistance vessels or whether the decrease in peripheral resistance is secondary to the fall in cardiac output; the latter possibility has been raised on the basis of autoregulation theory (Guyton *et al.*, 1970).

The evidence for a direct action of ARS on resistance vessels is circumstantial. In this context, both of the suggested mediators of the antihypertensive effect of the renal medulla (ARL and PG) have been shown to decrease peripheral resistance. Prewitt *et al.* (1979) have shown that APRL given intravenously to rats with chronic renal hypertension lower the blood pressure by decreasing peripheral resistance. In the same study, larger doses of APRL have been shown to lower cardiac output as well, most likely by inducing venodilatation. It is also well known that the hypotensive effect of PG is attributed to their vasodilator effect (McGiff *et al.*, 1974). The decrease in blood pressure induced by either transplants of renomedullary tissue or intravenous administration of either ANRL or APRL occurs in the absence of reflex tachycardia (Muirhead, 1976; Muirhead *et al.*, 1977; Prewitt *et al.*, 1979). Therefore, the antihypertensive effect of the medulla does not seem to be mediated via a sudden relaxation of resistance vessels. This, in itself, speaks against PG as mediators of this action. In fact, the absence of tachycardia under these conditions is compatible with the idea of central action of ARS. On the other hand, the blood-pressure-lowering action of renomedullary transplants and of medullary lipid extracts not containing PG is not instantaneous but progresses gradually over a period of several hours (Muirhead *et al.*, 1977). Therefore, if this effect involves a decrease in peripheral resistance, the vasodilatation must also proceed slowly. It is conceivable that the absence of tachycardia under these conditions may result from the adaptation of baroreceptors.

The precise mechanism by which ARS may decrease peripheral vascular resistance, i.e., induce arteriolar dilatation, remains unresolved. It has been shown that in both salt hypertension (Sušić *et al.*, 1976*a*) and one-kidney Goldblatt hypertension (Sušić *et al.*, 1978) renomedullary transplants do not exert antihypertensive activity by influencing plasma renin activity. However, it is possible that ARS antagonizes the peripheral effects of angiotensin and catecholamines, suggesting a relationship to vascular reactivity. Any other mechanism, such as interference with excitation–contraction coupling or so-called "water lodging" is also conceivable. Furthermore, Haddy and Overbeck (1976) recently proposed that altered concentrations of some humoral agent(s), opperating through the Na^+-K^+ pump in vascular smooth muscle cells, participate in the genesis of the volume-expanded hypertension. They also suggested that ANRL may be this agent. While reduced plasma concentration of ANRL would suppress the Na^+-K^+ pump, an elevated blood ANRL might exert a stimulatory effect.

5.3. The Effect of ARS on Cardiac Output

A recent report from our laboratory (Sušić *et al.*, 1978) supports the idea that the renal medulla exerts its antihypertensive action by preventing the rise in cardiac output in response to sodium–volume load. Thus, in the "early phase" (5 days after renal artery clipping) of one-kidney, renal-clip hypertension the blood pressure and cardiac output were found to be significantly lower in rats with medullary transplants than in those without any transplant or with renocortical transplants. Plasma volume was elevated to the same extent in all three groups. Later in the course of hypertension (35 days), significant reductions of blood pressure and total peripheral resistance were found in rats with medullary transplants when they were compared to other two groups. This course of events fits in well with the autoregulation theory of Guyton *et al.* (1970), and with the theory as modified by Folkow *et al.* (1973). Since cardiac output and blood pressure were significantly lower in the "early phase" of hypertension in animals with medullary transplants than in the other two groups, it is probable that neither autoregulatory vasoconstrictor response nor any structural changes in vascular walls occurred in the animals from this group. Therefore, peripheral resistance and blood pressure remained lower in the "chronic phase" of hypertension in this group. Yet the results do not exclude the possibility that ARS, in addition to its effect on cardiac output, also has a direct effect on vascular resistance.

The decrease in cardiac output observed in hypertensive animals with transplanted medullary tissue resulted from a decrease in stroke volume, because heart rate remained unchanged under these conditions (Sušić *et al.*, 1978). Theoretically, a decrease in stroke volume may be the result of either an inhibitory effect on myocardial contractility or a decrease in venous return. Results obtained in chronically instrumented, conscious dogs indicate that myocardial contractility is increased in saline-loaded anephric animals when compared to animals deprived of renal excretory function by ureterocaval anastomosis (Liard, 1976). On the basis of this study it is logical to assume that ARS might exert an antihypertensive function by decreasing contractility of cardiac muscle. Similarly, a reduced level of ARS (as in anephric subjects) may lead to an increase in myocardial contractility.

A decrease in venous return would also lead to a decrease in cardiac output as observed in hypertensive animals with renomedullary transplants. Although there are no reports that would unequivocally relate the renal medulla to this type of hemodynamic change, a growing body of evidence suggests the presence of a (antihypertensive) renal factor, the action of which ultimately leads to a decrease in venous return (Lucas and Floyer, 1973, 1974, Neubig and Hoobler, 1975; Bianchi *et al.*, 1978). Since the renal medulla does not exert its antihypertensive activity by affecting either renal excretory function or total body fluid volume (Muirhead *et al.*, 1972a, 1973; Sušić *et al.*, 1976a, 1978), it could theoretically decrease venous return either via an increase in venous capacitance or via an internal shift of fluid compartments, i.e., a shift of fluid from the intravascular to the interstitial space, or via both mechanisms. A decrease in venous compliance has been found in various forms of hypertension, including spontaneous and renal hypertension in rats (Simon, 1976, 1978) and essential hypertension in man (Ulrych, 1976). Therefore, it is possible that ARS exerts its antihypertensive effect by increasing venous capacitance, which in turn decreases venous pressure, venous return, end diastolic filling pressure, stroke volume, and cardiac output.

A very interesting suggestion concerning the mechanism of antihypertensive action of the kidney, especially of the medulla, has been made by Lucas and Floyer (1973, 1974). They have proposed that interstitial tissue compliance is controlled by a substance elaborated by the kidney. This proposal was based on the finding that the interstitial tissue pressure and the plasma extracellular fluid volume ratio were significantly higher in saline-loaded bilaterally nephrectomized rats than in saline-loaded animals deprived of renal excretory function by ureterocaval anastomosis (Lucas and Floyer, 1973). Similarly, an increase in both variables was found in rats with one-kidney Goldblatt hypertension (Lucas and Floyer, 1974). One study in saline-loaded dogs in which either bilateral nephrectomy or ureterocaval anastomosis was performed did not confirm these findings (Liard, 1976), but a report of Bianchi *et al.* (1978), who found an increase in plasma extracellular fluid volume ratio in bilaterally nephrectomized patients on maintenance hemodialysis, supports the proposal of Lucas and Floyer. A low tissue compliance, produced in anephric and renal hypertensive subjects by the absence of renal factor, would lead to an exaggerated plasma volume expansion upon fluid loading, which would in turn increase venous pressure (actually found in the studies of Lucas and Floyer), and augment venous return, cardiac output, and eventually blood pressure. It is tempting to propose that the antihypertensive function of the renal medulla is mediated via this mechanism.

Lucas and Floyer (1973) also proposed that changes in interstitial tissue compliance caused by a substance secreted by the kidney may be a part of the mechanism by which plasma volume is maintained constant under different conditions of hydration. In this context, it is of interest to note that the renomedullary interstitial cells, positioned in the part of the kidney exposed to changes in volume and osmolality that are brought about by changes in renal blood flow, are likely to be involved in the control of volume homeostasis, rather than in the regulation of blood pressure itself.

6. CONCLUDING REMARKS

Up to now there have not been many studies on the mechanism(s) of renomedullary antihypertensive action; therefore, there are still many unanswered questions. Yet the data so far obtained allow certain conclusions to be drawn and also provide a basis for formulating several sound working hypotheses:

1. The renal medulla exhibits an endocrinelike antihypertensive function, which is most pronounced when hypertension is primarily dependent on an excess of sodium and/or volume.
2. There is some evidence indicating that the release of renomedullary antihypertensive substance(s) is stimulated by saline loading and inhibited by a decrease in renal blood flow and/or renal arterial pressure.
3. Recent studies suggest that this substance(s) exerts its effect by preventing hypertensive hemodynamic response to sodium–volume overload.
4. Furthermore, data indicate that renomedullary antihypertensive substance(s) prevents hypertension by abolishing the rise in cardiac output, possibly by increasing venous capacitance and/or interstitial tissue compliance.

REFERENCES

Albrecht, I., 1974, The hemodynamics of spontaneous hypertension in rats (Part 1). Male study, *Jpn. Circ. J.* **38**:985.

Atherton, J. C., 1978, Lability of renal papillary tissue composition in the rat, *J. Physiol.* **274**:323.

Bianchi, G., Pagetti, D., Ferrari, P., Ponticelli, C., Bear, P. G., and Romagnoni, M., 1978, Increase in plasma extracellular fluid volume ratio caused by bilateral nephrectomy in patients on maintenance hemodialysis, *Nephron* **20**:75.

Bohman, S.-O., 1977, Demonstration of prostaglandin synthesis in collecting duct cells and other cell types of the rabbit renal medulla, *Prostaglandins* **14**:729.

Borst, J. G. G., and Borst-DeGeus, A., 1963, Hypertension explained by Starling's theory of circulatory homeostasis, *Lancet* **1**:677.

Coleman, T. G., Manning, R. D., Jr., Norman, R. A., Jr., and DeClue, J., 1976, The role of the kidney in spontaneous hypertension, *Am. Heart J.* **89**:94.

Dahl, L. K., and Heine, M., 1975, Primary role of renal homografts in setting blood pressure level in rats, *Circ. Res.* **36**:692.

Danon, A., Knapp, H. R., Oelz, O., and Oates, J. A., 1978, Stimulation of prostaglandin biosynthesis in the renal papilla by hypertonic mediums, *Am. J. Physiol.* **234**:F64.

Folkow, B., Hallback, M., Lundgren, Y., Sivertsson, R., and Weiss, L., 1973, Importance of adaptive changes in vascular design for establishment of primary hypertension, studied in man and spontaneously hypertensive rats, *Circ. Res.* **32**(Suppl. I):2.

Ganguli, M., Tobian, L., and Dahl, L., 1976, Low renal papillary plasma flow in both Dahl and Kyoto rats with spontaneous hypertension, *Circ. Res.* **39**:337.

Grollman, A., Muirhead, E. E., and Vanatta, J., 1949, Role of the kidney in pathogenesis of hypertension as determined by a study of the effects of bilateral nephrectomy and other experimental procedures on the blood pressure of the dog, *Am. J. Physiol.* **157**:21.

Guyton, A. C., Coleman, T. G., Bower, J. D., and Granger, H. J., 1970, Circulatory control in hypertension, *Circ. Res.* **27**(Suppl. II):135.

Haddy, F. J., and Overbeck, H., 1976, The role of humoral agents in volume expanded hypertension, *Life Sci.* **19**:935.

Laborit, H., and Valette, N., 1973, The effect of arachidonic acid on experimental arterial hypertension in the rat, *Agressologie* **14**:387.

Laragh, J. M., 1974, Vasoconstrictor–volume analysis for understanding and treating hypertension, in: *Hypertension Manual* (J. H. Laragh, ed.), Dunn Donnelley, New York, pp. 823–849.

Leach, B. E., Armstrong, F. B., Jr., Germain, G. S., and Muirhead, E. E., 1973, Vasodepressor action of prostaglandins A_2 and E_2 in the spontaneously hypertensive rat (SH rat): Evidence for an action mediated by the vagus, *J. Pharmacol. Exp. Ther.* **185**:470.

Ledingham, J. M., and Cohen, R. D., 1963, Hypertension explained by Starling's theory of circulatory homeostasis, *Lancet* **1**:887.

Lee, J. B., 1972, The inter-relationship between renal prostaglandins and blood pressure regulation, *Am. J. Med. Sci.* **263**:334.

Leonards, J. R., and Heisler, C. R., 1951, Maintenance of life in bilaterally nephrectomized dogs and its relation to malignant hypertension, *Am. J. Physiol.* **167**:553.

Liard, J. F., 1976, Haemodynamics and body fluid volumes in response to fluid loading in conscious dogs: Non-excretory renal influences, *Clin. Sci. Mol. Med.* **51**:243.

Lozzio, B. B., Buonocore, E., and Kentera, D., 1972, Radiologic and functional studies in rats with hereditary hydronephrosis, *Invest. Urol.* **10**:84.

Lucas, J., and Floyer, M. A., 1973, Renal control of changes in the compliance of the interstitial space: A factor in the aetiology of renoprival hypertension, *Clin. Sci.* **44**:397.

Lucas, J., and Floyer, M. A., 1974, Changes in body fluid distribution and interstitial space compliance during the development and reversal of experimental renal hypertension in the rat, *Clin. Sci. Mol. Med.* **47**:1.

McGiff, J. C., Crowshaw, K., and Itskovitz, H. D., 1974, Prostaglandins and renal function, *Fed. Proc. Fed. Am. Soc. Exp. Biol.* **33**:39.

Manthorpe, T., 1973, The effect on renal hypertension of subcutaneous isotransplantation of renal medulla from normal or hypertensive rats, *Acta Pathol. Microbiol. Scand. Sect A* **81**:725.

Manger, W. M., Van Praag, D., Weiss, R. J., Hart, C. J., Hulse, M., Rock, T. W., and Farber, S. J., 1976, Effect of transplanting renomedullary tissue into spontaneously hypertensive rats (SHR), *Fed. Proc. Fed. Am. Soc. Exp. Biol.* **35**:556.

Moncada, R., Korbut, R., Bunting, S., and Vane, J. R., 1978, Prostacyclin is a circulatory hormone, *Nature* **273**:767.

Muirhead, E. E., 1976, Renomedullary antihypertensive function, *Acta Biol. Med. Ger.* **35**:1181.

Muirhead, E. E., and Stirman, J. A., 1958, Dietary protein and hypertension of the dog: Protection by ureterocaval anastomosis with a study of kidneys so treated, *Am. J. Pathol.* **34**:561.

Muirhead, E. E., Jones, F., and Stirman, J. A., 1960a, Hypertensive cardiovascular disease of dog. Relation of sodium and dietary protein to ureterocaval anastomosis and ureteral ligation, *Arch. Pathol.* **70**:108.

Muirhead, E. E., Stirman, J. A., and Jones, F., 1960b, Renal autoexplantation and protection against renoprival hypertensive cardiovascular disease and hemolysis, *J. Clin Invest.* **39**:266.

Muirhead, E. E., Brown, G. B., Germain, G. S., and Leach, B. E., 1970, The renal medulla as an antihypertensive organ, *J. Lab. Clin. Med.* **76**:641.

Muirhead, E. E., Leach, B. E., Byers, L. W., Brooks, B., Daniels, E. G., and Hinman, J. W., 1971, Antihypertensive neutral renomedullary lipids (ANRL), in: *Kidney Hormones* (J. W. Fisher, ed.), Academic Press, New York, pp. 485–506.

Muirhead, E. E., Brooks, B., Pitcock, J. A., Stephenson, P., and Brosius, W. L., 1972a, Role of the renal medulla in sodium-sensitive component of renoprival hypertension, *Lab. Invest.* **27**:192,

Muirhead, E. E., Germain, G., Leach, B. E., Pitcock, J. A., Stephenson, P., Brooks, B., Brosius, W. L., Daniels, E. G., and Hinman, J. W., 1972b, Production of renomedullary prostaglandins by renomedullary interstitial cells grown in tissue culture, *Circ. Res.* **31**(Suppl. II):161.

Muirhead, E. E., Brooks, B., and Brosius, W. L., 1973, Renomedullary deficiency. A permissive factor in renoprival hypertension, *Arch. Pathol.* **95**:77.

Muirhead, E. E., Germain, G. S., Armstrong, F. B., Brooks, B., Leach, B. E., Byers, L. W., Pitcock, J. A., and Brown, P., 1975, Endocrine type antihypertensive function of renomedullary interstitial cells, *Kidney Intern.* **8**(Suppl. 5):122.

Muirhead, E. E., Rightsel, W. A., Leach, B. E., Byers, L. W., Pitcock, J. A., and Brooks, B., 1977, Reversal of hypertension by transplants and lipid extracts of cultured renomedullary interstitial cells, *Lab. Invest.* **35**:162.

Neubig, R. R., and Hoobler, S. W., 1975, Reversal of chronic renal hypertension: Role of salt and water excretion, *Proc. Soc. Exp. Biol. Med.* **150**:254.

Pace-Asciak, C. R., Carrara, M. C., and Nicolau, K. C., 1978, Prostaglandin I_2 has more potent hypotensive properties than prostaglandin E_2 in the normal and spontaneously hypertensive rat, *Prostaglandins* **15**:999.

Pitcock, J. A., Rightsel, W. A., Brown, P., Brooks, B., and Muirhead, E. E., 1976, Functional–morphological correlates of renomedullary interstitial cells, *Clin. Sci. Mol. Med.* **51**:291s.

Prewitt, R. L., Leach, B. E., Byers, L. W., Brooks, B., Lands, W. E. M., and Muirhead, E. E., 1979, Antihypertensive polar renomedullary lipid, a semisynthetic vasodilator, *Hypertension* **1**:299.

Simon, G., 1976, Altered venous function in hypertensive rats, *Circ. Res.* **38**:412.

Simon, G., 1978, Venous changes in renal hypertensive rats: The role of humoral factors, *Blood Vessels* **15**:311.

Simon, G., Pamnani, M. B., and Overbeck, H. W., 1976, Decreased venous compliance in dogs with chronic renal hypertension, *Proc. Soc. Exp. Biol. Med.* **152**:122.

Solez, K., D'Agostoni, R. J., Buono, R. A., Vernon, N., Wang, A. L., Finer, P. M., and Heptinstall, R. H., 1976, The renal medulla and mechanism of hypertension in the spontaneously hypertensive rat, *Am. J. Pathol.* **85**:555.

Sušić, D., and Kentera, D., 1978, Resistance of a substrain of Wistar rats to salt hypertension, *Res. Commun. Chem. Pathol. Pharmacol.* **20**:175.

Sušić, D., and Kentera, D., 1980, Role of the renal medulla in the resistance of rats to salt hypertension, *Pflügers Arch. Eur. J. Physiol.* **384**:283.

Sušić, D., and Sparks, J. C., 1975, Physiological actions of renomedullary prostaglandins—A viewpoint, *IRCS Med. Sci.* **3**:363.

Sušić, D., Sparks, J. C., and Kentera, D., 1975, The renin–angiotensin system in rats with hereditary hydronephrosis, *Pflügers Arch. Eur. J. Physiol.* **358**:265.

Sušić, D., Sparks, J. C., and Machado, E. A., 1976a, Salt-induced hypertension in rats with hereditary hydronephrosis: The effect of renomedullary transplantation, *J. Lab. Clin. Med.* **87**:232.

Sušić, D., Sparks, J. C., and Machado, E. A., 1976b, Renomedullary deficiency. A contributory factor in the pathogenesis of experimental renal hypertension, *Experientia* **32**:354.

Sušić, D., Sparks, J. C., and Kentera, D., 1977, Suppressed antihypertensive function of the renal medulla in rats with spontaneous hypertension, *Pflügers Arch. Eur. J. Physiol.* **368**:173.

Sušić, D., Sparks, J. C., Machado, E. A., and Kentera, D., 1978, The mechanism of reno-medullary antihypertensive action: Haemodynamic studies in hydronephrotic rats with one-kidney renal-clip hypertension, *Clin. Sci. Mol. Med.* **54**:361.

Thurau, K., 1964, Renal hemodynamics, *Am. J. Med.* **36**:698.

Tobian, L., and Azar, S., 1971, Antihypertensive and other functions of the renal medulla, *Trans. Assoc. Am. Physicians* **84**:281.

Ulrych, M., 1976, The role of vascular capacitance in the genesis of essential hypertension, *Clin. Sci. Mol. Med.* **51**:203s.

Walker, L. A., Whorton, A. R., Smigel, M., France, R., and Frolich, J. C., 1978, Antidiuretic hormone increases renal prostaglandin synthesis in vivo, *Am. J. Physiol.* **235**:F180.

Whorton, A. R., Smigel, M., Oates, J. A., and Frolich, J. C., 1977, Evidence for prostacyclin production in renal cortex, *Prostaglandins* **13**:1021.

CHAPTER **4**

Vasodepressor Substances Extractable from Kidney Tissue

BASAB K. MOOKERJEE and RAM V. PATAK

1. INTRODUCTION

The concept that the kidneys exert two independent and opposing influences on the regulation of arterial blood pressure was formulated following the publication of the classical Goldblatt experiment (Goldblatt *et al.*, 1934; Fasciolo *et al.*, 1938; Braun-Menendez, 1958; Braun-Menendez and von Euler, 1947). The renal prohypertensive function conducive to the development of hypertension is thought to be related to at least two functional attributes of the kidneys, namely the retention of sodium and water, and the activation of the renin–angiotensin system. The renal antihypertensive function may also be exerted by a similar dual mechanism, e.g., the relief of sodium–volume loads brought about by renal excretion (natriuresis and diuresis) and probably also by activation of endocrine-type mechanisms that may act locally within the kidneys and possibly systemically on the peripheral vasculature as well (Grollman, 1959; Muirhead *et al.*, 1975).

The experimental evidence supporting these opposing renal influences on blood pressure regulation has been discussed in detail in the preceding chapters in this volume. In this chapter, we focus our attention on the different types of antihypertensive substances that can be extracted from the renal medullary tissue in various species of animals and discuss briefly the possible roles of each of these in the regulation of arterial blood pressure. Four groups of substances, including their roles, are presented here: (1) the

BASAB K. MOOKERJEE • State University of New York at Buffalo, Buffalo, New York 14215, and Medical Research Service, Veterans Administration Medical Center, Buffalo, New York 14218.   RAM V. PATAK • University of Kansas Medical Center, Kansas City, Kansas 66103, and Medical Research Service, Veterans Administration Medical Center, Kansas City, Missouri 64128.

renal prostaglandins (acidic lipids), (2) antihypertensive neutral renomedullary lipid, (3) phospholipid renin inhibitors and phospholipases, and
(4) the renal kinins.

First we recount briefly those specific experimental observations that
suggested the existence of a renal antihypertensive function of an endocrine
and/or humoral origin. With this background it will be easier for the reader
to understand how attempts were made to extract and isolate antihypertensive substances from renal tissue. The occurrence of hypertension following
total ablation of renal tissue (renoprival hypertension) suggested that the
existence of normal renal tissue somehow offers protection against the
development of hypertension (Braun-Menendez and von Euler, 1947;
Grollman et al., 1949). The exact pathogenesis of renoprival hypertension in
man and in experimental animals is controversial. One school holds the
view that expansion of body fluid volume (especially the expansion of blood
volume that occurs following total renal ablation) leads to hypertension,
and therefore it is not necessary to invoke the existence of antihypertensive
humoral substances of renal origin (Leonards and Heisler, 1951; Orbison et
al., 1952). In contrast, other workers point to the evidence of an increase in
peripheral vascular resistance and they have held the opinion that renoprival
hypertension can indeed occur in the absence of expanded extracellular fluid
volumes (Grollman et al., 1951). In subsequent years, additional evidence
on the prevention and even reversal of renoprival hypertension after the pro-
vision of normal renal tissue strengthened the concept of an antihypertensive action of this renal tissue, independent of the excretory function of the
kidney. More specifically it was observed that renoprival hypertension in
dogs could be reduced by perfusion of blood through "normal" dog without
a significant change in sodium and water excretion. Additionally, transplantation of a normal kidney can rapidly reverse renoprival hypertension
despite the maintenance of expanded extracellular fluid volumes (Kolff and
Page, 1954; Kolff, 1957; Murihead et al., 1956). Ureterocaval and ureterovenous anastomosis was then shown to be equally effective in lowering
blood pressure, despite the absence of renal excretory function (Muirhead,
1962). Later still, it was shown that normal renal tissue could protect
against or even reverse hypertensive states not dependent on extracellular
fluid volume expansion, e.g., renal and renovascular types of hypertension
(Gomez et al., 1960; Kolff et al., 1964; Ducrot et al., 1966). The proposal
that the renal medulla is the major site of this nonexcretory type of
antihypertensive effect was developed following the observations of Muirhead et al. (1960). Autoexplantation of renal medulla prevented accelerated
renoprival hypertension but the autoexplantation of renal cortex was ineffective. This set the stage for attempts by various workers to isolate and
identify antihypertensive substances in renal tissue.

2. EARLIER WORK ON ANTIHYPERTENSIVE EFFECTS OF EXTRACTS OF WHOLE KIDNEY TISSUE

Braun-Menendez and his associates attempted to extract antihypertensive substances from renal tissue in the 1930s (Braun-Menendez and von Euler, 1947). Grollman *et al.* (1940) and Page *et al.* (1940) first reported the successful preparation of extracts of whole kidney tissue that lowered blood pressure in hypertensive animals and man. These experiments could not be easily interpreted or reproduced in view of the pyrogenic and nonspecific effects of the rather crude preparations. Subsequent refinements in extraction and analytical techniques have made possible the resurgence of interest that this subject has enjoyed since the early 1960s.

The relationship between active extracts obtained from whole kidneys described in the early efforts to the better-characterized renomedullary substances isolated later (such as prostaglandins and ANRL) remains unresolved. The water-soluble antihypertensive principle isolated by Hamilton and Grollman (1958) from whole hog kidney and from renal cortex was thought to be a peptide. Milliez *et al.* (1966) reported the prevention and also correction of renovascular hypertension in rabbits with extracts of whole kidney, which may well have contained lipids. With refinements in fractionation of techniques, renewed efforts along these lines have led to the identification of two distinct groups of lipid substances from renomedullary tissue, i.e., the prostaglandins (acidic lipids) (PG) and the antihypertensive neutral renomedullary lipid (ANRL). In addition, a phospholipid renin inhibitor has also been extracted from whole-kidney tissue.

3. RENOMEDULLARY ANTIHYPERTENSIVE LIPIDS

3.1. Renal Prostaglandins

In 1961, Lee and his associates found that extracts of renal medulla lowered the blood pressure when injected into vagotomized rats treated with pentolinium after being anesthetized with pentobarbital (Lee *et al.*, 1962, 1963). In the earlier studies these workers were unaware of concomitant progress to identify and characterize the action of prostaglandins. Lee and associates (1965) isolated three distinct fatty acid components from extracts of rabbit kidneys and named them compounds 1 and 2 and medullin. Compound 1 was found to lack vasodepressor effects but did possess marked stimulatory activity on nonvascular smooth muscle. Compound 2 had vasodepressor and stimulatory activity. Medullin possessed potent vasodepressor activity but had no effects on nonvascular smooth muscle (Fig. 1).

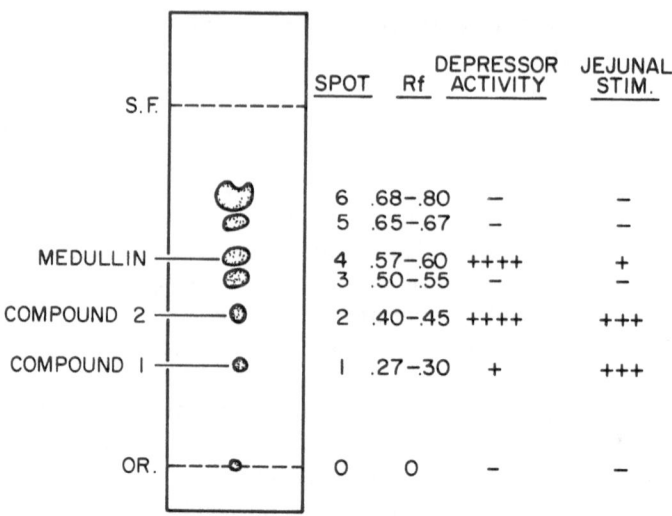

SPOT	Rf	DEPRESSOR ACTIVITY	JEJUNAL STIM.
6	.68–.80	–	–
5	.65–.67	–	–
4	.57–.60	++++	+
3	.50–.55	–	–
2	.40–.45	++++	+++
1	.27–.30	+	+++
O	O	–	–

FIGURE 1.   Isolation of medullin, compound 1, and compound 2 from rabbit renal medulla by thin-layer chromatography. Unlike compounds 1 or 2, medullin was devoid of nonvascular smooth muscle-stimulating activity. OR., Origin; S.F., solvent front. [From Lee *et al.* (1965), by permission of the American Heart Association, Inc.]

After becoming aware of developmental work on prostaglandins, Lee and his associates (1967) proceeded to show that compounds 1 and 2 and medullin were prostaglandins of the F, E, and A series, respectively. The structural features of some of these polar fatty acids and their metabolic synthetic pathways presently thought to occur in the kidney (Dunn and Hood, 1977) are depicted in Fig. 2.

Since the biosynthesis and metabolism of renal prostaglandins have been dealt with exhaustively elsewhere in this volume (Chapters 5 and 9), we briefly recount only a few features relevant to the contents of this chapter. The level of activity of the enzyme complex known as prostaglandin synthetase is known to be highest in the renal inner medulla and papilla, intermediate in the outer medulla, and lowest in the renal cortex (Larsson and Anggård, 1973a). The cell type believed by many to make the major contribution to renal prostaglandin synthesis was the renomedullary interstitial cell, but recent histochemical studies (Smith and Bell, 1978) have revealed that a number of different cells of renal origin, such as collecting duct cells, interstitial cells, and endothelial cells, can synthesize prostaglandins. The first step in the biosynthesis of prostaglandins is the conversion of the essential fatty acid linoleic acid, derived from phospholipid stores to the 20-carbon arachidonic acid (phospholipase A catalyzes the release of arachidonic acid from phospholipids). One oxygen atom is added to each carbon atom at positions 9 and 15 (catalyzed by prostaglandin

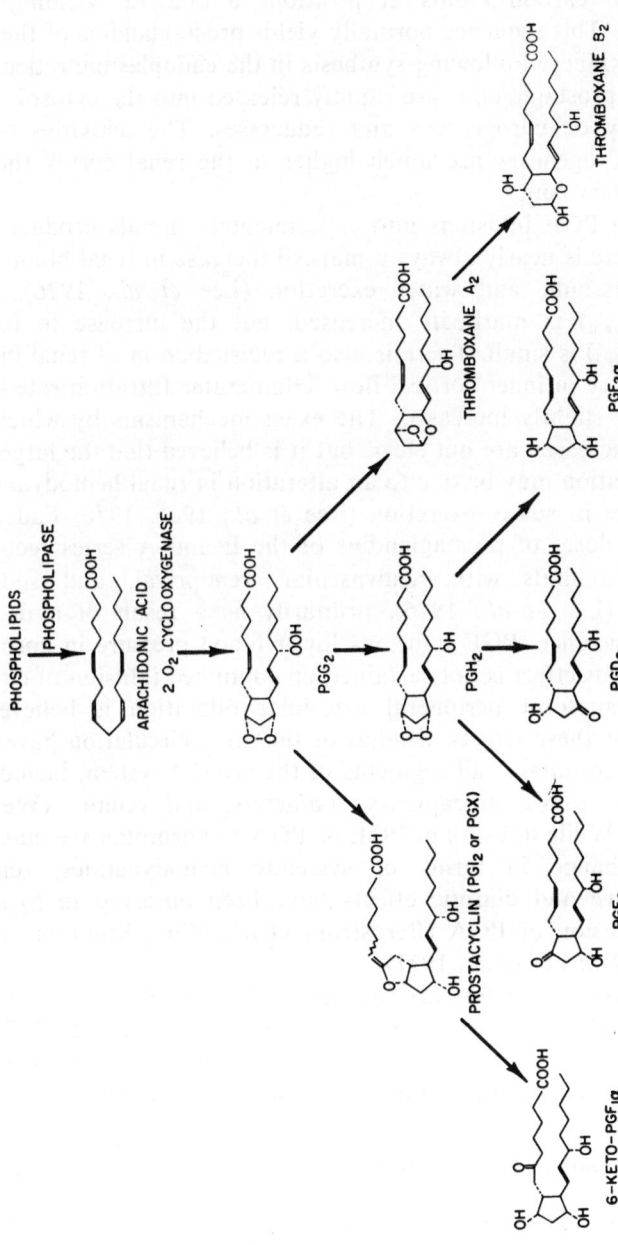

FIGURE 2. Sequence of biochemical synthetic pathways for prostaglandins and thromboxanes. All depicted conversions are thought to occur in the kidney. [From Dunn and Hood (1977), with permission from the publisher.]

synthetase) and the product undergoes cyclization by formation of a double bond between carbon atoms at positions 8 and 12, yielding a cyclic endoperoxide. This sequence normally yields prostaglandins of the E and F series in the kidney. Following synthesis in the endoplasmic reticulum, it is believed that prostaglandins are rapidly released into the cytosol. They are inactivated by dehydrogenases and reductases. The activities of prostaglandin dehydrogenases are much higher in the renal cortex than in the deeper medullary zones.

Although PGE infusions into experimental animals produce complex responses, there is nearly always a marked increase in renal blood flow and sodium, potassium, and water excretion (Lee et al., 1976). Osmolar clearance (C_{osm}) is markedly increased, but the increase in free water clearance (C_{H_2O}) is small. There is also a redistribution of renal blood flow with an increase in inner cortical flow. Glomerular filtration rate is usually unchanged or slightly increased. The exact mechanisms by which sodium excretion is increased are not clear, but it is believed that the large increase in urine formation may be due to an alteration in renal hemodynamics and to an increase in solute excretion (Lee et al., 1965, 1976; Fadem et al., 1977). Large doses of prostaglandins of the E and A series reduce blood pressure in animals with renovascular, renoprival, and spontaneous hypertension (Lee et al., 1976), primarily as a result of a decrease in peripheral resistance. PGE infusions lower blood pressure in normotensive animals, but this effect is not sustained on continued infusion of either PGE or PGA. Evanescent peripheral arteriolar dilatation is believed to be responsible for these effects. Studies of the microcirculation have revealed that PGE dilates almost all segments of the arterial system, including arterioles, metaarterioles, precapillary sphincters, and venules (Weiner and Kaley, 1969). While infusion of PGE or PGA in normotensive man leads to very little change in terms of systemic hemodynamics, remarkable antihypertensive and diuretic effects have been observed in hypertensive man after infusion of PGA (Bergstrom et al., 1965; Montgomery et al., 1973; Carr, 1973; Lee et al., 1971).

If renal prostaglandins are indeed involved in blood pressure regulation, what are the precise mechanisms that mediate such effects? To answer the question, we will discuss the three possible mechanisms that may mediate the antihypertensive function of renal prostaglandins.

3.1.1. *Regulation or Renovascular Reactivity*

Renal prostaglandins may exert an antihypertensive effect through their influence on renovascular reactivity and the intrarenal distribution of renal blood flow. The role of endogenous renal prostaglandins in the control of intrarenal distribution of blood flow in the resting state is controversial.

For reasons not well understood at this time, the administration of pharmacologic agents that inhibit prostaglandin synthesis (e.g., indomethacin) do not reproducibly reduce the output of prostaglandins from the kidneys of unanesthetized experimental animals (Zins, 1975; Itskovitz et al., 1973; Terrango et al., 1976). Nevertheless, there is much evidence to suggest that under "resting" conditions the distribution of renal blood flow between cortical and medullary zones may be regulated by a balanced intrarenal interaction between the local vasoconstrictor angiotensin II and the local vasodilator PGE_2 (Itskovitz and McGiff, 1974). Furthermore, renal prostaglandin, most likely PGE_2, has been observed to be primarily responsible for rapidly increasing renomedullary blood flow in response to certain stresses, e.g., trauma, hemorrhage, and hypotension (Itskovitz et al., 1973). Within kidneys, the vasoconstrictor–antinatriuretic forces (angiotensin, norepinephrine) are opposed by vasodilator–natriuretic forces (bradykinin, prostaglandins). According to this view, PGE_2 appears to be the penultimate regulator, since angiotensin, norepinephrine, and bradykinin seem to stimulate synthesis of PGE in renal medulla (Itskovitz and McGiff, 1974). Thus, normal function of the renal prostaglandin system would oppose the prohypertensive forces by favoring a relative distribution of renal blood flow that is conducive to natriuresis and diuresis. We consider here a sequence of events that might follow behaviorial or other hypertensive stimuli (e.g., stress, fright). Such a stimulus would lead to an increase in adrenergic activity with activation of the renin–angiotensin system to promote renal and systemic vasoconstriction. Indeed, it is well known that maneuvers that tend to cause renal ischemia (e.g., infusion of epinephrine or angiotensin, arterial occlusion, sympathetic renal nerve stimulation) readily increase the renal prostaglandins (McGiff et al., 1970). This increased production of prostaglandins also coincides with an increase in urine flow and with the recovery phase of the previously decreased renal blood flow (McGiff et al., 1970a,b). Thus, available evidence strongly supports the participation of endogenous renal prostaglandins in the regulation of renovascular reactivity by feedback opposition of vasoconstrictor and antinatriuretic effects of enhanced adrenergic activity and of vasopressor hormones.

Similarly, a relative deficiency in renal prostaglandin synthesis may contribute to the pathogenesis of hypertension since unopposed vasoconstriction would favor a redistribution of renal blood flow conducive to sodium retention. If indeed an absolute or relative deficiency or renal prostaglandins initiates or aggravates hypertension, then arterial blood pressure should become higher in hypertensive states after prolonged administration of drugs that inhibit prostaglandin synthesis. Experimental results from our laboratory provided strong support for this view (Patak et al., 1975). Normal subjects and patients with essential hypertension were placed on indomethacin, a nonsteroidal antiinflammatory drug that inhibits prostaglandin synthesis. Small, but significant increases in mean arterial blood pressure were observed in every normal and hypertensive subject (Fig. 3). This study also revealed remarkable blunting of the natriuretic effects of the loop diuretic agent furosemide, suggesting that the effects of this diuretic agent might be modulated by endogenous renal prostaglandins. Hypertension has also been observed to occur in rabbits and dogs after prolonged administration of nonsteroidal antiinflammatory agents (Lonigro *et al.*, 1973; Larsson and Änggård, 1973*b*; Colina-Chorio *et al.*, 1975). Vasopressor response to angiotensin II is enhanced after administration of indomethacin (Negus *et al.*, 1976). Urinary prostaglandin excretion, which is thought to reflect renal prostaglandin production (Frolich *et al.*, 1975*b*; Dunn *et al.*, 1978), is decreased in certain forms of hypertension (Tan and Murlow, 1978). In a recent study, although there was no significant increase in arterial pressure after indomethacin administration, a significant blunting of the antihypertensive action of diuretics and propranolol was observed (Lopez-Ovejero *et al.*, 1978). Taken together these observations tend to implicate a deficient response of renal prostaglandin synthesis in the pathogenesis of hypertension.

3.1.2. *Could Prostaglandins of Renal Origin, Acting on Peripheral Vasculature, Serve as a Circulating Antihypertensive Hormone?*

A role for renal prostaglandins as circulating antihypertensive hormones is considered to be unlikely, since a major portion of circulating

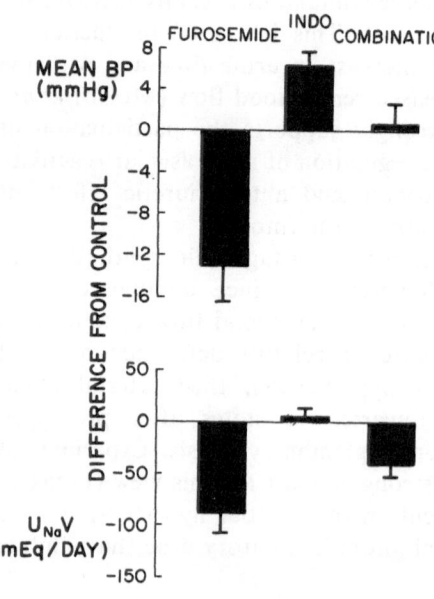

FIGURE 3. Effect of furosemide, indomethacin, and a combination of these agents on mean arterial pressure and sodium excretion in four normotensive and six essential hypertensive subjects. The subjects were placed on a controlled sodium (150 mEq/day) and potassium (50 mEq/day) diet, and given furosemide, indomethacin, and a combination of both agents following a 4-day equilibration period prior to administration of each agent. Bars denote mean increase or decrease as compared with that in the control period. The results were statistically significant except for: (1) the effect of combination of agents on mean arterial pressure and (2) effect of indomethacin on cumulative urinary sodium excretion. [From Patak *et al.* (1975), with permission from the publisher.]

PGE_2 is rapidly inactivated on a single pass through the lungs. The normal concentration of PGE_2 in peripheral blood may not reach a sufficiently high level for it to escape pulmonary degradation in amounts that may be biologically effective (McGiff *et al.*, 1969; Muirhead, 1976). While prostaglandins of the E series may thus be poor candidates for this role, PGA_2 is not inactivated by the lungs to a major extent (McGiff *et al.*, 1969). This resistance to pulmonary degradation made PGA_2 or one of its biologically active metabolites (e.g., 13,14-dihydro-PGA_2) a prime candidate as the circulating antihypertensive hormone (Lee, 1976). However, more current experimental evidence does not support such a proposal. Significant levels of circulating prostaglandins of the A series have not been demostrated to occur in the plasma (Frolich *et al.*, 1975*a*). Furthermore, PGAs have never been detected in fresh preparations of renal medulla even with the use of highly sensitive techniques (Larsson and Anggård, 1975). Some or all of the PGA_2 detectable in kidney extracts as reported in some studies probably was derived from the nonenzymatic dehydrogenation of PGE_2 during the extraction procedure (Lee *et al.*, 1967). A rigorous critique of the current controversy over the physiological role of prostaglandins of the A series is beyond the scope of the present chapter.

3.1.3. *Regulatory Effects on Other Renal Vasopressor and Vasodepressor Systems*

Renal prostaglandins may indirectly participate in blood pressure regulation by profoundly influencing the renin–angiotensin system as well as the renal kallikrein–kinin system. We have noted the remarkable suppression of plasma renin activity in normal and hypertensive human subjects given indomethacin (Patak *et al.*, 1975) in confirmation of earlier studies in rabbits (Larsson *et al.*, 1974; Romero *et al.*, 1973). The complex interrelationship between renal prostaglandins and the renin–angiotensin system is the subject of Chapter 10 of this volume. Additionally, renal prostaglandins may serve as modulators of renal kinins, a point we address later in this chapter.

3.2. Antihypertensive Neutral Renomedullary Lipid

Muirhead and his associates (Muirhead, 1976; Muirhead *et al.*, 1965, 1967) have detected an antihypertensive neutral lipid substance(s) in the renal medulla that is distinct from prostaglandins. Furthermore, the same group of workers have proposed that the well-documented antihypertensive effect of transplants of renal medulla or of renomedullary interstitial cells is mediated primarily by the secretion of ANRL. The hallmark of ANRL is that, unlike the acidic prostaglandins, the neutral lipid does not lower blood pressure acutely but requires a few hours to do so. Following the discontinuation of treatment of hypertensive animals with ANRL, the return of blood pressure to previous hypertensive levels is also slow (Fig. 4). Additionally, in contrast to prostaglandins, ANRL does not lower blood pressure of normotensive animals. In hypertensive animals, arterial pressue does not seem to be lowered much below normal (Muirhead, 1976; Muirhead *et al.*, 1975). A fraction has been separated that contains acidic lipids possessing acute vasodepressor effects, and another fraction has been found to contain neutral lipids, which show an antihypertensive effect of slow onset.

The details of the exact techniques used in preparing active ANRL preparations from renomedullary homogenates or from cultured interstitial cells cannot be presented here, but a summary of the procedure is shown in Fig. 5. Briefly, total lipids are extracted first from homogenates of fresh frozen rabbit renal medulla. The lipids are then subjected to Vitride reduction, a procedure designed to break all ester bonds and to reduce the lipids and fatty alcohols. This step is followed by florisil and lipophilic Sephadex chromatography. The interested reader is referred to reviews specifically dealing with these techniques (e.g., Muirhead, 1976). The ANRL preparations have been shown to be active in at least three types of experimental hypertension, e.g., canine renoprival hypertension induced by sodium-volume loading; renovascular hypertension in dog, rabbit and rat; and perinephritic hypertension induced by perinephric cellophane wrapping (Muirhead, 1976; Muirhead *et al.*, 1965, 1966). Relatively low doses of ANRL (30–300 μg/kg of a partially purified extract) were found to be very

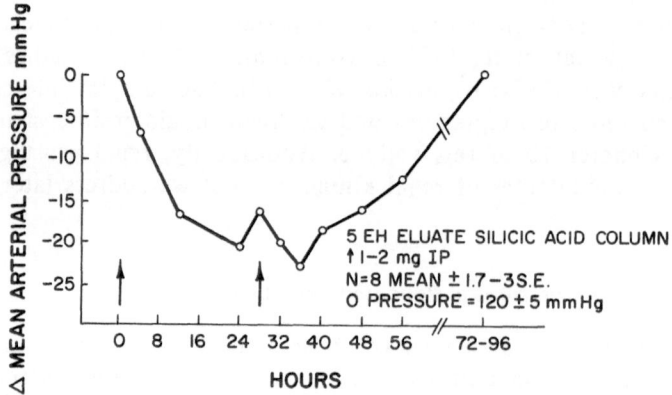

FIGURE 4. The antihypertensive action of ANRL in the hypertensive rabbit. Average values for eight experiments are included. The first dose of ANRL dropped the mean arterial pressure by 20 mm Hg within 24 hr; following the second dose, the pressure remained decreased for an additional 24 hr, then returned to preinjection hypertensive levels 72–96 hr after the first injection. [From Muirhead *et al.* (1971), with permission from the publisher.]

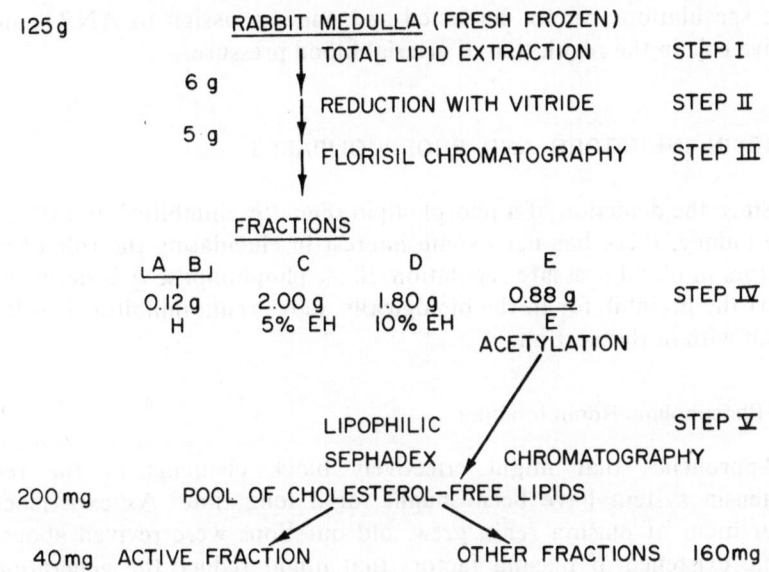

FIGURE 5. Flow chart of procedures for preliminary derivation of ANRL from renal medulla. [From Muirhead (1976), with permission from the publisher.]

effective in reducing mean arterial pressure in these experimental situations, whereas similar doses of PGE₂ were ineffective (Muirhead, 1976). As delineated in Fig. 4, a maximal effect was seen around 24–48 hr after initial treatment with ANRL in rabbits with one-kidney Goldblatt hypertension.

Unfortunately there has been no complete success in purifying and identifying the active principle of ANRL. The mechanism of action of ANRL must await purification and characterization of the active principle.

ANRL is known to lower blood pressure in the presence of substantial sodium–volume loads, yet this effect is not accompanied by natriuesis, diuresis, or reflex tachycardia (Muirhead, 1976). While ANRL ultimately should act by dilating vessels on the arterial side of the circulation, the exact mode of action is uncertain. A central action is possible, although vasodilatation does not occur acutely. Alternatively, ANRL might influence vascular reactivity by antagonizing the peripheral enhancement of the vasopressor effect of angiotensin mediated by sodium. It has also been hypothesized that cardiac output is reduced by an effect of ANRL on the heart or on venous compliance, followed by peripheral regulation at lower pressure (Muirhead, 1976). Finally, one should mention the unlikely possibility that a prostaglandin percursor (such as arachidonic acid) is esterified to a triglyceride in the neutral lipid and that hydrolysis *in vivo* (which takes time) eventually yields a vasodepressor prostaglandin. Until molecular indentification and full characterization of the ANRL is accomplished, the above speculations cannot be tested and one can assign to ANRL only a putative role in the regulation of arterial blood pressure.

4. RENIN INHIBITORS AND PHOSPHOLIPASES

Since the detection of a phospholipid renin "preinhibitor" in extracts of whole kidney, there has been some interest in elucidating the role of renin inhibitors in blood pressure regulation. Since phopholipase A is necessary to convert the preinhibitor to the biologically active renin inhibitor, it will also be dealt with in this section.

4.1. Phospholipid Renin Inhibitor

Approaches that might effectively block elements of the renin–angiotensin system have been sought for a long time. As experience in measurement of plasma renin grew, old questions were revived about the possible existence of plasma factors that might reduce the generation of angiotensin under conditions where concentrations of renin and of renin substrate in plasma remained constant. Boucher *et al.* (1964) had observed that under these conditions angiotensin generation was more rapid in some plasma samples than in others. Actually, it had been known for a long time that nephrectomized animals respond to renin with a greater and more sustained rise in arterial blood pressure than do normal controls (Tigerstedt and Bergman, 1898). Page and Helmer (1940) had shown that the increased sensitivity of nephrectomized dogs to renin could be lowered by transfusion of blood from normal dogs, a finding which suggested the existence of a renin inhibitor. The increase in rate of angiotensin generation for the first 24 hr following nephrectomy could be partially due to the parallel occurrence of a rise in renin substrate concentration. This concentration, however, does not rise any further after 24 hr, although the rate of angiotensin generation continues to rise (Sen *et al.*, 1967). Furthermore, the increase in renin reactivity (rate of angiotensin generation) in plasma from nephrectomized dogs was reversed by addition of normal dog plasma protein fractions. In plasma samples from patients with essential hypertension, the amount of angiotensin generated by the addition of a fixed amount of exogenous renin was independent of the renin–substrate concentration (Bumpus and Khosla, 1977). The existence of an inhibitor of renin appeared to be the best explanation for all these observations, and indeed Sen *et al.* (1967) obtained evidence that supported this concept (Sen *et al.*, 1968, 1969). Since the data on nephrectomized animals suggested that the substance was of renal origin, Sen *et al.* (1968, 1969) isolated a "phospholipid renin inhibitor" from whole canine kidneys. The substance was found to be very similar to phosphatidylserine but differed from it in fatty acid content and in amino acid structure. The substance powerfully inhibited the reaction of canine renin with substrate *in vitro*. Moreover, daily intramuscular injections of the inhibitor into hypertensive rats in does ranging from 2.6 to 6.7 mg/kg significantly reduced blood pressue (Zachariah *et al.*, 1975). Unlike with prostaglandins, the onset of the antihypertensive effect was relatively slow, as was the return of blood pressure to previous levels after discontinuation of therapy. The compound had no "acute" antihypertensive effect and had no effect on the blood pressue of the normotensive rat (Smeby *et al.*, 1967) (Fig. 6). The substance was believed to be distinct from the previously discussed antihypertensive factor isolated by Hamilton and Grollman in 1958 by aqueous acetone extraction of hog kidneys (Hamilton and Grollman, 1958), since the latter was described as insoluble in petroleum ether. The phospholipid is also distinct from ANRL, which is neutral and has a clearly different solubility profile in organic solvents. Similarly, it appears to be distinct from renal prostaglandins, which have a rapid onset of action and are acidic lipids. PGE_1 does not inhibit renin activities, although Kotchen and Miller (1974) have shown that PGA (10^{-6} M) can inhibit the generation of angiotensin I from renin substrate.

Interestingly, the renin inhibitor was found to be ineffective in animals other than the rat. The reason for this might be the presence in this species of very high levels of phospholipase A which plays an essential role *in vivo* in cleaving fatty acids from the phospholipid to yield the biologically active lysophospholipid. Hence, the phospholipid precursor has been named the "preinhibitor" whereas the lysophospholipid is the true "renin inhibitor." Inhibitory activity of the "preinhibitor" is lost when it is treated with

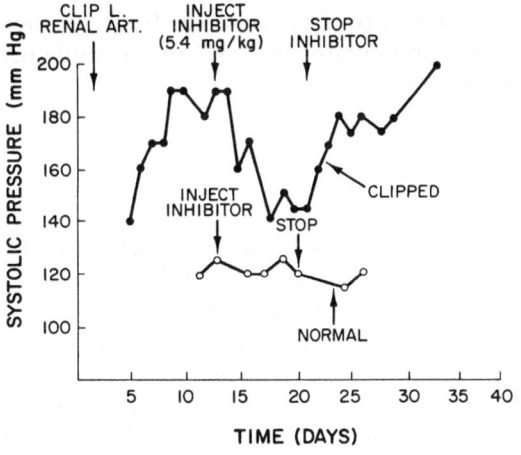

FIGURE 6. Typical response of a renal hypertensive (clipped) rat ●——● and a normotensive (control) rat ○——○ to single daily intramuscular injections of renin inhibitor. [From Smeby *et al.* (1967), by permission of the American Heart Association, Inc.]

phospholipase B (which removes both fatty acids from positions 1 and 2 of the phospholipid). It has recently been reported that the material has been successfully synthesized (Bumpus and Khosla, 1977). The synthetic material reportedly binds to renin with such a high specificity and affinity that it has even been used to purify renin by affinity chromatography. The role of this substance in the regulation of arterial blood pressure has not been established. The phospholipid does contain an unusually high amount of fatty acid migrating as arachidonic acid in gas chromatography, and biological activity is lost following reduction of this moiety (Sen et al., 1967).

4.2. Phospholipase A_2

It has been observed that after hypertension is induced by renal artery stenosis, plasma renin activity increases, although the renin protein concentration remains unchanged (Harris et al., 1973). Thus, the availability of renin could be controlled somehow by the renin inhibitor system. It was further shown by Osmond et al. (1969, 1973) that after bilateral nephrectomy the plasma concentration of the renin "preinhibitor" did not change, thereby eliminating changes in its concentration as a potential cause of increased renin reactivity. Since phospholipase A (PLA) is necessary to convert the inactive "preinhibitor" to the active "inhibitor" form, the possibility was considered that PLA might be a factor in regulating the availabiltiy of the inhibitor lysophospholipid. Indeed, in rats that have established spontaneous hypertension and renovascular hypertension, the activity of plasma PLA_2 is reduced. This reduction was dissociated from elevation in renin activity since PLA_2 was not reduced in rats placed on low-salt diet (Osmond et al., 1973). These observations suggest that other factors may regulate the availability of angiotensin peripherally. If future research continues to unravel the involvement of elements of this system in arterial blood pressure regulation, the basis for the establishment of the role of the "renin preinhibitor system" in the antihypertensive function of the kidneys will have been laid.

5. RENAL KININS

Although renal kinins are peptides and peptides and occur most abundantly in the renal cortex, a brief description of this system is appropriate in the light of present understanding of the very close functional relation of this system with the renal prostaglandins.

Kallikrein was the name given by Frey and co-workers (Frey and Kraut, 1926) to a protein found in urine and in pancreas, which acted on a plasma substrate (kininogen) to liberate a potent vasodepressor substance (kinin). The kallikreins in plasma appear to be somewhat different from those present in glands and organs. Plasma kallikrein is present in an inactive precursor form (prekallikrein). The precise mechanism of its activation is not well understood but the Hageman factor (clot-promoting factor XII) may be required for endogenous activation. A variety of kallikrein inhibitors normally protect against the potent effects of activated kinins. The best characterized plasma kallikrein releases brakykinin (a nonapeptide) on reaction with the circulating kininogen substrate (Rocha e Silva *et al.*, 1949), while the glandular kallikreins release kallidin (a decapeptide lysyl-bradykinin) from kininogen (Pierce and Webster, 1961). Bradykinin is a potent vasodilator peptide. Body fluids and organs also are rich sources of kininases and both bradykinin and kallidin are rapidly inactivated by pulmonary and vascular peptidases.

The precise cellular site of origin of urinary kallikrein has not been defined with certainty. Current evidence suggest that kallikrein resides along the more distal parts of the nephron and probably enters the urine at a distal site (Scicli *et al.*, 1978), whereas kininase II is present in the lining of the proximal tubule (Ward *et al.*, 1976; Scicli *et al.*, 1976; Orstavik *et al.*, 1976).

Could one of the kinins (e.g., bradykinin) serve as the circulating antihypertensive hormone of renal origin? This is considered unlikely in the light of the very large fractional inactivation of kinins after passage through the pulmonary circulation, and since very large quantitites of bradykinin are needed to produce significant peripheral vasodilation when infused into a vein (Rosas *et al.*, 1965). Therefore, it appears much more reasonable to consider that this kallikrein–kinin system may influence blood pressure regulation by primarily intrarenal effects (either tubular or renovascular events). The following intrarenal effects are worth mentioning:

1. The basal secretion of renal prostaglandins may be regulated in part by the activity of the renal kallikrein–kinin system (Terragno *et al.*, 1976). Since renal prostaglandins profoundly influence renal hemodynamics and intrarenal distribution of blood flow and thereby indirectly regulate excretion rates of sodium and water, the levels of activity of the renal–kinin system may be intimately involved in the regulation of blood pressure.
2. The renal kinin system may regulate the excretion of water. When sodium intake is held constant, variations in water intake were found to correlate directly and positively with urinary kallikrein excretion (Adetuyibi and Mills, 1972). The capacity of bradykinin to cause water excretion has been shown to be mediated by and dependent on its abiltiy to induce the synthesis of PGE_2 (McGiff and Nasjletti, 1976).

3. In addition to stimulating prostaglandin synthesis, presumably by
    activating phospholipases, kinins may actually determine the prin-
    cipal product of prostaglandin synthesis by regulating the activity
    of the enzyme PGE-9-ketoreductase, which converts PGE to PGF.
    The activity of the latter enzyme may in some way be influenced in
    an inverse way by the concentration of sodium ions. For example,
    under conditions of a sodium–volume deficit, kallikrein excretion is
    enhanced. But increased activity of PGE-9-ketoreductase, postu-
    lated to result from sodium depletion, leads primarily to an
    increase in PGF production, thereby attenuating the local vasodila-
    tor and diuretic effects of the peptide. PGF has no significant renal
    effect except in pharmacologic doses. Conversely, in the presence
    of significant sodium–volume loads, kinin cannot activate the
    reductase to the same extent, which leads to increased fractional
    release of PGE, creating conditions conducive to the excretion of
    salt (Terragno *et al.*, 1976). A selective increase in sodium load in
    the presence of constant normal water intake does not affect uri-
    nary kallikrein excretion (Adetuyibi and Mills, 1972). The relation-
    ship between kinins and sodium excretion is complex and
    bradykinin infusion does not consistently cause natriuresis unless
    prostaglandin synthesis is inhibited. There is evidence that
    under certain conditions, a prostaglandin released in response to
    increased intrarenal kinins may oppose natriuresis (Terragno *et al.*,
    1976).

In recent years, evidence has accumulated to suggest that a deficiency
in renal kallikreins may play a role in the pathogenesis of hypertension. The
precise mechanisms by which renal kinins control blood pressure are
unknown. Elliott and Nuzum, in 1934, reported a decrease in urinary
kallikrein excretion in hypertensive man (Elliott and Nuzum, 1934). Since
then, several other investigators have shown decreased urinary kallikrein
excretion in human hypertension (Margolius et al., 1971; Shimamoto *et al.*,
1978; Mitas *et al.*, 1978). Long-term studies of urinary kallikrein in normal
children have shown that kallikrein excretion is familially aggregated and is
markedly lower in black than in white children. Interestingly, kallikrein excretion was inversely related to blood pressure in both black and white
children (Zinner *et al.*, 1978). In renovascular hypertension in man,
kallikrein excretion from the stenotic kidney is reduced (Keiser *et al.*,
1976*a*). Although, as mentioned previously, several workers have repeatedly
confirmed the altered excretion of urinary kallikrein in various hypertensive
states, in primary aldosteronism there is a large increase in kallikrein excretion in the urine (Margolius *et al.*, 1974). Furthermore, recent studies show

that sodium and potassium intake may regulate urinary kallikrein excretion (Olshan *et al.*, 1978). Additionally, the same group of workers have shown that the degree to which sodium and potassium intake affects urinary kallikrein excretion is modulated by race and the level of blood pressure.

In spontaneously hypertensive rats, urinary kallikrein decreases only after hypertension becomes established (Keiser *et al.*, 1976*b*). In recent studies, a significant increase in blood concentration of kinins during long-term administration of converting enzyme inhibitor SQ14225 in conscious sodium-depleted dogs has been observed (McCaa *et al.*, 1978). A significant increase in plasma bradykinin concentration occurred following administration of a converting enzyme inhibitor, SQ20881, in hypertensive subjects, although no such increase in bradykinin was noted in normal subjects (Williams *et al.*, 1977).

All of these data support the notion that locally generated renal kallikreins do exert an important pathophysiological role in the regulation of systemic arterial pressure. However, still unanswered is the important question how these locally generated renal kinins modulate systemic arterial pressure. The kinins are among the most potent vasodilator substances known. On a molar basis, they are approximately ten times as potent as histamine. Intravenous infusion of kinins in humans or in the renal artery of dogs produces an increase in renal blood flow, urine flow, urinary sodium excretion, and urinary prostaglandin excretion (Barraclough *et al.*, 1965; Willis *et al.*, 1969; Stein *et al.*, 1972; Fadem *et al.*, 1977). The natriuretic action of kinins is thought to be due to alterations in renal hemodynamics, including redistribution of blood flow and changes in peritubular hydrostatic pressure (Willis *et al.*, 1969; Stein *et al.*, 1971, 1972). However, a direct or indirect action of kinins on tubular sodium transport, particularly distal tubular transport, cannot be excluded at the present time (Carretero *et al.*, 1976).

A deficiency in the renal kinin system may contribute to the genesis of hypertension by decreasing renal prostaglandin synthesis, particularly in the PGE_2 series. The PGE_2 compounds may mediate or modulate an important part of the renal antihypertensive function (McGiff and Nasjletti, 1976). All of these observations suggest the involvement of the renal kinin system in the pathophysiology of hypertension in man and experimental animals.

6. CONCLUDING REMARKS

A variety of substances having antihypertensive properties have been extracted from renal tissue. While intensive research continues to define the physiological roles of the renal prostaglandin and kinin systems, interest in

ANRL and the phospholipid renin inhibitor system may be expected to increase. The following concluding comments seem in order:

1. Renal prostaglandins appear to play an important role in the renal antihypertensive function. This role is exerted primarily by local effects, at or very near their sites of synthesis and most probably by PGE_2. Thus PGE_2 could be a major determinant of renovascular reactivity and of the intrarenal distribution of blood flow, which may secondarily influence the excretion of sodium–volume loads. There is insufficient evidence to support the view that a prostaglandin of renal origin serves as a circulating antihypertensive hormone acting peripherally. Incidentally, it has been shown that the mammalian kidney does have the capacity to synthesize prostacyclin (PGI_2) from exogenous arachidonic acid, although the isolated perfused rabbit kidney synthesizes predominately PGE_2 under baseline conditions (Needleman et al., 1978; Wong et al., 1979). Work in vitro with microsomes prepared from rabbit kidneys has revealed that the renal cortex but not the renal medulla is the site of prostacyclin synthesis (Whorton et al., 1978). Since prostacyclin is a potent vasodilator and is synthesized usually in the blood vessel walls, its potential role in blood pressure regulation cannot be overemphasized. It is likely that the function of prostacyclin in modifying blood pressure will be clarified by further work in the very near future.
2. The precise role of ANRL and of the phospholipid renin preinhibitor system in the regulation of blood pressure has not been fully elucidated at this time.
3. Renal kinins stimulate renal prostaglandin synthesis and may determine basal prostaglandin secretion by kidneys. The effects of renal kinins are probably mediated by varying renal prostaglandin output, and by the proportion of PGE to PGF synthesized. It is further likely that a renal vasodilator diuretic system consisting of the interacting kallikrein–kinin–prostaglandins may serve to oppose the vasoconstrictor–antinatriuretic–prohypertensive system of the adrenergic–renin–angiotensin–vasopressin system of neural and hormonal influences. These opposing influences act locally intrarenally.

Further work in determining the precise role of prostaglandins (especially prostacyclin) and of the other vasodepressors identified in the kidneys (such as ANRL and, renin inhibitors) will undoubtedly produce exciting new findings that will help to unravel the precise mode of operation of the renal antihypertensive functions.

ACKNOWLEDGMENT

The authors greatly appreciate the criticisms and suggestions of Dr. Jared Grantham, Professor of Medicine, University of Kansas Medical Center, Kansas City, Kansas, and the excellent secretarial assistance of Renee Russel. This work was supported by the Medical Research Service of the Veterans Administration.

REFERENCES

Adetuyibi, A., and Mills, I. H., 1972, Relation between Kallikrein and renal function, hypertension and excretion of sodium and water in man, *Lancet* **2**:203.

Barraclough, M. A., and Mills, I. H., 1965, Effects of bradykinin on renal function, *Clin. Sci.* **28**:69.

Bergstrom, S., Carlson, L. A., Eklund, L. G., and Oro, L., 1965, Cardio-vascular and metabolic response of PGE$_1$ in man, *Acta Physiol. Scand.* **64**:332.

Boucher, R., Veyrat, R., DeChamplain, D., and Genest, J., 1964, The measurement of renin by means of a new sensitive technique, *Can. Med. Assoc. J.***6**:1572.

Braun-Menendez, E., 1958, The pro-hypertensive and anti-hypertensive actions of kidney, *Ann. Int. Med.* **49**:717.

Braun-Menendez, E., and von Euler, V. S., 1947, Hypertension after bilateral nephrectomy in rat, *Nature* **160**:905.

Bumpus, F. M., and Khosla, M. C., 1977, Pathogenic factors involved in renovascular hypertension: State of art, *Mayo Clinic Proc.* **52**:417.

Carr, A. A., 1973, Effects of PGA$_1$ on renin and aldosterone in man, *Prostaglandins* **3**:621.

Carretero, O. A., and Scicli, A. G., 1976, Renal kallikrein: Its localization and possible role in renal function, *Fed. Proc. Fed. Am. Soc. Exp. Biol.* **35**:194.

Colina-Chorio, J., McGiff, J. C., and Nasjletti, A., 1975, Development of high blood pressure after inhibition of prostaglandin synthesis, *Fed. Proc. Fed. Am. Soc. Exp. Biol.* **34**:368.

Ducrot, H., Jungers, P., Funck-Brentano, J. L., Perrin, D., Crosnier, J., and Hamburger, J., 1966, l'Action de la transplantation renale sur l'hypertension anterielle, in: *l'Hypertension Arterielle* (P. Milliez and P. Tcherdakoff, eds.), Expansion Scientifique Francaise, Paris, pp. 208–222.

Dunn, M. J., and Hood, V. J., 1977, Prostaglandins and the kidney, *Am. J. Physiol.* **233**:F169.

Dunn, M. J., Liard, J. F., and Dray, F., 1978, Basal and stimulated rates of renal secretion and excretion of prostaglandin E$_2$, F and 13–14-dihydro-15-keto-F in the dog, *Kidney Int.* **13**:136.

Elliot, A. H., and Nuzum, F. R., 1934, Urinary excretion of a depressor substance (Kallikrein of Frey and Kraut) in arterial hypertension, *Endocrinology* **18**:462.

Fadem, S. F., Patak, R., Lifschitz, M., and Stein, J, 1977, Studies on the mechanism of increased sodium excretion during drug induced vasodilatation, *Kidney Int.* **12**:557 (abstr.).

Fasciolo, J. D., Houssay, B. A., and Taquini, A. C., 1938, The blood pressure raising secretion of the ischemic kidney, *J. Physiol.* **94**:281.

Frey, E. K., and Kraut, H., 1926, Über einen von der Niere ausgeschiedenen die Herztätigkeit anregenden Stoff, *Hoppe Seylers Z. Physiol. Chem.* **157**:32.

Frolich, J. C., Sweetman, B. J., Carr, K., Hollifield, J. W., and Oates, J. A., 1975a, Assessment of the levels of PGA$_2$ in human plasma by gas chromatography–mass spectroscopy, *Prostaglandins* **10**:185.

Frolich, J. C., Wilson, T. W., Sweetman, B. J., Smigel, M., Nies, A. S., Watson, J. T., and Oates, J. A., 1975*b*, Urinary prostaglandins: Identification and origin, *J. Clin. Invest.* **55**:763.

Goldblatt, H., Lynch, J., Hunzal, R. F., and Summerville, W. W., 1934, Studies on experimental hypertension. I. The production of persistent elevation of systolic blood pressure by renal ischemia, *J. Exp. Med.* **59**:347.

Gomez, A. H., Hoobler, S. W., and Blaquier, P., 1960, Effects of addition and removal of kidney transplant in renal and adrenocortical hypertensive rats, *Circ. Res.* **8**:464.

Grollman, A., 1959, Arterial hypertension of renal origin, *Perspect. Biol. Med.* **2**:208.

Grollman, A., Williams, J. R., and Harrison, T. R., 1940, Reduction of elevated blood pressure by administration of renal extracts, *J. Am. Med. Assoc.* **115**:1169.

Grollman, A., Muirhead, E. E., and Vanatta, J., 1949, Role of kidney in pathogenesis of hypertension as determined by the study of effects of bilateral nephrectomy and other procedures on the blood pressure of the dog, *Am. J. Physiol.* **157**:21.

Grollman, A., Turner, L. B., Levitch, M., and Hill, D., 1951, Hemodynamics of the bilaterally nephrectomized dog subjected to intermittent peritoneal lavage, *Am. J. Physiol.* **165**:167.

Hamilton, J. G., and Grollman, A., 1958, The preparation of renal extracts effective in reducing blood pressure in experimental hypertension, *J. Biol Chem.* **233**:528.

Harris, P. J., Munday, K. A., Noble, A. R., and Winch, M. N., 1973, Relationship between renin activity and concentration, *Proc. Physiol. Soc.* **72**:70.

Itskovitz, H. D., and McGiff, J. C., 1974, Hormonal regulation of renal circulation, *Circ. Res.* **34-35-1**(Suppl. 1):65.

Itskovitz, H. D., Terragno, N. A., and McGiff, J. C., 1973, Renal prostaglandins: Determinants of intrarenal distribution of blood flow, *Clin. Sci. Mol. Med.* **45**(Suppl. 1):321.

Keiser, H. R., Geller, R. G., Margolius, H. S., and Pisano, J. J., 1976*a*, Urinary kallikrein in hypertensive animal models, *Fed. Proc. Fed. Am. Soc. Exp. Biol.* **35**:199.

Keiser, H. R., Margolius, H. S., Brown, R., Rhamey, R., and Foster, J., 1976*b*, Urinary Kallikrein in patients with renovascular hypertension, in: *Chemistry and Biology. Biology of the Kallikrein–Kinin System in Health and Disease* (J. J. Pisano and K. F. Austen, eds.), U.S. Government Printing Office, Washington, D.C., pp. 423–426.

Kolff, W. J., 1957, Reduction of experimental renal hypertension by kidney perfusion, *Univ. Mich. Med. Bull.* **23**:238.

Kolff, W. J., and Page, I. H., 1954, Blood pressure reducing function of the kidney: Reduction of renoprival hypertension by kidney perfusion, *Am. J. Physiol.* **178**:75.

Kolff, W. J., Nakamoto, S., Poutasse, E. F., Straffon, R. A., and Figeroa, J. E., 1964, Effect of bilateral nephrectomy and kidney transplantation on hypertension in man, *Circulation* **30**(Suppl. 2):23.

Kotchen, T. A., and Miller, M. C., 1974, Effects of prostaglandins on renin reactivity, *Am. J. Physiol.* **266**:314.

Larsson, C., and Änggård, E., 1973*a*, Regional differences in the formation and metabolism of prostaglandins in rabbit kidney, *Eur. J. Pharmacol.* **21**:30.

Larsson, C., and Änggård, E., 1973*b*, Archidonic acid lowers and indomethacin increases the blood pressure of the rabbit, *J. Pharm. Pharmacol.* **25**:653.

Larsson, C., and Änggård, E., 1975, Mass spectrometric determination of prostaglandins in regions of rabbit kidney, in: Proceedings of the International Congress on Prostaglandins, Florence, Italy (May 26–30), p. 179 (abstr.).

Larsson, C., Weber, P., and Änggård, E., 1974, Arachidonic acid increases and indomethacin decreases plasma renin activity in the rabbit, *Eur. J. Pharmacol.* **28**:391.

Lee, J. B., 1976, The renal prostaglandins and blood pressure regulation in: *Advances in Prostaglandin and Thromboxane Research*, Vol. 2 (B. Samuelsson and R. Paoletti, eds.), Raven Press, New York, p. 573.

Lee, J. B., Hickler, R. B., Saravis, C. A., and Thorn, G. W., 1962, Sustained depressor effects of renal medullary extracts, *Circulation* **26**:747.

Lee, J. B., Hickler, R. B., Saravis, C. A., and Thorn, G. W., 1963, Sustained depressor effects of renal medullary extracts in the normotensive rat, *Circ. Res.* **13**:359.

Lee, J. B., Covino, B. G., Takman, B. H., and Smith, E. R., 1965, Renomedullary vasodepressor substance medullin. Isolation, chemical characterization and physiological properties, *Circ. Res.* **17**:57.

Lee, J. B., Crowshaw, K., Takman, B. H., Attrep, K. A., and Gongontas, J. Z., 1967, The identification of prostaglandins E_2, F_2 and A_2 from rabbit kidney medulla, *Biochem. J.* **105**:1251.

Lee, J. B., McGiff, J. C., and Kannegieser, H., 1971, Prostaglandin A_1: Anti-hypertensive and renal effects, *Ann. Intern. Med.* **74**:703.

Lee, J. B., Patak, R. V., and Mookerjee, B. K., 1976, Renal prostaglandins and the regulation of blood pressure, sodium and water homeostasis, *Am. J. Med.* **60**:798.

Leonards, J. R., and Heisler, C. R., 1951, Hypertension of renoprival origin, *Am. J. Physiol.* **167**:553.

Lonigro, A. J., Itskovitz, H. D., Crowshaw, K., and McGiff, J. C., 1973, Dependency of renal blood flow on prostaglandins in dog, *Circ. Res.* **32**:712.

Lopez-Ovejero, J. A., Weber, M. A., Dryer, J. I. M., Sealey, J. E., and Largh, J. H., 1978, Effects of indomethacin alone and during diuretic or adrenoreceptor blockage therapy on blood pressure and the renin system in essential hypertension, *Clin. Sci. Mol. Med.* **55**:203 S.

McCaa, R. E., Hall, J. E. and McCaa, C. S., 1978, The effects of angiotensin I-converting enzyme inhibitor on arterial blood pressure and urinary sodium excretion. Role of renal renin–angiotensin and kallikrein–kinin system, *Circ. Res.* **43**(Suppl. 1):32.

McGiff, J. C., and Nasjletti, A., 1976, Kinins, renal function and blood pressure regulation, *Fed. Proc. Fed. Am. Soc. Exp. Biol.* **35**:172.

McGiff, J. C., Terragno, N. A., Strand, J. C., Lee, J. B., Lonigro, A. J., and Ng, K. K. F., 1969, Selective passage of prostaglandins across the lung, *Nature* **223**:742.

McGiff, J. C., Crowshaw, K., Terragno, N. A., and Lonigro, A. J., 1970a, Renal prostaglandins: Possible regulators of renal actions of pressor hormones, *Nature* **227**:1255.

McGiff, J. C., Crowshaw, K., Terragno, N. A., Lonigro, A. J., Strand, J. C., Williamson, M. A., Lee, J. B., and Ng, K. K. F., 1970b, Prostaglandin-like substance appearing in blood during renal ischemia, *Circ. Res.* **27**:765.

Margolius, H. S., Geller, R. G., Pisano, J. J., and Sjordsma, A., 1971, Altered urinary kallikrein secretion in human hypertension, *Lancet* **2**:1063.

Margolius, H. S., Horwitz, D., Pisano, J. J., and Keiser, H. R., 1974, Urinary Kallikrein excretion in hypertensive man. Relationship to sodium intake and to sodium retaining steroids, *Circ. Res.* **35**:820.

Milliez, P., Meyer, Ph., Devaux, C. and Alexander, J. M., 1966, in: *l'Hypertension Arterielle* (P. Milliez and P. Tcherdakoff, eds.), Expansion Scientifique Francaise, Paris, pp. 203–207.

Mitas, J. A., Levy, S. B., Holle, R., Frigon, R. P., and Stone, R. A., 1978, Urinary Kallikrein activity in hypertension of renal parenchymal disease, *N. Engl. J. Med.* **299**:162.

Montgomery, R. G., Patel, N. C., and Lee, J. G., 1973, Comparison of diuretic effects of PGA_1, sodium ethacrynate and placebo, *Prostaglandins* **4**:381.

Muirhead, E. E., 1962, Protection against sodium overload hypertensive state, *Arch. Pathol.* **74**:214.

Muirhead, E. E., 1976, Renomedullary anti-hypertensive endocrine function, *Acta Biol. Med. Germ.* **35**:1181.

Muirhead, E. E., Stirman, J. A., Lesch, W., and Jones, F., 1956, The reduction of post-nephrectomy hypertension by renal homotransplants, *Surg. Gynecol. Obstet.* **103**:673.

Muirhead, E. E., Stirman, J. A., and Jones, F., 1960, Renal autoexplantation and protection against renoprival hypertensive cardiovascular disease and hemolysis, *J.Clin. Invest.* **39**:266.

Muirhead, E. E., Daniels, E. G., Booth, E., Freyberger, W. A., and Hinman, J. W., 1965, Renomedullary vasodepressor and anti-hypertensive function, *Arch. Pathol.* **80**:43.

Muirhead, E. E., Brooks, B., Kosinsky, M., Daniels, E. G., and Hinman, J. W., 1966, Reno-medullary anti-hypertensive principle in renal hypertension, *J. Lab. Clin. Med.* **67**:778.

Muirhead, E. E., Daniels, E. G., Pike, J. E., and Hinman, J. W., 1967, Renomedullary anti-hypertensive lipids and the prostaglandins, in: *The Prostaglandins: Nobel Symposium II, Uppsala* (S. Bergstrom and B. Samuelsson, eds.), Almquist and Wiksell, Stockholm, p. 183.

Muirhead, E. E., Leech, B. E., Byers, L. W., Daniels, E. G., and Hinman, J. W., 1971, Anti-hypertensive neutral renomedullary lipids, in: *Kidney Hormones* (J. W. Fisher, ed.), Academic Press, London, p. 485.

Muirhead, E. E., Germain, G. S., Armstrong, F. B., Brooks, B., Leech, B. E., Byers, L. W., Pitcock, J. A., and Brown, P., 1975, Endocrine type anti-hypertensive function of reno-medullary interstitial cells, *Kidney Int.* **8**(Suppl. 5):273.

Needleman, P., Bronson, S. D., Wyche, A., and Sinakoff, M., 1978, Cardiac and renal prosta-glandin I_2, *J. Clin. Invest.* **61**:839.

Negus, P., Tannen, R. L., and Dunn, M. J., 1976, Indomethacin potentiates the vasoconstric-tor actions of angiotensin II, *Prostaglandins* **12**:175.

Olshan, A., Mitas, J., Frigon, R. P., and Stone, R. A., 1978, The influence of dietary sodium, potassium and race on urinary kallikrein activity, *Kidney Int.* **14**:701 (abstr.).

Orbison, J. L., Christian, C. L., and Peters, E., 1952, Studies on experimental hypertension and cardiovascular disease, *Arch. Pathol.* **54**:185.

Orstavik, T. B., Nustad, K., Brandtzaeg, P., and Pierce, J. V., 1976, Cellular origin of urinary Kallikrein, *J. Histochem. Cytochem.* **24**:1037.

Osmond, D. H., Smeby, R. R., and Bumpus, F. M., 1969, Quantitative studies on renin pre-inhibitor, *J. Lab. Clin. Med.* **73**:795.

Osmond, D. H., McFadzen, P. A., and Ross, L. J., 1973, Plasma phospholipase A_2 activity in nephrectomized rats and question of renin inhibitor, *Proc. Soc. Exp. Biol. Med.* **144**:969.

Page, I. H., and Helmer, O. M., 1940, Angiotensin-activator, renin and angiotensin-inhibitor and mechanism of angiotensin tachyphylaxis in normal, hypertensive and nephrectomized animals, *J. Exp. Med.* **71**:495.

Page, I. H., Hebner, O., Hohlstaedt, K. G., Keinff, G. F., and Corchoran, A. C., 1940, Substance in kidneys and muscle eliciting prolonged reduction in blood pressure in human and experimental hypertension, *Proc. Soc. Exp. Biol. Med.* **43**:722.

Patak, R. V., Mookerjee, B. K., Bentzel, C. J., Hysert, P. E., Babej, M., and Lee, J. B., 1975, Antagonism of the effects of furosemide by indomethacin in normal and hypertensive man, *Prostaglandins* **10**:649.

Pierce, J. V., and Webster, M. E., 1961, Human plasma kallidins: Isolation and chemical studies, *Biochem. Biophys. Res. Commun.* **5**:353.

Rocha e Silva, M., Beraldo, W. T., and Rosenfeld, G., 1949, Bradykinin, a hypotensive and smooth muscle stimulating factor released from plasma globulin by snake venoms and by trypsin, *Am. J. Physiol.* **156**:261.

Romero, J. C., Strong, C. G., Torres, V. E., Ott, C., and Knox, F. G., 1973, Plasma, prosta-glandins, plasma renin activity and blood pressure in normal and renal hypertensive rabbits treated with indomethacin, Proceedings of the 6th Annual Meeting of the American Society of Nephrology, Washington, D.C., p. 89 (abstr.).

Rosas, R., Montaigne, D., Gross, M., and Bohr, D. R., 1965, Cardiac action of vasoactive peptides I. Bradykinin, *Circ. Res.* **16**:150.

Scicli, A. G., Carretero, O. A., Hampton, A., Cortes, P., and Oza, N. B., 1976, Site of kininogenase secretion in the dog nephron, *Am. J. Physiol.* **230**:533.

Scicli, A. G., Grandolfi, R., and Carretero, O. A., 1978, Site of formation of kinins in the dog nephron, *Am. J. Physiol.* **234**:F36.

Sen, S., Smeby, R. R., and Bumpus, F. M., 1967, Isolation of a phospholipid renin inhibitor from the kidney, *Biochemistry* **6**:1572.

Sen, S., Smeby, R. R., and Bumpus, F. M., 1968, Anti-hypertensive effect of an isolated phospholipid, *Am. J. Physiol.* **214**:337.

Sen, S., Smeby, R. R., and Bumpus, F. M., 1969, Plasma renin activity in hypertensive rats after treatment with "renin pre-inhibitor," *Am. J. Physiol.* **216**:499.

Shimamoto, K., Ando, T., Nakao, T., Tanaka, S., Sakuma, M., and Miyahara, M., 1978, A sensitive radioimmunoassay method for urinary kinins in man, *J. Lab. Clin. Med.* **91**:721.

Smeby, R. R., Sen, S., and Bumpus, F. M., 1967, A naturally occurring renin inhibitor. *Circ. Res.* **20-21**(Suppl. 2):129.

Smith, W. L., and Bell, T. G., 1978, Immunohistochemical localization of the prostaglandin-forming cyclo-oxygenase in renal cortex, *Am. J. Physiol.* **235**:F451.

Stein, J. H., Ferris, T. F., Huprich, J. E., Smith, T. C., and Osgood, R. W., 1971, Effect of renal vasodilation on the distribution of cortical blood flow in the kidney of the dog, *J. Clin. Invest.* **50**:1429.

Stein, J. H., Congbaley, R. C., Karsh, D. L., Osgood, R. W., and Ferris, T. F., 1972, The effect of bradykinin on proximal tubular sodium absorption in the dog: Evidence of functional nephron heterogeneity, *J. Clin. Invest.* **51**:1709.

Tan, Y. S., and Murlow, P. J., 1978, Impaired renal production of prostaglandin E_2: A newly identified lesion in human essential hypertension, *Prostaglandins* **15**:139.

Terragno, N. A., Malik, K. U., Nasjletti, A., Terragno, D. A., and McGiff, J. C., 1976, Renal prostaglandins, in: *Advances in Prostaglandin and Thromboxane Research*, Vol. 2 (B. Samuelsson and R. Paoletti, eds.), Raven Press, New York, p. 563.

Tigerstedt, R., and Bergman, P. G., 1898, Niere und Kreislauf, *Skand, Ark. Physiol.* **8**:223.

Ward, P. E., Erdos, E. G., Gudney, C. D., Dowen, R. M., and Reynolds, R. C., 1976, Isolation of membrane-bound renal enzymes that metabolize kinins and angiotensins, *Biochem. J.* **157**:643.

Weiner, R., and Kaley, G., 1969, Influence of PGE_1 on the terminal vascular bed, *Am. J. Physiol.* **217**:563.

Whorton, A. R., Smigel, M., Oates, J. A., and Frohlich, J. C., 1978, Regional differences in prostacyclin formation by the kidney, *Biochim. Biophys. Acta* **529**:178.

Williams, G. H., and Hollenberg, N. K., 1977, Accentuated vascular and endocrine response to SQ-20,881 in hypertension, *N. Eng. J. Med.* **297**:184.

Willis, L. R., Lundens, J. H., Hook, J. B., and Williamson, H. E., 1969, Mechanism of natriuretic action of bradykinin, *Am. J. Physiol.* **217**:1.

Wong, P. Y., McGiff, J. C., Cagan, L., Malik, K. U., and Sun, F. F., 1979, Metabolism of prostacyclin in the rabbit kidney, *J. Biol. Chem.* **254**:12.

Zachariah, N. Y., Smeby, R. R., Sen, S., Bumpus, F. M., and Singh, C., 1975, Phospholipase A_2 in experimental hypertension, *Am. J. Physiol.* **228**:1782.

Zinner, H. S., Margolius, H. S., Rosner, B., and Kass, E. H., 1978, Stability of blood pressure rank and urinary Kallikrein concentration in childhood: An eight year follow up, *Circulation* **58**:908.

Zins, G. R., 1975, Renal prostaglandins, *Am. J. Med.* **58**:14.

CHAPTER 5

Renal Prostaglandin Synthesis and Metabolism in Normal and Hypertensive States

CATHERINE LIMAS

1. INTRODUCTION

The impetus for studying prostaglandin synthesis and metabolism in hypertension derives largely from a consideration of their effects on the vascular system and the kidney. Through their actions on the vascular smooth muscle and water and electrolyte exchange in the kidney, prostaglandins may participate in the control of systemic blood pressure under physiological and/or pathological conditions.

The vascular smooth muscle tone, which determines systemic vascular resistance, is directly affected by prostaglandins through a modulation of Ca^{2+} movement across the plasma membranes (Altura and Altura, 1976). It is generally accepted that prostaglandins do not act as circulating hormones (Ferreira and Vane, 1967) but, rather, at or near their sites of synthesis; therefore, local biosynthesis within the vascular wall is probably the major determinant of their actions on the vessels. In fact, vascular tissue contains significant activity for prostaglandin synthesis as well as enzymes that degrade the active substances (Terragno et al., 1975; Limas, C. J., and Limas, 1977). It is also known that the response—dilatation or constriction—varies with different classes of prostaglandins and with different vascular beds (Messing et al., 1976). One can, then, visualize how the final effect of prostaglandin release within the vessel wall can be very specific,

CATHERINE LIMAS • Department of Pathology, Veterans Administration Hospital, and Departments of Laboratory Medicine and Pathology, University of Minnesota School of Medicine, Minneapolis, Minnesota 55455.

appropriately timed, and well localized to be of significance as a response to physiological needs or as an adaptation to abnormal circumstances.

Prostaglandins also interact with humoral and neural factors, such as angiotensin, kinins, and the sympathetic nervous system (Needleman et al., 1973; Davis and Horton, 1972; McGiff, 1978).

Within the kidney, the effects of prostaglandins on renal blood flow and salt and water exhange are relevant to blood pressure control. There is compartmentalization within the kidneys of the enzymes involved in prostaglandin synthesis and degradation, and this may be relevant to the physiological role of these substances. In general, the renal medulla, especially the papilla, is the major site of prostaglandin synthesis (Änggård et al., 1972; Crowshaw, 1973; Pong and Levine, 1976) whereas the bulk of degradation occurs in the renal cortex (Katzen et al., 1975; Pace-Asciak, 1975; Änggård et al., 1972). The cellular and subcellular localization of prostaglandin synthetase has been studied by histochemistry, immunofluorescence, and differential centrifugation. In the medulla, both renomedullary interstitial cells (RIC) and collecting ducts have been shown to possess prostaglandin synthetase by histochemical techniques (Bohman, 1977). Electron microscopy of subcellular fractions indicates that the endoplasmic reticulum (ER) (cytomembrane fraction II of Bohman and Larsson) (Fig. 1) is the predominant site of prostaglandin synthesis; since interstitial cells are the only

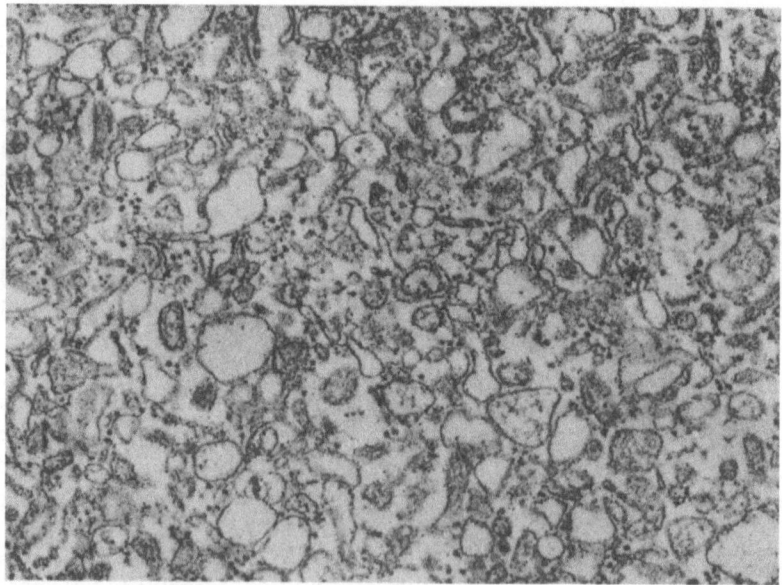

FIGURE 1. Electron microscopic appearance of microsomal fraction from rat renal medulla (×35,000).

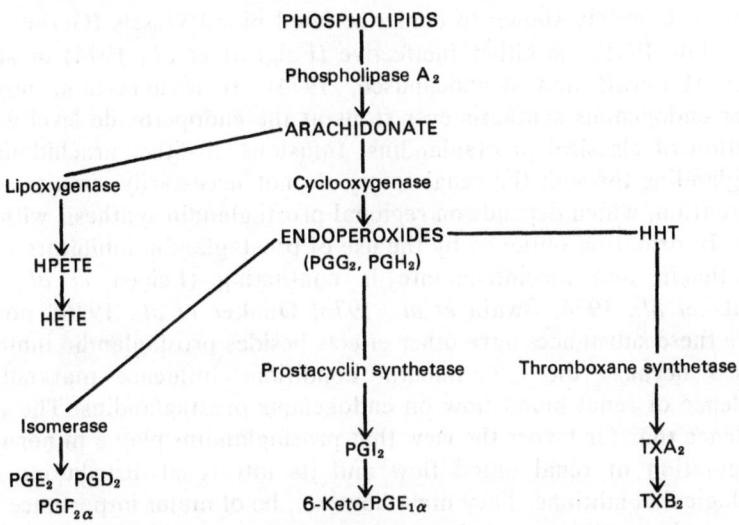

FIGURE 2. Pathways of arachidonate metabolism.

renomedullary cells with prominent endoplasmic reticulum, they may also be the major cellular component involved in prostaglandin synthesis (Bohman and Larsson, 1975). In fact, tissue culture experiments have unequivocally established the capacity of RIC for prostaglandin synthesis (Zusman and Keiser, 1977; Muirhead et al., 1972).

The pathway of prostaglandin synthesis from precursor fatty acids has been extensively reviewed (Maclouf et al., 1977). An outline of arachidonic acid metabolism in the kidney is given in Fig. 2. Prostaglandins (PG) E_2, $F_{2\alpha}$, I_2 and D_2 are synthesized by the medulla; under the usual experimental conditions, PGE_2 is by far predominant. Since PGE_2 has natriuretic and vasodilator properties, its synthesis may contribute to the antihypertensive function of the medulla.

2. RENAL EFFECTS OF PROSTAGLANDINS

The effect of locally synthesized prostaglandins on intrarenal blood flow distribution is, in part, predicated on the anatomy of the intrarenal vessels (Fourman and Moffat, 1971). For example, constriction or dilatation of the medullary vasa recta brought about by prostaglandins in the inner medulla will have secondary effects on the distribution of blood in the outer medulla and inner cortex.

Intrarenal infusion of prostaglandins of the E series or arachidonate induces dilation of inner cortical and medullary vessels. Only endoperoxides have been definitely shown to constrict renal blood vessels (Gerber *et al.*, 1977), while $PGF_{2\alpha}$ is either ineffective (Fulgraff *et al.*, 1974) or slightly dilatory (Fulgraff and Brandenbusch, 1974). It is uncertain, however, whether endogenous synthesis ever stops at the endoperoxide level without generation of classical prostaglandins. Infusions of either arachidonate or prostaglandins through the renal artery do not necessarily simulate the *in vivo* situation, which depends on regional prostaglandin synthesis within the kidney. Information obtained by the use of prostaglandin inhibitors such as indomethacin and meclofenamate is conflicting (Feigen *et al.*, 1976; Itskovitz *et al.*, 1974; Swain *et al.*, 1975; Donker *et al.*, 1976), not only because these substances have other effects besides prostaglandin inhibition, but also because the experimental conditions influence markedly the dependence of renal blood flow on endogenous prostaglandins. The weight of evidence thus far favors the view that prostaglandins play a minor role in the regulation of renal blood flow and its intrarenal distribution under physiological conditions. They may, however, be of major importance under pathological conditions—such as trauma, hypotension, anesthesia, or hypertension—which tend to disrupt normal regulation of blood flow. Under these circumstances, inhibition of prostaglandin synthesis may have easily demonstrable effects on the renal blood flow.

Prostaglandins influence salt and water balance both directly and indirectly. Indirect effects include those secondary to interference with (1) blood flow distribution and (2) antidiuretic hormone (ADH) action on the distal nephron (Grantham and Orloff, 1968; Berl *et al.*, 1977). Prostaglandins inhibit ADH-stimulated water reabsorption (Grantham and Orloff, 1968; Berl *et al.*, 1977), probably by antagonizing ADH-induced stimulation of adenylyl cyclase (Lum *et al.*, 1977).

Direct effects on tubular functions have been demonstrated by Kauker (1977), who observed inhibition of sodium reabsorption after injection of PGE_2 within the lumen of rat kidney tubules. Inhibition by PGE_2 of sodium transport by isolated perfused collecting ducts was shown in rabbits pretreated with mineralocorticoids (Stokes and Kokko, 1977).

3. REGULATION OF PROSTAGLANDIN METABOLISM IN THE KIDNEY

Regulation of the rate of renal prostaglandin synthesis and types of prostaglandins synthesized can be exerted at different points along the biosynthetic cascade.

3.1. Substrate Delivery

Fatty acids that serve as precursors for prostaglandin synthesis are incorporated within membrane phospholipids (Vonkeman and Van Dorp,

1968; Lands and Samuelsson, 1968) and must be released by the action of a membrane phospholipase (Flower and Blackwell, 1976) before being utilized by the prostaglandin synthetase complex. Substrate delivery is, therefore, regulated both by the lipid composition of ER membranes and by phospholipase activity.

3.1.1. *Lipid Composition of Renal Endoplasmic Reticulum Membranes*

Precursor fatty acids are incorporated into cellular membranes from the plasma free fatty acid pool (Hohenleitner and Spitzer, 1961), and evidence has been presented that dietary factors can influence the fatty acid composition of phospholipids in cell membranes, including those of the kidney (Danon *et al.*, 1975*a*,*b*). In addition, the fractional turnover rate of individual fatty acids varies (Hagenfeldt and Warner, 1975) and may be an important factor influencing membrane lipid composition. The renal medulla is particulary rich in arachidonate (Müller *et al.*, 1976) and this contributes to its high prostaglandin biosynthetic capacity.

3.1.2. *Phospholipase Activity*

Incorporation of labeled arachidonate into medullary phospholipids occurs predominantly into the 2-position of phosphatidylcholine (Isakson *et al.*, 1976; Limas, C., and Limas, 1979). Therefore, a membrane phospholipase A_2 is responsible for releasing arachidonate. Studies in platelets indicate that phosphatidylcholine is located on the outer surface of the cell membrane (Schick *et al.*, 1975) whereas phosphatidylserine, phosphatidylethanolamine, and phosphatidylethanolamine plasmalogen are largely at the inner surface. Phospholipase may also be located at the outer cell surface in close proximity to its substrate; such localization would make the enzyme highly accessible to regulatory influences from the extracellular milieu. Two such influences have so far been recognized, i.e., calcium ion concentration and hormonal stimuli. Calcium enhances phospholipase activity and any stimulus resulting in increased calcium ion concentration in the vicinity of the phospholipase will increase prostaglandin synthesis. It has, in fact, recently been shown that PGE_2 release from endogenous phospholipids by renomedullary slices *in vitro* is strongly dependent on Ca^{2+} concentration in the incubation medium (Zenser and Davis, 1978). Ionophores, which facilitate movement of calcium across plasma membrane, also enhance phospholipase activity (Knapp *et al.*, 1977). Since increased concentration of Ca^{2+} has a direct inhibitory effect on the cyclooxygenase (Kunze *et al.*, 1974) there must be a specific calcium pool that is utilized for phospholipase activation. Some of the hormonal stimuli that have been shown to enhance phospholipase may also act through Ca^{2+}, the primary example being angiotensin (Danon *et al.*, 1975*a,b*; Baudouin *et al.*, 1972).

It should be noted that activation of lysosomal phospholipases could also participate in the regulation of prostaglandin synthesis. In this instance, however, the spatial organization of phospholipid classes within the cell membrane makes phosphatidylethanolamine and phosphatidylserine more accessible substrates for phospholipase. Consequently, the nature of the fatty acid released and the effects on prostaglandin synthesis may be quite different since some fatty acids are inhibitory. Such activation of lysosomal phospholipases may occur under ischemic conditions, e.g., in the later stages of hypertensive vascular damage.

3.2. Cyclooxygenase Activity

Cyclooxygenase activity may be modulated through the following mechanisms:

3.2.1. *Levels of Enzyme*

Cyclooxygenase has a short half-life and its levels depend on continuous protein synthesis. Interference at this level influences prostaglandin synthesis by determining the total number of enzyme molecules. This is exemplified by the observation that enhancement of prostaglandin synthesis after ureteral ligation requires RNA and protein synthesis (Morrison *et al.*, 1978).

3.2.2. *Availability of Oxygen*

Since the initial steps of prostaglandin synthesis involve addition of a singlet oxygen |O| by a dioxygenase mechanism (Hemler and Lands, 1977), oxygen availability may become a limiting factor. Renal medulla normally has a low partial oxygen pressure and any interference with the latter can profoundly affect prostaglandin synthesis. A positive correlation has been reported between P_{O_2} and changes in medullary cyclic AMP induced through endogenous prostaglandin synthesis (DeRubertis *et al.*, 1976) by renomedullary slices.

3.2.3. *Availability of Cofactors*

A number of compounds are required for optimal prostaglandin synthesis *in vitro* and many of these are normally present within the cell, e.g., reduced glutathione (GSH), hemoproteins, and aminoacids (Blackwell *et al.*, 1975; Tai *et al.*, 1976). Cyclooxygenase is a hemoprotein (Van derOuderaa *et al.*, 1979) and hematin is required for conversion of the apoenzyme to the holoenzyme. Routine addition of cofactors in assay mixtures makes comparisons of results from different laboratories difficult and inferences about the situation *in vivo* tenuous.

3.2.4. *Presence of Activators and Inhibitors*

It has recently been recognized that activators and inhibitors of prostaglandin synthesis are normally present within cells. For example, a heat-stable nondialyzable cytoplasmic factor from the kidney stimulates PGI_2 and, to a lesser extent, PGE_2 synthesis by medullary microsomes (Morita and Murota, 1979). Cook and Lands (1975) have postulated the existence of a peroxide activator that regulates cyclooxygenase activity and is, in turn, degraded by GSH peroxidase. The presence of inhibitors is especially relevant in the case of the renal cortex, which has been consistently shown to have a low apparent biosynthetic activity (Crowshaw, 1973; Larsson and Änggård, 1974). Indeed, we have found that incubation of cortical slices together with medullary slices significantly inhibits prostaglandin synthesis by the latter. We have pursued the question further and have shown the existence in renocortical cytosol of an inhibitor of prostaglandin synthesis that is heat-labile, nondialyzable, and trypsin-sensitive. The fact that it inhibits the synthetase from aorta, medulla, and seminal vesicles without signficantly affecting the type of prostaglandins synthesized suggests that it acts at an early step. The inhibitory substance is strongly dependent on the presence of GSH in the incubation mixture, and *N*-ethylmaleimide, which blocks the active mercaptan group of GSH, prevents or reverses the inhibition. These results indicate that the cytoplasmic cortical inhibitor is related to GSH peroxidase. Activation of this inhibitor could influence the amount of prostaglandins synthesized by the cortex.

3.3. Postsynthetic Modifications of Prostaglandins

The products of the cyclooxygenase reaction may be modified through the activities of enzymes that act distal to the formation of endoperoxides. PGE_2 isomerase (which shifts the reaction to PGE_2) and PGE 9-ketoreductase (which converts PGE_2 to $PGF_{2\alpha}$) are primary examples. The activities of these enzymes are dependent on cofactors, such as GSH for E_2 isomerase (Ogino *et al.*, 1977) and NADP for 9-ketoreductase (Lee and Levine, 1974), which therefore regulate the type of prostaglandins ultimately synthesized. The activities of prostaglandin-inactivating enzymes may influence the duration and site of action of the synthesized prostaglandins and thus amplify or minimize prostaglandin output. Evidence has been presented that, in genetic hypertension, decreased renal prostaglandin catabolism may be an early change (Armstrong *et al.*, 1976; Pace-Asciak, 1976; Limas, C. J., and Limas, 1977*a,b*).

4. PROSTAGLANDINS IN HYPERTENSION

Three approaches have been used in studying the implications of prostaglandins for the physiopathology of hypertension: (1) measurement of prostaglandin levels in fluids (blood, urine) and tissue of normal and hypertensive subjects, (2) comparison *in vitro* of rates of prostaglandin synthesis and degradation, and (3) administration of prostaglandin inhibitors and observation of their effects on the course of hypertension. A number of studies, in humans experimental animals, have been published and the results are listed in Table 1. It is obious that conclusions about the role of prostaglandins differ widely even in studies using the same hypertensive model. These discrepancies may be accounted for by a number of variables:

1.   The experimental model of hypertension
2.   Duration and severity of hypertension
3.   Animal species
4.   Anesthesia or prior manipulation of animals
5.   Tissue preparations studied
6.   Protocol for extracting and assaying prostaglandins
7.   Protocol for handling tissues and incubating subcellular fractions
8.   Purity of subcellular fractions

A critical evaluation of the literature requires familiarity with the limitations of the experimental design and methodology. Unless standardized methodology is used and extreme care is taken during handling of tissues, spurious or uninterpretable results will be obtained. Determination of peripheral blood or plasma concentrations of prostaglandins as an indicator of their involvement in hypertension is probably of little value because several cell types (unrelated to blood pressure control) contribute to this pool of prostaglandins and because the major effects of prostaglandins are exerted locally. Urinary prostaglandins are preferable in this regard since their origin is primarily intrarenal (Frölich *et al.*, 1975). However, the cell population involved in prostaglandin synthesis within the kidney is heterogeneous and measurement of urinary prostaglandins does not include the fraction secreted directly into the renal venous blood or excreted as metabolites (Granström and Kindahl, 1976; Samuelsson *et al.*, 1978).

The potential for error is even greater when tissue concentrations are used as an index of prostaglandin synthesis. Since these substances are not stored, there is no *a priori* reason for the validity of this approach. Moreover, tissue handling and homogenization activate endogenous phospholipases and result in release of variable but substantial amounts of prostaglandins, thus making interpretation of tissue levels erroneous (Samuelsson *et al.*, 1978).

The methodology for extraction and quantitation of prostaglandins is of obvious importance. Insensitive methods not amenable to reliable quantitation, such as the recently reported use of the immunofluorescence of cyclooxygenase (Stygles *et al.*, 1978), should be used only for assessing the topographical distribution of enzymes. Among the multitude of methods used, gas chromatography–mass spectrometry is probably the best for identification of prostaglandins (Samuelsson *et al.*, 1978); radioimmunoassay is also useful provided that the specificity and sensitivity are carefully validated. A combination of radioisotopic and chromatographic techniques using labeled precursors has the advantage of being suitable for dynamic studies of prostaglandin synthesis and degradation.

Release of prostaglandins from tissue slices *in vitro* has been used as an index of prostaglandin synthesis *in vivo*. In general, prostaglandin release from radiolabeled precursors in the incubation medium is preferable to extraction of unlabeled prostaglandins. In any case, one should compare "basal" release rates after the initial nonspecific burst of prostaglandin release has plateaued. An extended equilibration period prior to actual measurements may be needed for this purpose. Differences in the incubation protocol may, in part, explain the disparate results reported for the spontaneously hypertensive rats (SHR) in two separate studies by the same group of investigators (Stygles *et al.*, 1976, 1977).

Subcellular fractionation and characterization of individual steps in prostaglandin synthesis has the advantage that it lends itself to the study of regulatory mechanisms not otherwise possible. The usual precautions about subcellular studies apply here. Each fraction should be characterized for morphological and enzymatic purity and relative yields from different tissues or different animals models should be given. It should be kept in mind that the conditions for assays *in vitro* are selected by the investigator to give maximum activity and may not reflect the situation *in vivo*. Once the regulatory components (activators, inhibitors, substrate concentration) of the system have been identified it is important to measure their concentrations *in vivo*. Only then are comparisons between different experimental models meaningful.

5. RENOMEDULLARY INTERSTITIAL CELLS AND PROSTAGLANDINS

RIC are strategically located between the limbs of Henle, collecting ducts, and capillaries, with their cytoplasmic processes closely apposed to the basement membranes of these structures. They have been shown to

TABLE 1

Prostaglandins in Hypertension

Experimental model	References	Tissue	Method[a]	Result
SHR	Zusman et al. (1973)	Kidney, plasma	RIA	↑PGA
	Sirois and Gagnon (1974)	Medullary slices	Bioassay	↓PGE
	Dunn (1976)	Medullary microsomes	TLC	↑PGE$_2$
	Greenberg (1976)	Portal vein	Bioassay	↑PGE
	Stygles et al. (1976)	Medullary slices	RIA	↓PGE$_2$
	Stygles et al. (1977)	Medullary slices	RIA	No change
	C. J. Limas and Limas (1977a)	Medullary microsomes	TLC	↑PGE$_2$
	Ahnfeld-Ronne and Arrigoni-Martelli (1977)	Urine	RIA	↑PGF$_{2\alpha}$
	Rioux et al. (1977)	Aorta	Bioassay	↑PGE$_2$
	Stygles et al. (1978)	Medulla	Immunofluorescence	No change
	C. J. Limas and Limas (1977b)	Aorta, vein	TLC	↑PGE$_2$
	Quirion et al (1978)	Aorta	Bioassay	↑PGE$_2$
	Pace-Asciak et al. (1978)	Aorta	Bioassay	↑PGI$_2$
	C. J. Limas and Limas (1979)	Medullary slices	TLC	↑PGE$_2$
	Pace-Asciak (1976)	Kidney	RIA	↑PGE

Salt–DOCA	Tobian and Azar (1971)	Papilla slices	Bioassay	↑PGE_2
	Leary et al. (1974)	Medullary slices	Bioassay	↓PGE_2
	Stygles et al. (1976)	Medullary slices	RIA	↓PGE_2
Goldblatt	Nekrasova et al. (1970)	Medullary slices	Bioassay	↓PGE_2
	Sirois and Gagnon (1974)	Medullary slices	Bioassay	↓PGE_2
	Grodzinska et al. (1974)	Medullary slices	Bioassay	
	Pugsley et al. (1975)	Medullary slices	Gas chromatography–electron capture	↓PGE_2
	Smith and Somova (1976)	Renal vein	Column chromatography–mass spectrometry	↑PGE_2
Human	Abe et al. (1976)	Plasma, kidneys	RIA	↓PGE_2
	Papnicolaou et al. (1976)	Urine	Bioassay	↓PGE_2
	Hornych et al. (1975)	Plasma	Bioassay	↑PGA
	Hornych et al. (1976a,b)	Plasma	RIA	↑PGA
	Ripka (1976)	Plasma	RIA	↑PGF
	Tan et al. (1978)	Urine	RIA	↓PGE_2
	Tandon et al. (1978)	Plasma	RIA	↑PGE_2

[a] RIA, radioimmunoassay; TLC, thin-layer chromatography.

generate prostaglandins in tissue culture (Muirhead *et al.*, 1972; Zusman and Keiser, 1977). Their morphological hallmark is the presence within their cytoplasm of lipid-laden droplets or granules. These lipid granules have not been conclusively shown to contain prostaglandins. A correlation between granularity of RIC and renomedullary prostaglandin synthesis was initially suggested on the assumption that the granules represent storage sites for arachidonate. This assumption is probably erroneous since the granules contain very little arachidonate, most of which is esterified in triglycerides (Änggård *et al.*, 1972). Furthermore, arachidonate incorporated into membrane phospholipids is a more likely substrate for the cyclooxygenase.

Conflicting data had appeared in the literature concerning the granularity of RIC in hypertensive states. Decreased granularity was thought to reflect either accelerated release or exhaustion of antihypertensive material. We decided, therefore, to reinvestigate the problem by observing the effects of indomethacin (Limas, C., *et al.*, 1976a). Short-term administration of indomethacin in doses that were shown to inhibit medullary prostaglandin synthesis affected morphological appearance and granularity of RIC as well as [^{14}C]arachidonate incorporation into medullary phospholipids. In contrast to previous suggestions, we found that indomethacin significantly depressed the granularity of RIC. Ultrastructural studies revealed other concomitant changes such as ballooning of the cisternae of the rough ER. These changes may be important in view of biochemical evidence suggesting that the ER is the major site of prostaglandin synthesis (Bohman and Larsson, 1975).

Although [^{14}C]arachidonate was incorporated into microsomal lipids of both cortex and medulla, only the latter had decreased radioactivity after indomethacin. Furthermore, there was good correlation between microsomal [^{14}C]arachidonate incorporation and RIC granularity in the treated animals. These results indicated a positive correlation between granularity and prostaglandin synthesis although the nature of the relationship was not clear. We suggested that the granules might contain by-products of the phospholipase activity (e.g., nonutilized fatty acids), which would slow down the synthetase reaction unless sequestered and removed. Direct evidence for or against this suggestion is still lacking.

RIC were then studied in the SHR (Limas, C., *et al.*, 1976b). Compared to that of normotensive Wistar–Kyoto rats (WKY) or SHR whose blood pressure was brought to normal levels with antihypertensive drugs, the granularity of the RIC of untreated SHR was significantly increased. Granule counts increased in the presence of mild to moderate degrees of arteriolar sclerosis but decreased in long-standing hypertension with severe, extensive vascular lesions and secondary ischemic damage of the renal parenchyma. We interpreted these results as showing an adaptive response of the renal medulla to hypertension in the form of enhanced production of antihypertensive substances. Clearly, no evidence was found to support the contention that prostaglandin deficiency is involved in the initiation of genetic hypertension in SHR. Moreover, this adaptive response is not sufficient to prevent the development of vascular damage. In long-standing hypertension with severely affected vessels, ischemic changes supervene and granularity of RIC declines, perhaps reflecting diminished capacity for prostaglandin synthesis.

6. RENAL PROSTAGLANDIN METABOLISM IN THE SPONTANEOUSLY HYPERTENSIVE RAT

A more direct approach to the question of renal prostaglandin metabolism is the comparison of activities of enzymes concerned with the synthesis and degradation of these substances. We therefore compared the ability of isolated microsomes from the renal medulla of SHR and WKY to synthesize prostaglandins *in vitro* (Limas, C. J., and Limas, 1977a). In the age groups studied (6–22 weeks), SHR had enhanced synthetic capacity (Fig. 3), which increased with age (Fig. 4); these results were similar to those reported by Dunn (1976) in a comparable assay system. The *in vitro* activities of 15-hydroxy-prostaglandin dehydrogenase, both NAD^+- and $NADP^+$-dependent forms, were lower in the SHR (Fig. 5), so that the net effect would be increased prostaglandin output from the kidney. Depression of the activities of degrading enzymes has also been reported in the genetically hypertensive rat of the New Zealand strain (Armstrong *et al.*, 1976).

Since the initial (and, possibly, rate-limiting) step in prostaglandin

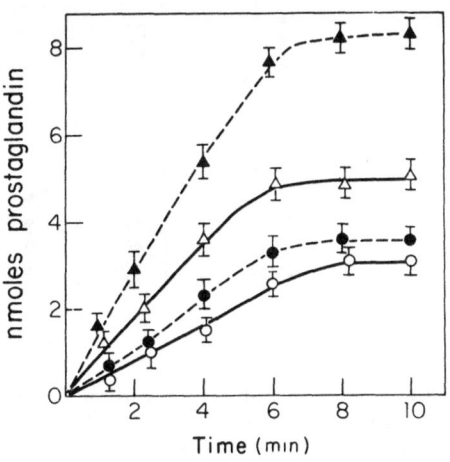

FIGURE 3.   Time course of prostaglandin synthesis by medullary microsomes of 20-week-old SHR (▲,●) and WKY (△,○). results are given as nmoles PGE_2 (▲,△) or $PGF_{2\alpha}$ (●,○) per mg protein. Each value represents mean ± SE from six experiments. [Reproduced from C. Limas *et al.* (1976b) by permission from the American Physiological Society.]

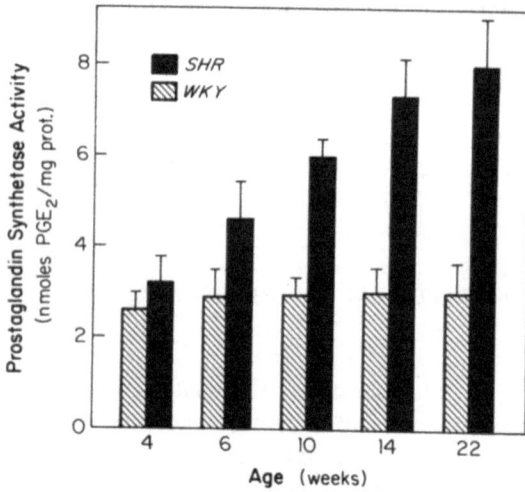

FIGURE 4. Age dependence of medullary microsomal prostaglandin synthesis by SHR and WKY. [Reproduced from C. Limas *et al*. (1976*b*) by permission from the American Physiological Society.]

biosynthesis is activation of phospholipase A_2, which releases precursor fatty acids from membrane phospholipids, the activity of this enzyme was also compared in hypertensive and normotensive animals (Limas, C., and Limas, 1979). In addition, the effects of vasoactive substances such as bradykinin and angiotensin on the release of [^{14}C]arachidonate from renomedullary phospholipids was studied. The rate of prostaglandin synthesis from phosphatidylcholine and prostaglandin release by renomedullary slices of SHR was higher than that in age-matched WKY. These differences were accentuated when [^{14}C]arachidonate-labeled tissues were challenged with

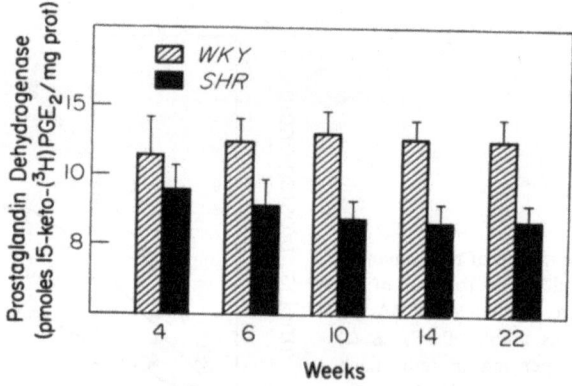

FIGURE 5. Effect of age on cortical NAD^+-dependent 15-hydroxyprostaglandin dehydrogenase from SHR and WKY. [Reproduced from C. Limas *et al*. (1976*b*) by permission from the American Physiological Society.]

TABLE 2

Comparison of the Effects of Bradykinin and Angiotensin II on Release of
Arachidonate and Prostaglandins from Renomedullary Slices of
20-Week-Old WKY and SHR[a]

Additions	^{14}C radioactivity released (cpm)[b]		
	Arachidonate	PGE_2	$PGF_{2\alpha}$
None			
WKY	1349 ± 122	103 ± 26	44 ± 11
SHR	1951 ± 167	$132 \pm 22*$	58 ± 18
Bradykinin			
WKY	62997 ± 488	8769 ± 207	876 ± 72
SHR	87752 ± 674^c	$11385 \pm 411*$	$989 \pm 84*$
Angiotensin II			
WKY	84235 ± 517	10011 ± 378	1155 ± 103
SHR	$109377 \pm 622*$	$14643 \pm 488*$	$1392 \pm 101*$

[a] From C. Limas and Limas (1979).
[b] Results represent means $\pm$ SE for six experiments.
[c] Increased release of labeled arachidonate in response to bradykinin and angiotensin II
is a result of phospholipase A_2 stimulation. There is a small difference in baseline
(unstimulated) phospholipase activity between SHR and WKY, which is magnified in
the presence of bradykinin and angiotensin II.
* $p < 0.01$ compared to WKY.

bradykinin or angiotensin II (Table 2), suggesting that phospholipase A_2
activity in hypertensive animals is more responsive to certain stimuli.

7. CONCLUSIONS AND FUTURE DIRECTIONS

The vascular wall and the kidney represent sites of both synthesis and
action of prostaglandins. Under the usual experimental conditions, PGE_2 is
the major prostaglandin synthesized by the renal medulla. In most animal
species, PGE_2 acts as a vasodepressor, diuretic, and natriuretic substance
and, on this basis, renomedullary synthesis is expected to have an antihypertensive effect.

The amounts, types, and actions *in vivo* of synthesized prostaglandins
can be regulated by factors such as availability of substrate, cofactors,
inhibitors, oxygen tension, and activities of specific enzymes. The com-
plexity of the system makes interpretation of experimental results difficult
and open to error. Studies *in vitro* can focus on a limited number of variables at a time and are usually designed to demonstrate optimal activities,
which may not reflect conditions *in vivo*. Studies *in vivo*, on the other hand,
are subject to a great variety of influences that cannot be easily controlled,
and the results are often not reproducible.

To date there is no convincing evidence that a primary deficiency of prostaglandins is causally related to the development of hypertension. On the contrary, the early phase of blood pressure elevation in the SHR is associated with increased synthesis of prostaglandins, which may represent an adaptive process. This process may attenuate the rate of blood pressure increase until other more permanent protective changes occur in the vessels. Our understanding of the role of prostaglandins in hypertension could be improved by a multidisciplinary approach. For example, correlation of enzymatic activities with morphologic changes in the tissues under study will help distinguish primary changes from those secondary to hypertensive vascular damage. Sequential studies of prostaglandin synthesis in various stages of hypertension will also test the hypothesis that modifications of prostaglandin metabolism represent a biologically important adaptive phenomenon.

REFERENCES

Abe, K., Saito, T., Otsuka, Y., Seino, M., and Yasujima, M., 1976, An evaluation of plasma and renal prostaglandins in hypertension, in: *Advances in Prostaglandin and Thromboxane Research*, Vol. 2 (B. Samuelsson and R. Paoletti, eds.), Raven Press, New York, p. 599.

Ahnfeld-Ronne, I., and Arrigoni-Martelli, E., 1977, Renal prostaglandin metabolism in spontaneously hypertensive rats, *Biochem. Pharmacol.* **26**:485.

Altura, B. M., and Altura, B. T., 1976, Vascular smooth muscle and prostaglandins, *Fed. Proc. Fed. Am. Soc. Exp. Biol.* **35**:2360.

Änggård, E., Bohman, S.-O., Griffin, J. E., III, Larsson, C., and Maunsbach, A. B., 1972, Subcellular localization of the prostaglandin system in the rabbit renal papilla, *Acta Physiol. Scand.* **85**:237.

Armstrong, J. M., Blackwell, G. J., Flower, R. J., McGiff, J. C., Mullane, K. M., and Vane, J. R., 1976, Genetic hypertension in rats is accompanied by a defect in renal prostaglandin metabolism, *Nature* **260**:582.

Baudouin, M., Meyer, P., Fermandjian, S., and Morgat, J. L., 1972, Calcium release induced by interaction of angiotensin with its receptors in smooth muscle cell microsomes, *Nature* **235**:336.

Berl, P., Raz, A., Wald, H., Horowits, J., and Czaczkes, W., 1977, Prostaglandin synthesis inhibition and the action of vasopressin: Studies in man and rat, *Am. J. Physiol.* **232**:F529.

Blackwell, G. J., Flower, R. J., and Vane, J. R., 1975, Some characteristics of the prostaglandin synthesizing system in rabbit kidney microsomes, *Biochim. Biophys. Acta* **398**:178.

Bohman, S.-O., 1977, Demonstration of prostaglandin synthesis in collecting duct cells and other cell types of the rabbit renal medulla, *Prostaglandins* **14**:729.

Bohman, S.-O., and Larsson, C., 1975, Prostaglandin synthesis in membrane fractions from rabbit renal medulla, *Acta Physiol. Scand.* **94**:244.

Cook, H. W., and Lands, W. E. M., 1975, Evidence for an activating factor formed during prostaglandin biosynthesis, *Biochem. Biophys. Res. Commun.* **65**:464.

Crowshaw, K., 1973, The incorporation of [1-^{14}C]arachidonic acid into the lipids of rabbit renal slices and conversion to prostaglandins E_2 and $F_{2\alpha}$, *Prostaglandins* **3**:607.

Danon, A., Chang, L. C., Sweetman, S. J., Nies, A. S., and Oates, J. A., 1975a, Synthesis of prostaglandins by the rat renal papilla *in vitro;* mechanism of stimulation by angiotensin II, *Biochim. Biophys. Acta* **388**:71.

Danon, A., Heimberg, M., and Oates, J. A., 1975b, Enrichment of rat tissue lipids with fatty acids that are prostaglandin precursors, *Biochim. Biophys. Acta* **388**:318.

Davis, H. A., and Horton, E. W., 1972, Output of prostaglandins from the rabbit kidney, its increase on renal nerve stimulation and its inhibition by indomethacin, *Br. J. Pharmacol.* **46**:658.

DeRubertis, F. R., Zenser, T. V., Craven, P. A., and Davis, B. B., 1976, Modulation of the cyclic AMP content of rat renal inner medulla by oxygen: Possible role of local prostaglandins, *J. Clin. Invest.* **58**:1370.

Donker, A. J., Ausz, L., Brentjens, J. R., Van DerHem, G. K., and Hollemans, H. J., 1976, The effect of indomethacin on kidney function and plasma renin activity in man, *Nephron* **17**:288.

Dunn, M. J., 1976, Renal prostaglandin synthesis in the spontaneously hypertensive rat, *J. Clin. Invest.* **58**:862.

Feigen, L. P., Klainer, E., Chapnick, B. M., and Kadowitz, P. J., 1976, The effect of indomethacin on renal function in pentobarbital-anesthetized dogs, *J. Pharmacol. Exp. Ther.* **198**:457.

Ferreira, S. H., and Vane, J. R., 1967, Prostaglandins: Their disappearance from and release into the circulation, *Nature* **216**:868.

Flower, R. J., and Blackwell, G. J., 1976, Importance of phospholipase A_2 in prostaglandin biosynthesis, *Biochem. Pharmacol.* **25**:285.

Fourman, J., and Moffat, D. B., 1971, *Blood Vessels of the Kidney*, Oxford, Blackwell Scientific Publications, p. 58.

Frölich, J. C., Wilson, T. W., Sweetman, B. J., Smigel, M., Nies, A. S., Carr, K., Watson, J. T., and Oates, J. A., 1975, Urinary prostaglandins: Identification and origin, *J. Clin. Invest.* **55**:763.

Fulgraff, G., and Brandenbusch, G., 1974, Comparison of the effects of the prostaglandins A_1, E_2, and F_{2a} on kidney function in dogs, *Pfluegers Arch.* **349**:9.

Gerber, J. G., Ellis, E. F., and Nies, A. S., 1977, The effect of endoperoxide analogues on renal function and hemodynamics, *Fed. Proc. Fed. Am. Soc. Exp. Biol.* **36**:402.

Granström, G., and Kindahl, H., 1976, Radioimmunoassay for urinary metabolites of prostaglandin $F_{2\alpha}$, *Prostaglandins* **12**:759.

Grantham, J. J., and Orloff, J., 1968, Effect of prostaglandin E_1 on the permeability response of the isolated collecting tubule to vasopressin, adenosine 3',5'-monophosphate, and theophylline, *J. Clin. Invest.* **47**:1154.

Greenberg, S., 1976, Evidence for enhanced venous smooth muscle turnover of prostaglandin-like substance in portal veins from spontaneously hypertensive rats, *Prostaglandins* **11**:163.

Grodzinska, L., Schor, K., Wartner, V., Forster, W., and Gryglewski, R., 1974, Prostaglandin synthesis activity in the renal medulla of normal and hypertensive rats, *Pol. J. Pharmacol. Pharm.* **26**:229.

Hagenfeldt, L., and Warner, J., 1975, Turnover of plasma free arachidonic and oleic acids in resting and exercising human subjects, *Metabolism* **24**:799.

Hemler, M. E., and Lands, N. E. M., 1977, Biosynthesis of prostaglandins, *Lipids* **13**:591.

Hohenleitner, F. J. and Spitzer, J. J., 1961, Changes in plasma free fatty acid concentrations on passage through the dog kidney, *Am. J. Physiol.* **200**:1095.

Hornych, A., Bedrossian, J., Bariety, J., Menard, J., Corvol, P., Safar, M., Fontaliran, F., and

Fillier, P., 1975, Prostaglandins and hypertension in chronic renal diseases, *Clin. Nephrol.* **4**:144.

Hornych, A., Safar, M., Weiss, Y., Menard, J., Corvol, P., Bariety, J., and Millez, P., 1976a, Prostaglandins and essential hypertension, *Eur. J. Clin. Invest.* **6**:314.

Hornych, A., Weiss, Y., Safar, M., Menard, J., Corvol, P., Fontaliran, E., Bariety, J., and Milliez, P., 1976b, Prostaglandins A and B in the peripheral blood of hypertensive patients, *Prostaglandins* **12**:383.

Isakson, P. C., Raz, A., and Needleman, P., 1976, Selective incorporation of ^{14}C-prostaglandins, *Prostaglandins* **12**:739.

Itskovitz, H. D., Terragno, N. A., and McGiff, J. C., 1974, Effect of a renal prostaglandin on distribution of blood flow in the isolated kidney, *Circ. Res.* **34**:770.

Katzen, D. R., Pong, S. S., and Levine, L., 1975, Distribution of prostaglandin E 9-ketoreductase and NAD-dependent and NADP-dependent 15-hydroxyprostaglandin dehydrogenase in the renal cortex and medulla of various species, *Res. Commun. Chem. Pathol. Pharmacol.* **12**:781.

Kauker, M. L., 1977, Prostaglandin E_2 effect from the luminal side on renal tubular ^{22}Na efflux: Tracer microinjection studies, *Proc. Soc. Exp. Biol. Med.* **154**:272.

Knapp, H. R., Oelz, O., Roberts, L. J., Sweetman, B. J., Oates, J. A., and Reed, P. W., 1977, Ionophores stimulate prostaglandin and thromboxane biosynthesis, *Proc. Natl. Acad. Sci. USA* **74**:4251.

Kunze, H., Bohn, E., and Vogt, W., 1974, Effects of local anesthetics on prostaglandin biosynthesis *in vitro*, *Biochim. Biophys. Acta* **360**:260.

Lands, W. E. M., and Samuelsson B., 1968, Phospholipid precursors of prostaglandins, *Biochim. Biophys. Acta* **164**:426.

Larsson, C., and Anggard, E., 1974, Regional differences in the formation and metabolism of prostaglandins in the rabbit kidney, *Eur. J. Pharmacol.* **21**:30.

Leary, W. P., Ledingham, J. G., and Vane, J. R., 1974, Impaired prostaglandin release from the kidneys of salt-loaded and hypertensive rats, *Prostaglandins* **7**:425.

Lee, S. C., and Levine, L., 1974, Prostaglandin metabolism I. Cytoplasmic reduced nicotinamide adenine dinucleotide phosphate-dependent and microsomal reduced nicotinamide adenine dinucleotide-dependent prostaglandin E 9-ketoreductase activities in monkey and pigeon tissues, *J. Biol. Chem.* **249**:1369.

Limas, C., and Limas, C. J., 1979, Enhanced renomedullary prostaglandin synthesis in SHRs: Possible role of a membrane phospholipase, *Am. J. Physiol.* **236**:H65.

Limas, C., Limas, C. J., and Gesell, M, 1976a, Effects of indomethacin on renomedullary interstitial cells, *Lab. Invest.* **34**:522.

Limas, C., Limas, C. J., Ragan, D., and Freis, E. D., 1976b, Renomedullary interstitial cells in the spontaneously hypertensive rat, *Lab. Invest.* **34**:606.

Limas, C. J., and Limas, C., 1977a, Prostaglandin metabolism in the kidneys of spontaneously hypertensive rats, *Am. J. Physiol.* **233**:H87.

Limas, C. J., and Limas, C., 1977b, Vascular prostaglandin synthesis in the spontaneously hypertensive rat, *Am. J. Physiol.* **233**:H493.

Lum, G. M., Aisenbrey, G. A., Dunn, M. J., Berl, T., Schrier, R. W., and McDonald, K. M., 1977, *In vivo* effect of indomethacin to potentiate the renal medullary cyclic AMP response to vasopressin, *J. Clin. Invest.* **59**:8.

McGiff, J. C., 1978, Prostaglandins and the kidney, *Contrib. Nephrol.* **13**:461.

Maclouf, J., Sors, H., and Rigaud, M., 1977, Recent aspects of prostaglandin biosynthesis. A review, *Biomedicine* **26**:362.

Messing, E. J., Weiner, R., and Kaley, G., 1976, Prostaglandins and local circulatory control, *Fed. Proc. Fed. Am. Soc. Exp. Biol.* **35**:2367.

Morita, I., and Murota, S. I., 1979, Tissue specific regulation of prostaglandin production.

Stimulation of 6-ketoprostaglandin $F_{1\alpha}$ biosynthesis by rat kidney cytosol, *Biochim. Biophys. Acta* **582**:173.

Morrison, A. R., Moritz, H., and Needleman, P., 1978, Mechanisms of enhanced renal prostaglandin biosynthesis in uteteral obstruction. Role of *de novo* protein synthesis, *J. Biol. Chem.* **253**:8210.

Muirhead, E. E., Germain, G., Leach, B. E., Pitcock, J. A., Stephenson, P., Brooks, B., Brosius, W. L., Daniels, E. G., and Ninman, J. W., 1972, Production of renomedullary prostaglandins by interstitial cells grown in tissue culture, *Circ. Res.* **31**(Suppl. 2):161.

Müller, M. M., Kaiser, E., Bauer, P., Scheiber, V., and Hohenegger, M., 1976, Lipid composition of the rat kidney, *Nephron* **17**:41.

Needleman, P., Kauffman, A. H., Douglas, J. R., Jr, Johnson, E. M., Jr, and Marshall, G. R., 1973, Specific stimulation and inhibition of renal prostaglandin release by angiotensin analysis, *Am. J. Physiol.* **224**:1415.

Nekrasova, A. A., and Lantsberg, L. A., 1969, Role of renal prostaglandins in the pathogenesis of hypertension, *Kardiologiya* **9**:86.

Nekrasova, A. A., Paleseva, F. M., and Khundadze, S. S., 1970, Content of depressor prostaglandin-like substances and renin activity in the kidneys of patients with renovascular hypertension, *Kardiologiya* **10**:88.

Ogino, N., Miyamoto, T., Yamamoto, S., Hayaishi, O., 1977, Prostaglandin endoperoxide E isomerase from bovine vesicular gland microsomes, a glutathione-requiring enzyme, *J. Biol. Chem.* **252**:890.

Pace-Asciak, C., 1975*a*, Prostaglandin 9-hydroxydehydrogenase activity in the adult rat kidney, *J. Biol. Chem.* **250**:2789.

Pace-Asciak, C., 1975*b*, Activity profiles of prostaglandin 15- and 9-hydroxydehydrogenase and 13-reductase in the developing rat kidney, *J. Biol. Chem.* **250**:2795.

Pace-Asciak, C., 1976, Decreased renal prostaglandin catabolism precedes onset of hypertension in the developing spontaneously hypertensive rat, *Nature* **263**:510.

Pace-Asciak, C. R., Carrara, M. C., Rangaraj, G., and Nicolaou, K. C., 1978, Enhanced formation of PGI_2, a potent hypotensive substance, by aortic rings and homogenates of the spontaneously hypertensive rat, *Prostaglandins* **15**:1005.

Papanicolaou, N., Mountokalakis, T., Safar, M., Bariety, J., and Milliez, P., 1976, Deficiency of renomedullary prostaglandin synthesis related to the evolution of essential hypertension, *Experientia* **32**:1015.

Pong, S. S., and Levine, L., 1976, Biosynthesis of prostaglandins in rabbit renal cortex, *Res. Commun. Chem. Pathol. Pharmacol.* **13**:115.

Pugsley, D. J., Beilin, L. F., and Reto, R., 1975, Renal prostaglandin synthesis in the Goldblatt hypertensive rat, *Circ. Res.* **36–37**(Suppl. 1):81.

Quirion, R., Rioux, F., and Regoli, D., 1978, Effects of arachidonic acid and indomethacin on the *in vitro* release of prostaglandins by aortic, strips of spontaneously hypertensive rats, *Can. J. Physiol. Pharmacol.* **56**:509.

Rioux, F., Quiron, R., and Regoli, D., 1977, The role of prostaglandins in hypertension: I. The release of prostaglandins by aorta strips of renal, DOCA–salt, and spontaneously hypertensive rats, *Can. J. Physiol. Pharmacol.* **55**:1330.

Ripka, O., Kucerova, K., Linhartova, J., Ort, J., and Peleska, J., 1976, Radioimmunoassay of renal venous prostaglandins in essential hypertension, *Acta. Biol. Med. Ger.* **35**:1221.

Samuelsson, B., Granström, E., Green, K., Hamberg, M., and Hammaratröm, S., 1978, Prostaglandins, *Annu. Rev. Biochem.* **44**:669.

Schick, P. K., Kuricka, K., and Chacko, G. K., 1975, Structural organization of platelet membrane phospholipids, *Fed. Proc. Fed. Am. Soc. Exp. Biol.* **34**:126.

Sirois, P., and Gagnon, D. J., 1974, Release of renomedullary prostaglandins in normal and hypertensive rats, *Experientia* **30**:1418.

Smith, G. W., and Somova, L. I., 1976, Renal function and renal venous prostaglandin concentrations during different stages of experimental renal hypertension in the rat, *Br. J. Pharmacol.* **58**:253.

Stokes, J. B. and Kokko, J. P., 1977, Inhibition of sodium transport by prostaglandin E_2 across the isolated, perfused rabbit collecting tubule, *J. Clin. Invest.* **59**:1099.

Stygles, V. G., Reinke, D. A., and Hook, J. B., 1976, Prostaglandin E_2 production by renomedullary tissue of DOCA, Goldblatt, and spontaneously hypertensive rats, *Res. Commun. Chem. Pathol. Pharmacol.* **15**:753.

Stygles, V. G., Reinke, D. A., Rickert, D. E., and Hook, J. B., 1977, Increased blood pressure in the SHR is not related to a deficit in renomedullary PGE_2, *Experientia* **34**:1025.

Stygles, V. G., Smith, W. L., Reinke, D. A, and Hook, J. B., 1978, Prostaglandin-forming cyclooxygenase in renal medulla of spontaneously hypertensive rats during development, *Biol. Neonate* **33**:709.

Swain, J. A., Heyndricks, G. R., Boettcher, D. H., and Vatner, S. F., 1975, Prostaglandin control of renal circulation in the unanesthetized dog and baboon, *Am. J. Physiol.* **229**:826.

Tai, H. H., Tai, C. W., and Hollander, C. S., 1976, Biosynthesis of prostaglandins in rabbit kidney medulla, *Biochem. J.* **154**:257.

Tan, S. Y., Sweet, P., and Mulrow, P. J., 1978, Impaired renal production of PGE_2: A newly identified lesion in human essential hypertension, *Prostaglandins* **15**:139.

Tandon, A. K., Singh, R. H., and Udupa, K. N., 1978, Plasma prostaglandins in essential hypertension and ischemic heart disease, *Indian J. Med. Res.* **67**:490.

Terragno, D. A., Crowshaw, K., Terragno, N. A., and McGiff, J. C., 1975, Prostaglandin synthesis by bovine mesenteric arteries and veins, *Circ. Res.* **36**–**37**(Suppl. 1):76.

Tobian, L., and Azar, S., 1971, Antihypertensive and other function of the renal papilla, *Trans. Assoc. Am. Phys.* **84**:281.

Van derOuderaa, F. J., Buytenhek, M., Slikkerveer, F. J., and Van Dorp, D. A., 1979, On the haemoprotein character of prostaglandin endoperoxide synthetase, *Biochim. Biophys. Acta* **572**:29.

Vonkeman, H., and Van Dorp, D. A., 1968, The action of prostaglandin synthetase on 2-arachidonyl lecithin, *Biochim. Biophys. Acta* **164**:430.

Whorton, A. R., Smigel, M., Oates, J. A., and Frölich, J. C., 1978, Regional differences in prostacyclin formation by the kidney. Prostacyclin is a major prostaglandin of renal cortex, *Biochim Biophys. Acta* **529**:176.

Zenser, T. V., and Davis, B. B., 1978, Effects of calcium on prostaglandin E_2 synthesis by rat inner medullary slices, *Am. J. Physiol.* **235**:F213.

Zusman, R. M. and Keiser, H. R., 1977, Prostaglandin biosynthesis by rabbit renomedullary interstitial cells in tissue culture, *J. Clin. Invest.* **60**:215.

Zusman, R. M., Forman, B. H., Schneider, G., Caldwell, B. R., Speroff, L., and Mulrow, P. J., 1973, The effect of chronic sodium loading and sodium restriction on plasma and renal concentrations of prostaglandin A in normal Wistar and spontaneously hypertensive Aoki rats, *Clin. Sci.* **45**:325s.

CHAPTER 6

Fatty Acid Composition and Depot Function of Lipid Droplet Triacylglycerols in Renomedullary Interstitial Cells

INGE NORBY BOJESEN

1. INTRODUCTION

Although the renin–angiotensin system is known to play an important role in renal hypertension, data have accumulated suggesting that a renal factor besides this system and besides sodium balance is responsible for blood pressure regulation. The question of whether this factor is a vasopressor or a vasdepressor substance has been much discussed. Several lines of evidence have been presented to support the theory that it has a hypotensive action. The theory that hypertension could result from a deficiency of such a vasodepressor substance has recently been supported by studies of Dietz *et al.* (1978) on the reversibility of experimental renal hypertension.

Several types of lipids have been proposed as renal antihypertensive factors since it was possible to extract different lipid fractions with a vasodepressor effect from the kidney, in particular from the renal papilla. The interest in these studies increased with the rediscovery, in the interstitium of the renal papilla, of a cell type characterized by a high content of intracellular lipid droplets, a well-developed Golgi complex, and much rough endoplasmic reticulum. An important physiological role for these interstitial cells was considered highly probable in view of the findings that their lipid droplet content varied considerably with the physiological state of the kidney.

INGE NORBY BOJESEN • Institute of Experimental Hormone Research, University of Copenhagen, DK-2100 Copenhagen Ø, Denmark.

However, the question still remains of whether any of the antihypertensive lipids previously isolated from the renal papilla (Muirhead *et al.*, 1971; Sen *et al.*, 1967; Lee *et al.*, 1965) is important in the prevention of hypertension. This situation prompted us to study renal papillary lipogenesis, not only from the point of view of hypertension but also to provide basic information about the lipid metabolism of the renal papilla.

This chapter describes the isolation and characterization of the lipid droplets of the renomedullary interstitial cells from four different species. In addition, some recent biochemical studies are reported, which provide new information about lipid synthesis and metabolism in the rat renal papilla. On the basis of these studies a theory is put forward about the local significance of the lipogenesis of the renal papillary interstitial cells. On the other hand, the results do not support the contention that the papilla produces a lipid of systemic significance.

2. ISOLATION AND CHARACTERIZATION OF PAPILLARY LIPID DROPLETS

Primary fluorescing particles in the cytoplasm of rat renal papillary cells were observed by Nissen and Bojesen (1969). In contrast to other papillary cells the interstitial cells are very rich in primary fluorescing particles, and these correspond in distribution and localization to the lipid droplets in these cells as revealed by phase-contrast fluorescence microscopy. Homogenization of the tissue followed by ultracentrifugation permitted the isolation of a floating layer containing spherical primary fluorescing particles. Other cellular particles in the renal papilla show some primary fluorescence, but of an intensity dissimilar to that of the lipid droplets. Furthermore, the density of these cellular components in a centrifugation system is much higher than that of the lipid droplets. Therefore, the isolated floating layer was considered to consist of interstitial cell lipid droplets.

2.1. Qualitative Studies

2.1.1. *Lipid Classes in the Interstitial Cell Lipid Droplets*

Chemical analyses of isolated lipid droplets from rats (Nissen and Bojesen, 1969) confirmed the results obtained by histochemical methods (Nissen, 1967), which suggested that the droplets contain simple saturated and unsaturated lipids. Further studies were carried out by Bojesen (1974*a*) on lipid droplets isolated from dog, pig, rabbit, and rat papillary homogenates. In all four species, the isolated lipid droplet layer was composed of 80–98% triacylglycerols, a few percent phospholipids and free fatty acids, and only trace amounts of cholesteryl esters. Similar results have been obtained by other investigators using analogous isolation procedures for rabbit papillary lipid droplets. Änggård et al. (1972) found 84% of the lipid droplet fraction in the form of nonpolar lipids and Comai et al. (1975) found 72% triacylglycerols.

Less than 5% (0.8–4.8%) free fatty acids was found by Bojesen in all species (Bojesen, 1974a). The percentage is not given by Änggård et al., whereas Comai et al. found as much as 25% in the lipid droplet fraction from rabbit. The divergent results probably reflect differences in the amount of fatty acids liberated during homogenization. The actual content of free fatty acids in the floating layer is necessarily determined by phase distribution of fatty acids in the homogenate.

With regard to the amount of phospholipids in the droplets, it should be noted that the lipid droplet preparations are not completely pure. Contamination by small amounts of membrane fragments was often seen under the microscope (Bojesen, 1974a; Bohman and Maunsbach, 1972); the fragments probably come mainly from the endoplasmic reticulum. Therefore, a considerable variation in the amount of phospholipids in the isolated fraction is not unexpected, and the phospholipid contents found must be regarded as maximum values.

Rat papillae are much less resistant to homogenization than are papillae from the other species and they therefore allow the isolation of a cleaner droplet preparation. However, even in these preparations up to 5% phospholipids was found (Bojesen, 1974a).

In lipid droplet preparations from rabbit papillae Änggård et al. (1972) found 17% polar lipids (phospholipids, sphingolipids, and ceramides), compared to the 2.6–14% found by Bojesen (1974a) and the 1.1% reported by Comai et al. (1975).

Fractionation of phospholipids by thin-layer chromatography revealed that phosphatidyl cholines were the principal phospholipids. The amount of phosphatidyl ethanolamines was usually very small and no other phospholipids could be detected (Bojesen, 1974a).

2.1.2. Protein Determinations

As is the case with phospholipids, the proteins in the floating droplet layer may be constituents of the droplets themselves or of adherent membrane contaminations. Therefore, the measured protein content does not necessarily indicate surface proteins of lipid droplets. The amount of protein found by Comai et al. (1975) in lipid droplets isolated from rabbit papillae corresponds to a lipid/protein ratio of about 8:1 by weight, which is compatible with flotation in water.

Although the available data on the protein and phospholipid composition of the droplets are somewhat ambiguous, they suggest a resemblance of these droplets to chylomicrons in serum (Zilversmit, 1969). Accordingly, it might be assumed that the lipid droplets are not surrounded by a complete membrane. Electron microscopic studies support this view (Bohman, 1974; Bulger and Trump, 1966; Osvaldo-Decima, 1973). These studies showed that the droplets are not surrounded by a triple-layered or complete membrane, but by a thin electron-dense zone, which is similar in ultrastructure to the zone surrounding chylomicrons.

2.1.3. *Fatty Acid Composition of Droplet Triacylglycerols**

The fatty acid composition of droplet triacylglycerols was not the same in the various species, but in all animal groups it differed distinctly from that of triacylglycerols from other tissues and from plasma of the same species (Fig. 1) (Bojesen, 1974a). This observation was confirmed by Comai *et al.* (1975) in the rabbit papilla. The most conspicuous feature of the lipid droplet triacylglycerols in rats, rabbits, and dogs is the rather high percentage of polyunsaturated fatty acids, especially the prostaglandin precursor arachidonic acid. Also remarkable is the large proportion of adrenic acid in papillary triacylglycerols from these animals. Only small amounts of this acid have previously been found in triacylglycerols from other tissues, namely in testes (Oshima and Carpenter, 1968) and in ovaries (Carney and Walker, 1972). However, this fatty acid is characteristic of cholesteryl esters in adrenal lipid droplets from rat (Gidez and Feller, 1969), rabbit (Comai *et al.*, 1975), human (Takayasu *et al.*, 1970), and dog (Lo Chang and Sweeley, 1963).

Lipid droplets isolated from rat hepatocytes (Diaugustine *et al.*, 1973), like the droplets from renal papillae, consisted mainly of triacylglycerols, but the long-chain fatty acid composition was markedly different. Only linoleic acid, oleic acid, and palmitic acid were found.

2.2. Quantitative Studies

Several authors have found alterations in the number of lipid droplets of rat renomedullary interstitial cells, especially in connection with hypertension and prolonged water diuresis. More acute alterations in

---

* The following fatty acids appear in the text, figures, and tables; they are listed in the form trivial name (carbon number:number of double bonds) chemical name: Myristic acid (14:0) *n*-tetradecanoic acid, palmitic acid (16:0) *n*-hexadecanoic acid, palmitoleic acid (16:1) *cis*-9-hexadecenoic acid, stearic acid (18:0) *n*-octadecanoic acid, oleic acid (18:1) *cis*-9-octadecenoic acid, linoleic acid (18:2) *cis*-9:12-octadecadienoic acid, linolenic acid (18:3) *cis*-6,9,12-octadecatrienoic acid, arachidic acid (20:0) *n*-eicosanoic acid, —— (20:1) *cis*-11-eicosenoic acid, —— (20:2) *cis*-11,14-eicosadienoic acid, homo-γ-linolenic acid (20:3) *cis*-8,11,14-eicosatrienoic acid, arachidonic acid (20:4) *cis*-5,8,11,14-eicosatetraenoic acid, and adrenic acid (22:4) *cis*-7,10,13,16-docosatetraenoic acid.

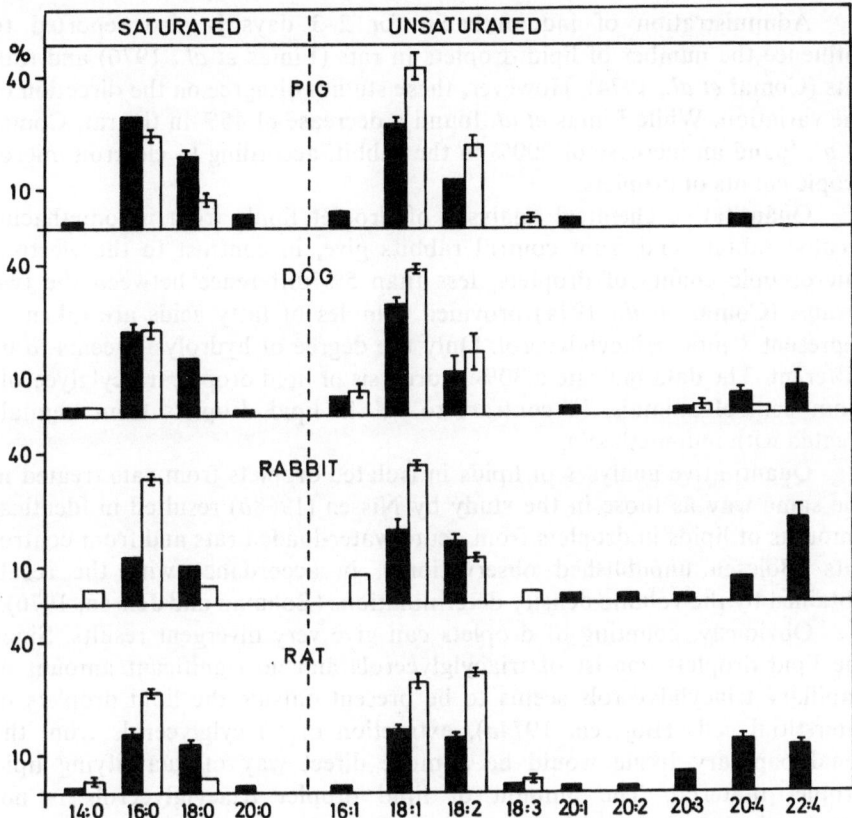

FIGURE 1. The fatty acid composition of renal papillary triacylglycerols (solid bars) from four species compared with the fatty acid composition of corresponding plasma triacylglycerols (open bars).

response to salt and water loading were reported by Nissen (1968a,b) using light microscopic counts of the number of lipid droplets per interstitial nucleus. A sharp increase was observed following a short period of hydration in dehydrated rats (number of lipid droplet per nucleus increased from 6.9 to 34.2). Bohman and Jensen (1976) have been unable to reproduce the findings of Nissen by means of a more accurate electron microscopic stereological method, but they found that rats water-loaded for 5 hr had a significantly higher value than dehydrated rats (4.2% compared to 1.9% of cell volume). Attainment of a proper hydrated state by the dehydrated rats seems to be the crucial point in these investigations. It is possible that Nissen had in some way obtained a hydrated state in his rats (urine osmolality was not measured) although Bohman and Jensen, in an attempt to reproduce the experiments of Nissen, were unable to obtain low urine osmolality as an indication of a hydrated state.

Administration of indomethacin for 2–3 days is also reported to influence the number of lipid droplets in rats (Limas et al., 1976) and rabbits (Comai et al., 1974). However, these studies disagree on the direction of the variation. While Limas et al. found a decrease of 45% in the rat, Comai et al. found an increase of 200% in the rabbit, according to electron microscopic counts of droplets.

Quantitative chemical analyses of droplet lipids from indomethacin-treated rabbits and from control rabbits give, in contrast to the electron microscopic counts of droplets, less than 5% difference between the two groups (Comai et al., 1974) provided 3 moles of fatty acids are taken to represent 1 mole triacylglycerol. Only the degree of hydrolysis seems to be different. The data indicate a 30% hydrolysis of lipid droplet triacylglycerols from control animals, in contrast to 0% in lipid droplets from animals treated with indomethacin.

Quantitative analyses of lipids in isolated droplets from rats treated in the same way as those in the study by Nissen (1968b) resulted in identical amounts of lipids in droplets from acute water-loaded rats and from control rats (Bojesen, unpublished observations), in accordance with the result obtained by the volume density determinations (Bohman and Jensen, 1976).

Obviously, counting of droplets can give very divergent results. Since the lipid droplets consist of triacylglycerols and no significant amount of papillary triacylglycerols seems to be present outside the lipid droplets of interstitial cells (Bojesen, 1974a), extraction of triacylglycerols from the renal papillary tissue would be a more direct way of quantifying lipid droplet material. The amount of lipid droplet triacylglycerols is not necessarily correlated with the number of droplets per cell. Comparison of the two parameters requires knowledge of the size distribution of droplets. Only if this is the same within the different states studied can parallel variations be expected.

An increase in size as well as in number was, however, found by Bohman and Jensen (1976) in response to water loading, whereas the study of Comai et al. (1974) suggests a decrease of droplet size after indomethacin administration.

Quantitative determinations of triacylglycerols extractable from papillae of rats in different states of water balance have recently been made (Fig. 2) (Bojesen, unpublished data). The amount of triacylglycerols was found to increase with increasing diuresis in three groups of rats (untreated, water-deprived, and saline-diuretic rats) whereas the amount in papillae from water-diuretic rats was outstandingly low. The difference between untreated and water-deprived rats was highly significant ($p < 0.001$), and a significant correlation between diuresis and the ratio of triacylglycerols to phospholipids in the saline diuretic rats was found, with a correlation coefficient of 0.94. These results suggest a functional correlation between the diu-

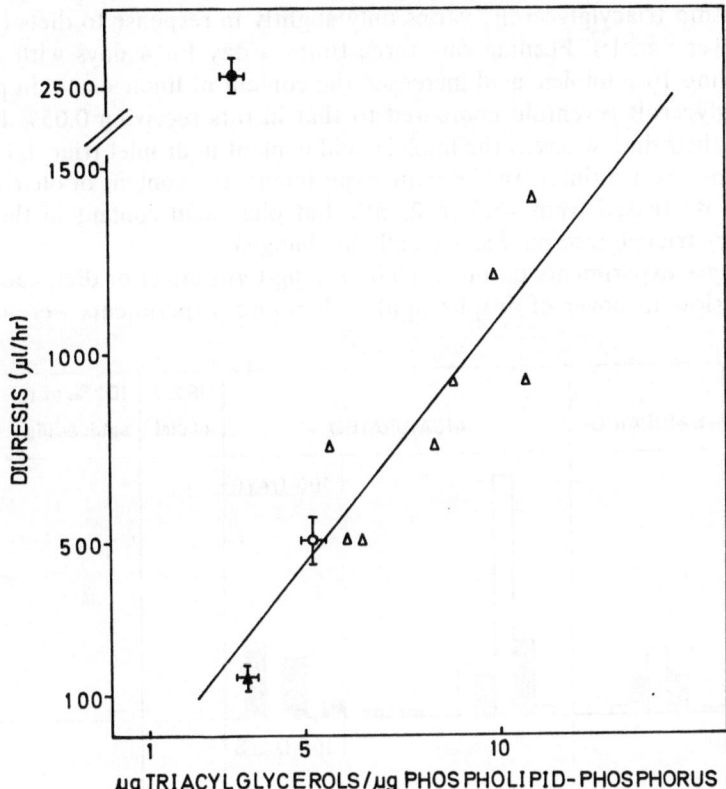

FIGURE 2.   Triacylglycerol content [expressed as µg triacylglycerols (molecular weight 884)/µg phospholipid–phosphorus] of rat renal papillae as a function of diuresis (µl/hr). Triacylglycerols were isolated from lipid extracts of papillary homogenates and hydrolyzed, and the liberated glycerol was then determined. Phospholipids were quantified by phosphorus analyses. Papillae from four different groups of rats were studied. O , Group I: rats with free access to water; ▲ , group II: rats deprived of water for 24 hr, △ , group III: rats with only 1% NaCl solution to drink for 48 hr; ● , group IV: rats with only 5% dextrose water to drink for 24 hr. The line is drawn by the method of least squares.

retic state of rats and the lipid droplets in the interstitial cells. The variations in amount of lipid seem smaller than those suggested by the counting procedure of Nissen, but in reasonable agreement with the results of Bohman and Jensen (1976).

2.3.   Influence of Diet on the Fatty Acid Composition of the Renal Papillary Droplets

Experiments with rats on different diets demonstrate that the fatty acid composition of the papillary droplet triacylglycerols, in contrast to that of the plasma triacylglycerols, varies only slightly in response to diets (Fig. 3, two lower panels). Feeding rats three times a day for 4 days with a meal containing 10% linoleic acid increased the content of linoleic acid in plasma triacylglycerols sevenfold compared to that in rats receiving 0.05% linoleic acid in their diet, whereas the linoleic acid content in droplet triacylglycerols changed only 1.6 times. In the same experiments the content of oleic acid in plasma decreased from 45.5 to 25.5%, but oleic acid content in the renal papillary triacylglycerols was virtually unchanged.

These experiments do not exclude a long-term effect of diet, caused by a very slow turnover of droplet lipids. Therefore, experiments were carried

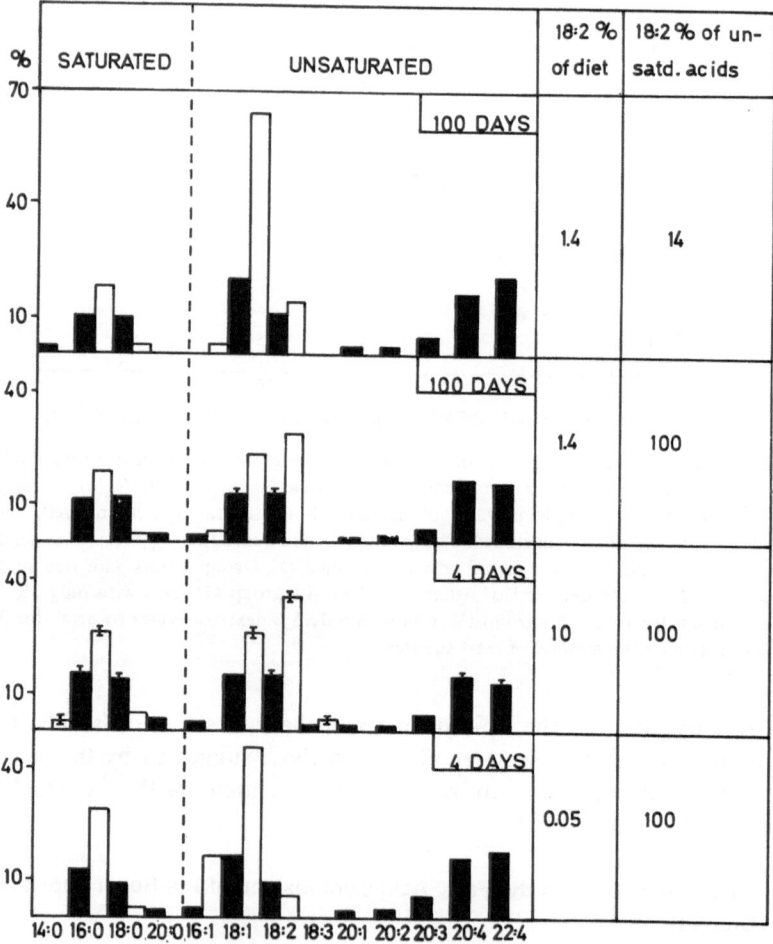

FIGURE 3. The fatty acid composition of triacylglycerols from renal papillae (solid bars) and from plasma (open bars) of rats fed different diets for different periods of time.

out in which groups of five rats were fed from the age of 3 weeks to the age of 15 weeks with a diet containing 1.4% linoleic acid and 8.4% oleic acid and compared to a control group of rats receiving a diet with a low oleic acid content. The ratio of saturated to unsaturated fatty acids of the food was 0.2 for the experimental group and 1.7 for the control group. When animals were given a high-oleic-acid diet the content of oleic acid in plasma increased by a factor of 2.8, but the content in droplet triacylglycerols increased only from 12% to 19% (a factor of 1.6) (Fig. 3, two upper panels).

The fatty acid composition of droplet triacylglycerols in rat papillae thus does not simply reflect dietary lipids, a result confirmed by Comai *et al.* (1975) in rabbits. This indicates that the fatty acid composition of droplet triacylglycerols is a species- and tissue-specific characteristic rather than a result of different diets. Moreover, it indicates that the accumulation of lipid droplets in the interstitial cells is not the result of a simple accumulation of plasma triacylglycerols. Instead a local synthesis of triacylglycerols from locally synthesized fatty acids or from fatty acids selectively taken up from plasma appears likely. The presence of adrenic acid in high proportion indicates that a chain elongation of the abundant arachidonic acid occurs in the renal papilla.

3. BIOCHEMICAL INVESTIGATIONS OF THE RENAL PAPILLA

3.1. Energy Metabolism

Studies in the dog by Kean *et al.* (1969) and by Bernanke and Epstein (1965) as well as in the rabbit by Lee *et al.* (1962) have shown that, in contrast to the renal cortex, the major source of energy for the renal papilla is glucose. The net glucose uptake by the papilla is three times that of the cortex. While almost all the glucose taken up by the cortex *in vitro* is incorporated into CO_2, only 20% of the papillary glucose uptake appears as CO_2. In the *in vitro* experiments mentioned above it was demonstrated that the renal papillae have an unusually large capacity for anaerobic glycolysis, but even more remarkable is the persistent formation of large amounts of lactic acid from glucose in the presence of oxygen. Besides this anaerobic and aerobic glycolysis a significant proportion of glucose is processed through the phosphogluconate shunt. The results obtained by these biochemical methods are in excellent agreement with those obtained by enzyme–histochemical methods: the activity of all enzymes that participate in glucose metabolism via the glycolytic and phosphogluconate oxidative pathway was demonstrated in the renal inner medulla and particularly in the interstitial cells (Guder and Schmidt, 1976; Szokol and Soltész, 1973).

Together with the information gathered on the specific composition of droplet triacylglycerols, these studies suggest a vivid lipogenesis in the renomedullary interstitial cells, a synthesis which may be intimately connected with their function. In order to substantiate this suggestion, studies of papillary lipogenesis were initiated.

3.2. Lipid Metabolism

3.2.1. Synthesis of Papillary Lipids in Vitro from Acetate Glucose

The biosynthesis of long-chain fatty acids from the precursors [14C]acetate (Bojesen et al., 1976) and [14C]glucose (Bojesen, 1980a), and their incorporation into droplet triacylglycerols, was investigated in rat renal papillary slices in vitro.

A very efficient incorporation of the two precursors into lipid droplet triacylglycerols was seen since 21–37% of the incorporated radioactivity was present in this lipid fraction. When [14C]acetate was the lipogenic precursor all the radioactivity was present in the fatty acid moiety, whereas only 26% was found in this moiety when [14C]glucose was the precursor. Glucose was incorporated mainly into the glycerol part of the papillary glycerolipids (Bojesen, 1980a). Radio gas–liquid chromatography of the triacylglycerol fatty acids synthesized from the two substrates showed very similar patterns. An example is given in Table 1.

Schmidt degradation [a decarboxylation procedure (Bojesen et al., 1976)], applied to the [1-14C]-labeled fatty acids formed, revealed that a de novo synthesis as well as a chain elongation process had taken place. The

TABLE 1

Relative Amount of Radioactivity Incorporated into Major Long-Chain Fatty Acids of Triacylglycerols after 4 hr Incubation with [1-14C]Acetate and [1-14C]Glucose[a]

| Fatty acid (number of carbon atoms:number of double bonds) | Renal papillary triacylglycerols | | | |
| | [1-14C]Acetate (8.6 µM) | | [1-14]Glucose (5 mM) | |
	rat I (%)	rat II (%)	rat A (%)	rat B (%)
Palmitic acid (16:0)	15.5	15.0	24.4	16.0
Stearic acid (18:0)	14.1	18.0	16.2	14.9
Arachidic acid (20:0)	16.1	14.5	13.7	21.3
Adrenic acid (22:4)	54.5	52.5	46.0	48.0

[a] Papillary slices (25 mg tissue/2 ml medium) were incubated at 37°C in Krebs–Ringer phosphate buffer (pH = 7.4) containing 5 mM [1-14C]glucose (specific activity 0.1 Ci/mole) and 8.6 µM [1-14C]acetate (specific activity 58 Ci/mole). Triacylglycerols were isolated from lipid extracts of the papillary slices, after incubation for 4 hr, by thin-layer chromatography. After transesterification, the resulting methyl esters were separated by radio gas–liquid chromatography and the percentage distribution of radioactivity was calculated from the gas–liquid chromatograms by triangulation with a [14C]fatty acid methyl ester standard for calibration. The fatty acids included in the table together contained more than 82% of the total methyl ester radioactivity.

saturated fatty acids, myristic acid and palmitic acid, were synthesized almost entirely by a *de novo* pathway, but the major part of the radioactive acetate was found to be incorporated by a chain elongation of preexisting fatty acids, and the major product was demonstrated to be adrenic acid. *In vitro* the radioactivity of this acid accounted for 40% of total radioactivity in triacylglycerol fatty acids (lipid droplet fraction) and 20% of total radioactivity in fatty acids from membrane phospholipids extracted from the precipitate after isolation of lipid droplets.

From glucose as well as from acetate the fraction of fatty acid equivalences synthesized by the chain elongation pathway is 20- to 30-fold greater than the fraction of fatty acids synthesized by the *de novo* pathway. By comparing the contributions of acetate and glucose to the fatty acid synthesis it is found that acetate in concentrations of 9 μM is diluted about 30–50 times by acetate synthesized from 5 mM glucose.

The synthesis of adrenic acid is not a unique property of the renal papilla. It has been demonstrated in lymphocytes (Blomstrand, 1966), in brain mitochondria (Yatsu and Moss, 1970; Aeberhard and Menkes, 1968) and microsomes (Aeberhard and Menkes, 1968), as well as in adrenal microsomes (Stoffel and Ach, 1964).

The intracellular organelle involved in the fatty acid synthesis of the renal papilla has not been determined directly and it can not be inferred from the available information. A microsomal elongation pathway, as described by Stoffel and Ach (1964) in adrenals, in combination with a cytoplasmic *de novo* synthesis could account for the pattern of fatty acid synthesized in the renal papilla. The fact that radioactive 11,14-eicosadienoic acid is synthesized by the papilla *in vivo* as well as *in vitro* from [^{14}C]acetate, whereas arachidonic acid remains unlabeled in both situations (Bojesen *et al.*, 1976), could be interpreted in terms of a pure chain elongation of linoleic acid, with the microsomal desaturation pathway being unimportant in the renal papilla. In many tissues the activity of the microsomal desaturase decreases rapidly with increasing chain lengths above 18 atoms (Brett *et al.*, 1971). On the other hand, the spectrum of fatty acids synthesized by the mitochondria from rabbit heart and aorta (Whereat, 1971) is also in accordance with our data on renal papilla (Bojesen *et al.*, 1976).

The percentage renewal of triacylglycerols and phospholipids can be calculated from experiments *in vitro* with [^{14}C]glucose on basis of the specific activity of glycerol in these glycerolipids and the specific activity of added glucose, assuming that the intracellular glucose store is negligible. Incubations carried out with [^{32}P]Na$_2$HPO$_4$ and [^{14}C]choline as substrates confirm this assumption, since the fractional renewal of phospholipids is the same, independent of the precursor used (Bojesen, unpublished results). Of the glycerol in triacylglycerols and phospholipids, 14.5% $\pm$ 3.8% ($N = 7$)

and $7.2\% \pm 0.7\%$ ($N = 6$), respectively, was renewed during 4 hr of incubation.

The percentage renewal of the individual fatty acids in the triacylglycerol and phospholipid molecules can also be calculated on the basis of the specific activity of the fatty acids and that of the precursors, [1-^{14}C]acetate and [U-^{14}C]glucose. It turns out that, compared to synthesized glycerol, only three per thousand of the corresponding acid equivalences are synthesized *de novo* from glucose. No fatty acids or nitrogen-containing bases were present in the incubation media. Thus, a corresponding amount of lipid was hydrolyzed to supply "building blocks" for the synthesis of new glycerolipids. Consequently, the percentage renewal of glycerol in papillary lipids indicates that the turnover rate of these lipids is fast.

Although the rate of triacylglycerol synthesis *in vitro* is high, it is too small to account for the rapid increment in number of lipid droplets of unchanged size distribution, as suggested by Nissen (1968*b*). The observed *in vitro* rate of synthesis is, however, compatible with the changes in triacylglycerol content found after variations of state of hydration maintained over longer periods of time (24 or 48 hr) (Fig. 2).

3.2.2.   *Synthesis of Papillary Lipids from Acetate in Vivo*

To investigate the lipogensis of the papillary tissue *in situ* [1-^{14}C]acetate was administered to three eviscerated rats (Bojesen *et al.*, 1976). This preparation was chosen since it excludes the large contribution of the entire portal system to acetate production and metabolism.

The relationship between the rate of acetate incorporation into fatty acids and acetate concentration used was the same as that *in vitro*. Furthermore the distribution of radioactivity in total fatty acids synthesized by the tissue *in vivo* closely resembles the synthesis *in vitro* (Bojesen *et al.*, 1976), indicating that the information obtained by studies *in vitro* is of physiological significance. It is noteworthy that arachidonic acid remains unlabeled in both situations. Thus, it is not synthesized by the tissue from linoleic acid. However, in some cases, *in vivo* as well as *in vitro*, an unidentified fatty acid, both heavier and more unsaturated, made up for less than 8% of the total fatty acid radioactivity. Thus, it is possible that the tissue possesses a low desaturase activity under certain conditions.

Interestingly, analyses of the fatty acids from the outer medulla after the experiments *in vivo* with [^{14}C]acetate revealed no detectable radioactivity or mass at the positions of adrenic acid and arachidic acid at the instrumental settings used for papillary samples. Only radioactive palmitic and stearic acid were present (Bojesen *et al.*, 1976). Electron microscopic investigations show that the lipid-laden interstitial cells become sparse toward the outer medullary zone. This finding, together with the observations mentioned above, supports the contention that the important chain elongation process of papillary tissue takes place mainly in the papillary interstitial cells.

3.2.3. Synthesis of Papillary Lipids from Fatty Acids in Vitro

The uptake of exogenous fatty acids was studied in incubation experiments using two of the major components of the fatty acids in papillary triacylglycerols, namely [1-^{14}C]palmitic and [1-^{14}C]arachidonic acid (Bojesen, unpublished observations). The rate of incorporation of these two long-chain fatty acids into papillary lipids (membrane phospholipids and droplet triacylglycerols) increased with increasing concentration of total added fatty acids over a dose range of 100 (Figs. 4 and 5). As the exogenous fatty acid concentration increased, the rate of incorporation into papillary triacylglycerols increased faster than the rate of incorporation into phospholipids.

The distribution of incorporated fatty acids in the different lipid classes of the renal papilla is given in Table 2. Note that the distribution is dependent on the concentration of added fatty acids but that the pattern is different in phospholipids and triacylglycerols. The percentage incorporation of both of the two acids into phospholipids decreases when the fatty acid concentrations are increased, while the opposite is true for triacylglycerols.

TABLE 2

Percentage Distribution of ^{14}C in Lipids Extracted from Papillary Slices after Incubations with Different Concentrations of [1-^{14}C]Palmitic Acid (16:0) and [1-^{14}C]Arachidonic Acid (20:4) for 2 hr[a]

Lipids[b]	16:0				20:4			
	10 μM	23 μM	113 μM	517 μM	1.2 μM	12 μM	92 μM	450 μM
Pl	75.2	75.0	71.6	56.0	85.3	84.4	78.0	63.5
MG	1.0	1.1	0.9	1.1	0.2	0.2	—	0.3
DG	5.6	6.2	5.7	6.7	4.2	3.8	3.6	3.5
FFA	5.6	4.1	5.4	13.7	2.6	2.4	3.4	8.7
TG	12.6	13.7	16.1	22.2	7.5	9.1	14.5	23.8
SE	0.1	0.1	0.3	—	0.2	0.3	0.4	0.5

[a] Papillary slices were incubated (see Table 1) in buffers prepared as described in Fig. 4. After extraction the papillary lipids were separated by thin-layer chromatography together with a mixture of reference compounds. The different components were localized under a 254 mμ lamp after spraying with dichlorofluorescein. The distribution of radioactivity in the different spots was determined by liquid scintillation counting, as described in Fig. 4. Recovery of phospholipids was 72%, recovery of free fatty acids and neutral lipids was 98% to 100%.
[b] Pl, phospholipids; MG, monoacylglycerols; DG, diacylglycerols; FFA, free fatty acids; TG, triacylglycerols; SE, steryl esters.

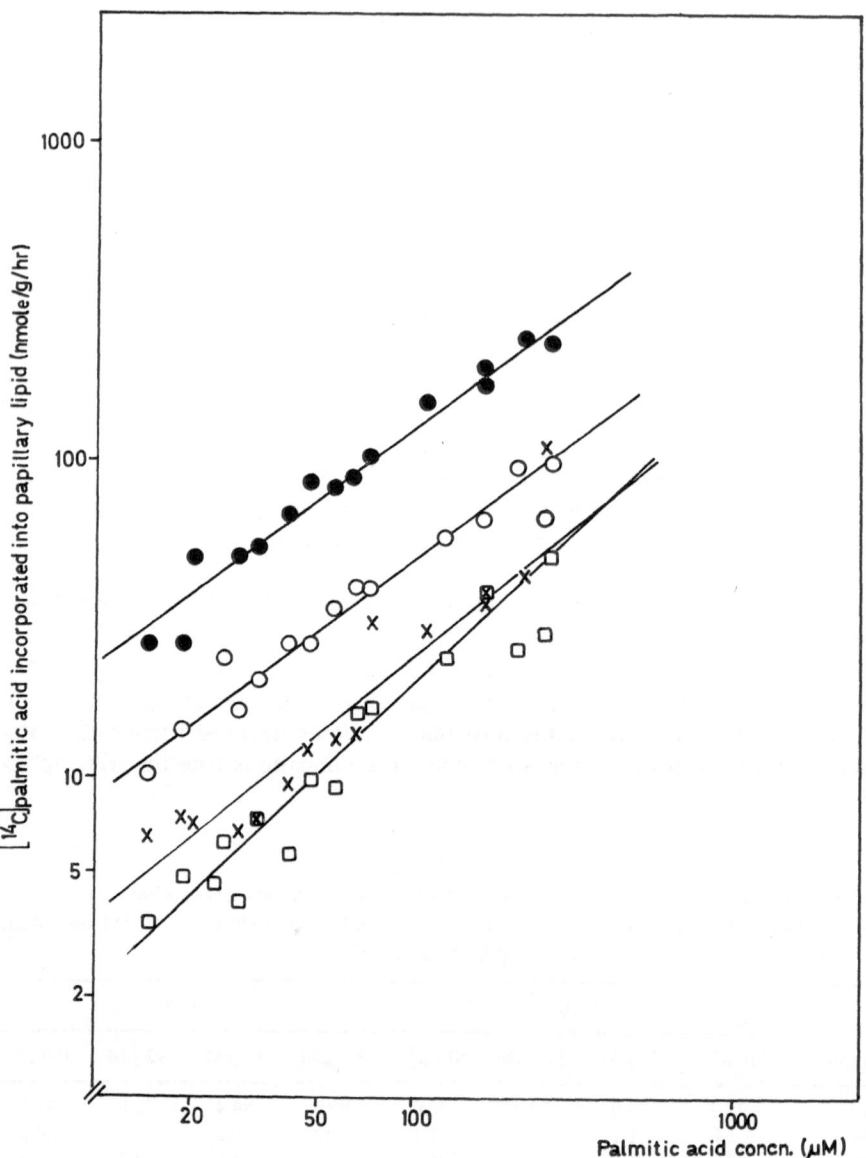

FIGURE 4. The relationship between rate of [1-^{14}C]palmitic acid incorporation into papillary triacylglycerols and phospholipids and the total medium concentration of palmitic acid at two different osmolalities. Renal papillary slices were incubated 2 hr at 37°C in phosphate buffer (pH 7.4, 340 mosmole/kg H$_2$O) with and without urea containing 5 mM glucose and 150 μM bovine serum albumin. Complexation of fatty acids to albumin was performed by gently shaking a buffer solution containing defatted albumin for 15 min at 37°C with glass spheres (diameter 90 μm) on which the fatty acids were deposited. Papillary lipids were extracted by homogenizing the slices with CH$_2$Cl$_2$:CH$_3$OH (2:1, v/v) and separated by thin-layer chromatography. The distribution of incorporated activity was determined by liquid scintillation counting directly on a suspension of the silica gel scraped from the thin-layer plate in 5 ml Luma Gel. Recovery of phospholipids was 72%; recovery of triacylglycerols was 100%. The lines were drawn by the method of least squares, ×, Incorporation into triacylglycerols at 340

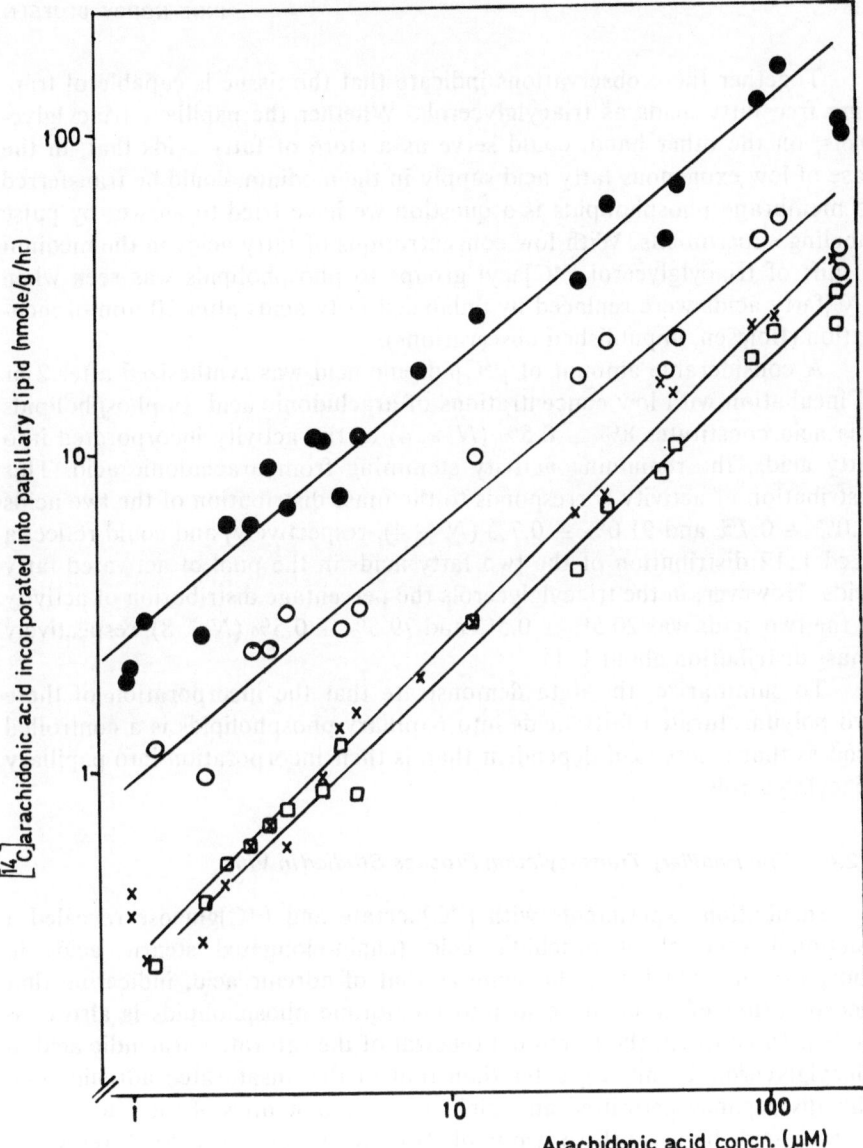

FIGURE 5. The relationship between rate of [1-^{14}C]arachidonic acid incorporation into papillary triacylglycerols and phospholipids and the total medium concentration of arachidonic acid at two different osmolalities. Experimental conditions as in Fig. 4. The lines were drawn by the methods of least squares. ×, Incorporation into triacylglycerols at 340 mosmole/kg H$_2$O; □, incorporation into triacylglycerols at 1370 mosmole/kg H$_2$O; ●, incorporation into phospholipids at 340 mosmole/kg H$_2$O; ○, incorporation into phospholipids at 1370 mosmole/kg H$_2$O.

mosmole/kg H$_2$O; □, incorporation into triacylglycerols at 1370 mosmole/kg H$_2$O; ●, incorporation into phospholipids at 340 mosmole/kg H$_2$O; ○, incorporation into phospholipids at 1370 mosmole/kg H$_2$O.

Together these observations indicate that the tissue is capable of trapping free fatty acids as triacylglycerols. Whether the papillary triacylglycerols, on the other hand, could serve as a store of fatty acids that, in the case of low exogenous fatty acid supply in the medium, could be transferred to membrane phospholipids is a question we have tried to answer by pulse labeling experiments. With low concentrations of fatty acids in the medium a shift of triacylglycerol [^{14}C]acyl groups to phospholipids was seen when [^{14}C]fatty acids were replaced by unlabeled fatty acids after 20 min of incubation (Bojesen, unpublished observations).

A considerable amount of [^{14}C]adrenic acid was synthesized after 2 hr of incubation with low concentrations of arachidonic acid. In phospholipids this acid constitutes 8% $\pm$ 0.5% (N = 4) of the activity incorporated into fatty acids, the remaining activity stemming from arachidonic acid. This distribution of activity corresponds to the mass distribution of the two acids [9.0% $\pm$ 0.7% and 91.0% $\pm$ 0.7% (N = 4), respectively] and could reflect a fixed 1:12 distribution of the two fatty acids in the pool of activated fatty acids. However, in the triacylglycerols the percentage distribution of activity of the two acids was 20.5% $\pm$ 0.5% and 79.5% $\pm$ 0.5% (N = 8), respectively (mass distribution about 1:1).

To summarize, the data demonstrate that the incorporation of these two polyunsaturated fatty acids into papillary phospholipids is a controlled process that is less load-dependent than is their incorporation into papillary triacylglycerols.

3.2.4. *The Papillary Transacylation Process Studied in Vitro*

Incubation experiments with [^{14}C]acetate and [^{14}C]glucose revealed a fractional renewal of arachidic acid (chain-elongated stearic acid) in phospholipids, which was the same as that of adrenic acid, indicating that incorporation of arachidic acid into membrane phospholipids is also controlled. In contrast, the fractional renewal of the saturated arachidic acid in triacylglycerols is much greater than that of the unsaturated adrenic acid. This discrepancy permitted an insight into the dynamics of the interchange of fatty acids between these two pools (Fig. 6) (Bojesen,1974*b*). After about 6 hr of incubation the two acids had roughly the same specific activity in lipid droplet triacylglycerols as in membrane phospholipids. The initial preferential incorporation of the two fatty acids in phospholipids and triacylglycerols, respectively, does not correspond to the preformed amounts nor does it result in a progressively increasing discrepancy. On the contrary, it gradually decays. Both facts are easily explained by a rapidly equilibrating transacylation process. The specific activity of palmitic and stearic acid of the lipid classes was the same during the entire periods of incubation. The hypothesis that a rapidly equilibrating transacylation takes place is further

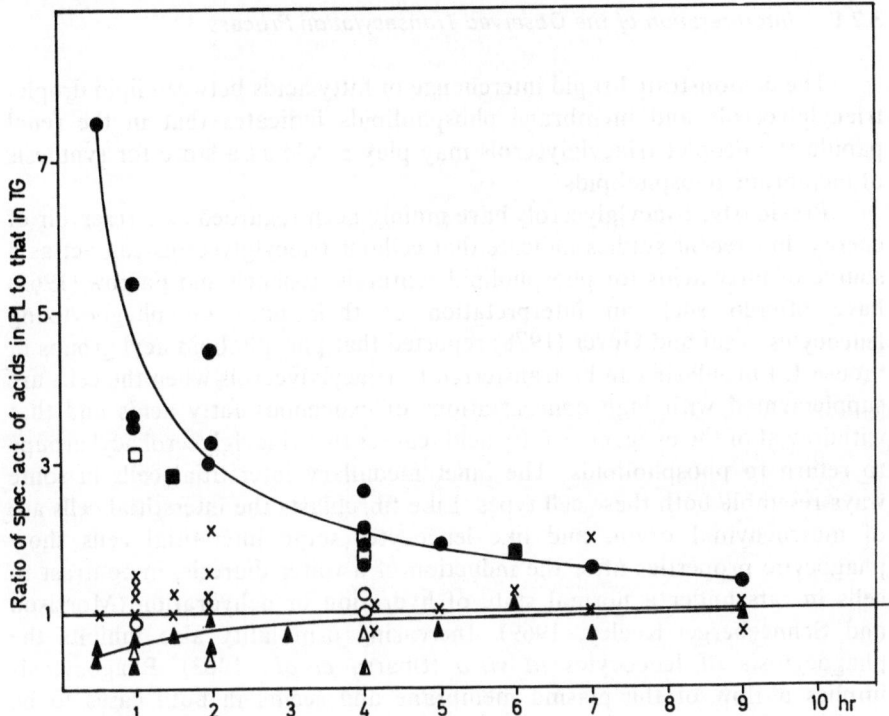

FIGURE 6. Changes in the ratio of specific activities of locally synthesized docosa-7,10,13,16-tetraenoic acid and eicosanoic acid in phospholipids to those in triacylglycerols during incubation of rat renal papillary slices with [^{14}C]acetate and [^{14}C]glucose in media of 340 mosmole/kg H$_2$O and 1370 mosmole/kg H$_2$O. ●, [^{14}C]docosa-7,10,13,16-tetraenoic acid synthesized from [^{14}C]acetate at 340 mosmole/kg H$_2$O; □, [^{14}C]docosa-7,10,13,16-tetraenoic acid synthesized from [^{14}C]glucose by incubation at 340 mosmole/kg H$_2$O; ■, [^{14}C]docosa-7,10,13,16-tetraenoic acid synthesized from [^{14}C]acetate in a pulse-labeling experiment by incubation at 340 mosmole/kg H$_2$O; ○, [^{14}C]docosa-7,10,13,16-tetraenoic acid synthesized from [^{14}C]acetate by incubation at 1370 mosmole/kg H$_2$O; ▲, [^{14}C]eicosanoic acid synthesized from [^{14}C]acetate by incubation at 340 mosmole/kg H$_2$O; △, [^{14}C]eicosanoic acid synthesized from [^{14}C]glucose by incubation at 340 mosmole/kg H$_2$O; ▲, [^{14}C]eicosanoic acid synthesized from [^{14}C]acetate by incubation at 1370 mosmole/kg H$_2$O, ×, [^{14}C]palmitic and stearic acid synthesized from acetate and glucose by incubation at 340 and 1370 mosmole/kg H$_2$O.

supported by a pulse-labeling experiment with [^{14}C]acetate (Fig. 6) and by experiments with [1-^{14}C]arachidonic acid. After 2 hr of incubation with [1-^{14}C]arachidonic acid the specific activity of adrenic acid was 0.336 and 0.034 μCi/μmole in phospholipids and in triacylglycerols, respectively, giving a ratio of 10:1. After 4 hr this ratio was decreased to 6:1 (0.67/0.11). The corresponding ratios for arachidonic acid were 1.8:1 after 2 hr and 1.3:1 after 4 hr (Bojesen, unpublished data).

3.2.5. *Interpretation of the Observed Transacylation Process*

The demonstrated rapid interchange of fatty acids between lipid droplet triacylglycerols and membrane phospholipids indicates that in the renal papilla the droplet triacylglycerols may play a role as a store for synthesis of membrane phospholipids.

Previously, triacylglycerols have mainly been regarded as a reservoir of energy, but recent studies indicate that cellular triacylglycerols can act as a source of fatty acids for phospholipid synthesis. Elsbach and Farrow (1969) have offered such an interpretation of their data on phagocytizing leucocytes. Tsai and Geyer (1978) reported that phospholipid acyl groups in mouse L fibroblasts can be transferred to triacylglycerols when the cells are supplemented with high concentrations of exogenous fatty acids and that withdrawal of the exogenous fatty acids causes the triacylglycerol acyl groups to return to phospholipids. The inner medullary interstitial cells in some ways resemble both these cell types. Like fibroblasts the interstitial cells are of mesenchymal orgin, and like leucocytes some interstitial cells show phagocytic properties after the induction of a water diuresis, in contrast to cells in rats under a normal state of hydration or dehydration (Morrison and Schneeberger-Keeley, 1969). Increasing osmolality also inhibits the phagocytosis of leucocytes *in vitro* (Sbarra *et al.*, 1963). Phagocytosis implies a flow of the plasma membrane and seems in both cases to be associated with a turnover of membrane phospholipids in equilibrium with triacylglycerols with respect to fatty acids.

The chief objection to the above interpretation of the results, i.e., one in analogy with the phenomenon seen in leucocytes and mouse L fibroblasts, is that the renal papilla represents a composite tissue. The lipid droplets (triacylglycerols) are present only in the interstitial cells, whereas the analyzed phospholipids originate from membranes in all papillary cells. Thus, all cells contribute to the fatty-acid-specific activities of phospholipids, whereas only interstitial cells contribute to triacylglycerol data. For an understanding of the problem it is important to recall that the amount of phospholipids (9.4 mg/g tissue wet weight) is about 4 times the amount of triacylglycerols (2.3 mg/g tissue wet weight). The fraction of papillary phospholipids present in the interstitial cells is unknown. However, a crude evaluation on the basis of morphology suggests that it may be rather large. Interstitial cells constitute 25–30% of the total cellular volume in rat papilla (Bohman and Jensen, 1976). They are described as stellate flat cells with many long cytoplasmic processes. Therefore the ratio of surface to volume may be as large as that of capillary endothelial cells and cells of the loop of Henle. More important, however, is the presence of a very prominent intracellular membrane system.

Provided that the phospholipids in the interstitial cells do not entirely dominate the results described indicate that the lipogenesis of the interstitial cells is able to influence the fatty acid composition of the phospholipids in adjacent cells by an intercellular exchange. A phospholipid exchange between biological membranes and between membranes and lipoproteins is a well-known phenomenon. An exchange of phospholipids between fibroblasts in culture has been reported (Peterson and Rubin, 1970), and the data of Joist *et al.* (1976) suggest a direct exchange of phosphatidylcholine between plasma and platelets, a mechanism known to be operative also in erythrocyte–plasma systems. Kibel *et al.* (1976) report that lipids (phospholipids and triacylglycerols) are genuine constituents of basement membranes isolated from glomeruli and that these lipids have a fast turnover rate due to exchange with adjacent cells. Proximity of membranes seems to be important and close contact between the basement membrane of capillaries and loops of Henle and the cytoplasmic processes of the interstitial cells has been demonstrated morphologically.

The transacylation is observed in media of 340 mosmole/kg H_2O, corresponding to the osmolality of the papilla in highly diuretic rats, and therefore coincides with the appearance of phagocytic properties of the interstitial cells (Morrison and Schneeberger-Keeley, 1969). Assuming that the fatty acid exchange is confined to this physiological state of the papilla, it should then be expected to disappear in hyperosmotic media. Unfortunately, under these conditions the specific activity of the polyunsaturated adrenic acid in the two lipid classes was the same independent of incubation time (Fig. 6). Thus, the lipogenesis in hyperosmotic media did not offer the opportunity for observing the exchange phenomenon, although it may still occur.

3.2.6. *The Influence of Medium Osmolality upon Papillary Lipogensis*

3.2.6a. In Vitro Lipogenesis from Glucose. Increasing the osmolality of the medium from 340 mosmole/kg H_2O to 1370 mosmole/kg H_2O resulted in a decrease of the acetate incorporation into fatty acids of papillary glycerolipids by a factor of 7 to 9 (Bojesen, 1980*b*). This effect of the osmolality of the medium was further studied with [^{14}C]glucose as the substrate and urea as the variable solute. The osmolality of the papillary interstitium varies considerably in response to external influences due to variable concentrations of electrolytes and urea. However, in the normal antidiuretic state the contribution of urea predominates.

The incorporation rate of glucose carbon into papillary lipids decreased by a factor of 4.5 within the physiological range of osmolalities from 400 to 2000 mosmole/kg H_2O (Fig. 7) (Bojesen, 1980*b*). However, the possibility

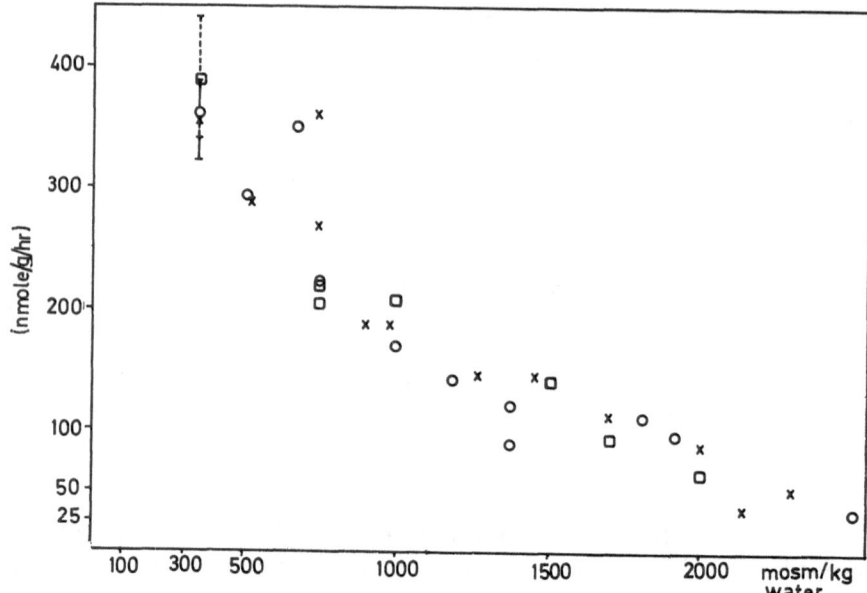

FIGURE 7. Osmolality dependency of glucose incorporation *in vitro* into papillary lipids. Papillary slices from three different groups of rats were incubated for 2 hr at 37°C with air as the gas phase in Krebs–Ringer phosphate buffer (340 mosmole/kg H_2O) containing 5 mM glucose and different amounts of urea in order to obtain different osmolalities. ×, Group I: rats with free access to water (normal rats); O, group II: rats deprived of water for 24 hr (dehydrated rats); □, group III: rats with only 1% NaCl solution to drink for 48 hr (saline-diuretic rats).

exists that the observed behavior is merely a consequence of an adaptation when papillae of a certain osmolality are transferred to a medium of a quite different osmolality. This possibility could, however, be countered by the fact that the curves were identical for tissue from normal, dehydrated, and diuretic rats and that no minimum around zero was found by plotting the incorporation rate as a function of the relative change in osmolality.

The major lipid classes, triacylglycerols and phospholipids, contain more than 90% of the incorporated ^{14}C activity from [^{14}C]glucose. The glycerol backbone contains 73.7% and 82.2% of the activity found in triacylglycerol and phospholipid, respectively, after incubation in isotonic medium. These percentages gradually increase with increasing osmolality so that at 750 mosmole/kg H_2O they are 93% and 96%, at 1000 mosmole/kg H_2O they are 96.5% and 97.5% and from 1800 mosmole/kg H_2O and upwards they are 99.0% and 99.5%. This shows that the synthesis of fatty acids from glucose via acetyl-CoA decreases by a factor of 10 when the osmolality is increased from 400 to 1800 mosmole/kg H_2O. This finding is in accordance with the observation mentioned above that the lipogenesis from acetate is decreased by a factor of 7 to 9 when the osmolality is increased from 340 to 1370 mosmole/kg H_2O, and demonstrates that the acetate equivalence of glucose does not change with the osmolality.

3.2.6b. *In Vitro Lipogenesis from Fatty Acids.* The effect of adding urea to the incubation media on the incorporation rate of exogenous fatty acids has been studied in a series of experiments (Figs. 4 and 5) (Bojesen, unpublished results). The rate at which arachidonic acid and palmitic acid were incorporated into papillary phospholipids was 2.6-fold lower at 1370 mosmole/kg H_2O than at 340 mosmole/kg H_2O for all concentrations of fatty acids studied. However, the rate of incorporation into papillary triacylglycerols was much less dependent on medium osmolality.

The relationship between the incorporation rate into papillary triacylglycerols and phospholipids and the fatty acid concentration can be represented by the regression line $\log y = \alpha \log x + \beta$ with correlation coefficients higher than 0.94 in all cases.

3.2.6c. *In Vitro Prostaglandin Synthesis.* The effect of hypertonic buffers on the prostaglandin production has been reported by Danon *et al.* (1978). Media made hypertonic with sucrose and with NaCl in high, unphysiological concentrations strongly stimulated the prostaglandin output from renal papillary slices, while physiological concentrations of urea (100–1000 mM) and NaCl (130–350 mM) also stimulated the output, although to a smaller extent. Studies on interstitial cells in culture (Zusman and Keiser, 1977) also show that PGE_2 synthesis increases when the osmolality of the medium is increased with mannitol.

Independent studies of the effect of urea on the rate of PGE_2 biosynthesis in renal papillary slices were carried out in our laboratory (unpublished data) to elucidate a possible connection between prostaglandin production and the production of glycerolipids. As in the study of Danon *et al.* (1978), the rate of PGE_2 biosynthesis was found to increase 2–3 times when the medium osmolality was increased from 340 to 1370 mosmole/kg H_2O. The inverse relation between the osmolality effects on the synthesis of glycerolipids and prostaglandins suggested the participation of prostaglandins in regulation of glycerolipid biosynthesis. However, participation of prostaglandins in such an intracellular control could not be substantiated. *De novo* synthesis of papillary glycerolipids from [^{14}C]glucose and fatty acid synthesis from [^{14}C]glucose and [^{14}C]acetate in hypertonic media were not effected by 72% and 90% inhibition of prostaglandin synthesis by aspirin and indomethacin, respectively, *in vitro*.

An apparent stimulating effect of prostaglandins on lipogenesis could be inferred from the study of Limas *et al.* (1976). These authors observed a decrease (45%) in the incorporation of arachidonic acid into rat papillary phospholipids after administration of indomethacin for 48 hr. The animals also had a significantly lower number of lipid droplets in the interstitial cells of the papilla (5.6 vs. 9.9), suggesting that the overall rate of lipogenesis was lowered. This could be a direct effect of the drug, but a more likely explanation can be offered on the basis of the effect of osmolality upon lipogenesis described above, since it is known that indomethacin enhances the effect of vasopressin (Fejes-Tóth *et al.*, 1977; Berl *et al.*, 1977).

4. COMPARISON BETWEEN *IN VITRO* AND *IN VIVO* DATA

Fatty acid synthesis from acetate in rat renal papillae was qualitatively as well as quantitatively the same in eviscerated rats as in slices incubated *in vitro* when the medium was isotonic (Bojesen *et al.*, 1976). This seemed somewhat surprising in view of the demonstrated importance of extracellular osmolality for papillary lipogenesis *in vitro* and since the osmolality in normal rat papillae is highly hypertonic. However, the problem disappeared when it was found that the osmolality of papillary interstitium in eviscerated rats was as low as 463 ± 47 mosmole/kg H_2O ($N = 4$) (Bojesen, 1980*b*), a value at which lipogenesis is affected insignificantly (Fig. 7).

Thus the present investigations indicate that the extracellular osmolality *in vitro* as well as *in vivo* is an important regulating factor for papillary lipogenesis. The prostaglandins are probably not the mediators of this effect. The effects of osmolality on lipogenesis and prostaglandin production are thus parallel phenomena.

Comparison of the fatty acid composition of papillary phospholipids isolated from water-diuretic rats (group IV in Fig. 2) with the fatty acid composition of phospholipids from water-deprived rats (group II in Fig. 2) did not reveal any significant difference. However, in contrast to this observed constancy in phospholipid fatty acid composition in different states of water balance, the percentage amount of arachidonic acid in lipid droplet triacylglycerols decreased to $9.9\% \pm 0.3\%$ ($N = 4$) after 24-hr water loading from $17.0\% \pm 0.2\%$ ($N = 4$) after water deprivation. Since the amount of total triacylglycerols was the same in the two groups of rats (Fig. 2) the amount of arachidonic acid containing triacylglycerols was about halved in response to water diuresis.

5. CONCLUSION: THE PHYSIOLOGICAL ROLE OF THE LIPID DROPLETS OF RENOMEDULLARY INTERSTITIAL CELLS

Several possible functions of the interstitial cells of the renal papilla have been suggested, including production of the ground substance, a mechanical function in relation to the countercurrent system, and the production of a hormone. The latter suggestion implies that the lipid droplets are stores of the product itself or of a precursor, since no other obvious storage organelles are present in these cells. From the *in vitro* data presented here it can be calculated that the rate of *de novo* synthesis of papillary droplet triacylglycerols in rat is about 60 nmoles per 24 hr (50 mg papillary tissue) at the tonicity corresponding to the normal state of dehydration. Thus, from a purely quantitative point of view it is extremely unlikely that the droplets are stored products to be secreted. The similarity of the droplets to chylomicrons makes this possibility even more unlikely and thus only the precursor possibility is left open.

The investigations of renal papillary lipogenesis *in vivo* and *in vitro* presented here have not revealed the synthesis of any unique lipid. Thus, these studies do not directly support the proposal that the antihypertensive effects of the renal medulla observed by others result from the production of an organ-specific lipid in this tissue.

On the other hand they point to a specific function of the lipid droplets of the renomedullary interstitial cells that has not been proposed previously, namely, as a depot for fatty acids that are transferable to membrane phospholipids. This local significance of the lipid droplets is rendered probable on the basis of following observations:

1. Fatty acids are apparently shuttling back and forth between phospholipids and triacylglycerols.
2. The tissue has the capacity to trap exogenous fatty acids as triacylglycerols.
3. The turnover rate of papillary phospholipids *in vitro* is fast at low tonicity, compared to the relatively slow turnover rate known for membrane renewal in general.
4. The extracellular osmolality is an important regulator of papillary lipogenesis, as indicated by studies *in vitro* and substantiated by studies *in vivo*.

The observed increase in the turnover rate of papillary phospholipids in response to decreased osmolality is obviously not solely caused by a direct labilization of the papillary membranes, since the synthesis of intracellular triacylglycerols is also increased. The mechanism of the observed effect must involve a regulation of the metabolism of the total tissue glycerolipids, perhaps through changes in the intracellular ionic conditions. Parallel to the increased turnover of papillary glycerolipids, the incorporation into phospholipids of exogenous palmitic acid and arachidonic acid is also increased. However, the fatty acid composition of papillary phospholipids is completely independent of the functional state of the kidney. In water- and saline-diuretic rats the papillary interstitium is approximately isotonic

(Atherton *et al.*, 1968, 1970) and in water-deprived rats it is hypertonic. The fatty acid composition of papillary phospholipids is thus maintained constant over a wide range of osmolality. This constancy of the phospholipid composition independent of the water balance might be essential for the proper functioning of the papillary structures. It was found that the fatty acids stored as triacylglycerols can be used in phospholipid synthesis. In a transition state the droplets therefore ensure an adequate supply of those fatty acids necessary for papillary phospholipid production, independent of which exogenous fatty acids are available.

The increased requirement for fatty acids as a result of the metabolic change that occurs following the transition from an antidiuretic to a diuretic state will obviously be most critical for those fatty acids that are present in plasma at low concentrations (i.e., arachidonic acid). During such a transition a deficit may result unless a depot is present in the form of intracellular lipid droplets. The significance of such a depot function during a steady state is difficult to assess at present, since we do not know the stoichiometry of the cellular uptake and release of fatty acids.

The tissue has a high capacity to elongate arachidonic acid and to incorporate the product (adrenic acid), as well as arachidonic acid, into triacylglycerols. Provided that a retroconversion of adrenic acid to arachidonic acid also occurs in the renal papilla, as has been described by Stoffel *et al.* (1970) for rat liver, this ready elongation suggests the existence of a deposition and trapping mechanism for arachidonic acid.

The ability of the tissue to trap arachidonic acid and adrenic acid as triacylglycerols is apparently regulated by the local osmolality. At high osmolality the capacity of the tissue to elongate and trap arachidonic acid is low and may be inadequate. In this case the concentration of free arachidonic acid would be expected to increase, with a subsequent increase in the production of prostaglandins. Such a mechanism is in full agreement with the observed reciprocal relationship between the turnover rate of glycerolipids and the production of prostaglandins when the osmolality is varied.

REFERENCES

Aeberhard, E., and Menkes, J. H., 1968, Biosynthesis of long chain fatty acids by subcellular particles of mature brain, *J. Biol. Chem.* **243**:3834.

Änggård, E., Bohman, S.-O., Griffin, J. E., Larsson, C., and Maunsbach, A. B., 1972, Subcellular localization of the prostaglandin system in the rabbit renal papilla, *Acta Physiol. Scand.* **84**:231.

Atherton, J. C., Hai, M. A., and Thomas, S., 1968, The time course of changes in renal tissue composition during water diuresis in the rat, *J. Physiol.* **197**:429.

Atherton, J. C., Green, R., and Thomas, S., 1970, Effects of 0.9% saline infusion on urinary and renal tissue composition in the hydropaenic normal and hydrated conscious rat, *J. Physiol.* **210**:45.

Berl, T., Raz, A., Wald, H., Horowitz, J., and Czaczkes, W., 1977, Prostaglandin synthesis inhibition and the action of vasopressin: Studies in man and rat, *Am. J. Physiol.* **232**:F529.

Bernanke, D., and Epstein, F. H., 1965, Metabolism of the renal medulla, *Am. J. Physiol.* **208**:541.

Blomstrand, R., 1966, Fatty acid synthesis in human lymphocytes, *Acta Chem. Scand.* **20**:1122.

Bohman, S.-O., 1974, The ultrastructure of the renal medulla as observed after improved fixation methods, *J. Ultrastruct. Res.* **47**:329.

Bohman, S.-O., and Jensen, P. K. A., 1976, Morphometric studies on the liquid droplets of the interstitial cells of the renal medulla in different states of diuresis, *J. Ultrastruct. Res.* **55**:182.

Bohman, S.-O., and Maunsbach, A. B., 1972, Ultrastructure and biochemcial properties of subcellular fractions from rat renal medulla, *J. Ultrastruct. Res.* **38**:225.

Bojesen, I., 1974a, Quantitative and qualitative analyses of isolated lipid droplets from interstitial cells in renal papillae from various species, *Lipids* **9**:835.

Bojesen, I., 1974b, Interconversion of lipids in renal papillae, Proceedings of the 17th International Conference on the Biochemistry of Lipids, Milan (September 1974), p. 27.

Bojesen, I., 1980a, In vitro and in vivo lipogenesis of the rat renal papillae from glucose, *Biochem. Biophys. Acta* (in press).

Bojesen, I., 1980b, The influence of urea upon lipogenesis in renal papillae of rats, *Lipids* (in press).

Bojesen, I., Bojesen, E., and Capito, K., 1976, *In vitro* and *in vivo* synthesis of long-chain fatty acids from [1-¹⁴C]acetate in the renal papillae from rats, *Biochem. Biophys. Acta* **424**:8.

Brett, D., Howling, D., Morris, L. J., and James, A. T., 1971, Specificity of the fatty acid desaturases: The conversion of saturated to monoenoic acid, *Arch. Biochem. Biophys.* **143**:535.

Bulger, R. E., and Trump, B., 1966, Fine structure of the rat renal papilla, *Am. J. Anat.* **118**:685.

Carney, J. A., and Walker, B. L., 1972, Ovarian lipids from normal and essential fatty acid-deficient rats during oestrus and dioestrus, *Comp. Biochem. Physiol.* **41**:137.

Comai, K., Prose, P., and Farber, S. J., 1974, Correlation of renal medullary prostaglandin content and renal interstitial cell lipid droplets, *Prostaglandins* **6**:375.

Comai, K., Farber, S. J., and Paulsrud, J. R., 1975, Analyses of renal medullary lipid droplets from normal, hydronephrotic and indomethacin treated rabbits, *Lipids* **10**:555.

Danon, A., Knapp, H. R., Oelz, O., and Oates, J. A., 1978, Stimulation of prostaglandin biosynthesis in the renal papilla by hypertonic mediums, *Am. J. Physiol.* **234**:F64.

Diaugustine, R. P., Schaefer, J. M., and Fouts, J. R., 1973, Hepatic lipid droplets; Isolation, morphology and composition, *Biochem. J.* **132**:323.

Dietz, R., Mast, G. J., Schomig, A., Luth, J. B., and Rascher, W., 1978, Reversal of renal hypertension: Effects on renin, salt and water balance, *Klin. Wochenschr.* **56**(Suppl. I):23.

Elsbach, P., and Farrow, S., 1969, Metabolsim of phospholipids by phagocytic cells IV. Cellular triacylglycerols as a source of fatty acids for lecithin synthesis during phagocytosis, *Biochim. Biophys. Acta* **176**:438.

Fejes-Tóth, G., Magyar, A., and Walter, J., 1977, Renal response to vasopressin after inhibition of prostaglandin synthesis, *Am. J. Physiol.* **232**:F416.

Gidez, L. I., and Feller, E., 1969, Effect of the stress of unilateral adrenalectomy on the depletion of individual cholesteryl esters in the rat adrenal, *J. Lipid Res.* **10**:656.

Guder, W. G., and Schmidt, U., 1976, Enzymatic organization of carbohydrate metabolism along the nephron, in: *Proceedings of the 6th International Congress on Nephrology, Florence 1975* (S. Giovannetti, V. Bonomini, and G. D'Amico, eds), Karger, Basel, p. 187.

Joist, J. H., Dolezel, G., Lloyd, J. V., and Mustard, J. F., 1976, Phospholipid transfer between plasma and platelets *in vitro*, *Blood* **48**:199.

Kean, E. L., Adams, P. H., Winters, R. W., and Davies, R. E., 1961, Energy metabolism of the renal medulla, *Biochim. Biophys. Acta* **54**:474.

Kibel, G., Heilhecker, A., and van Bruchhausen, F., 1976, Lipid associated with bovine kidney glomerular basement membranes, *Biochem. J.* **155**:535.

Lee, J. B., Vance, V. K., and Cahill, G. F., Jr., 1962, Metabolism of ^{14}C-labelled substrates by rabbit kidney cortex and medulla, *Am. J. Physiol.* **203**:27.

Lee, J. B., Covino, B. G., Takman, B. H., and Smith, E. R., 1965, Renomedullary vasodepressor substance medullin: Isolation, chemical characterization and physiological properties, *Circ. Res.* **17**:57.

Limas, C., Limas, C. J., and Gesell, M. S., 1976, Effects of indomethacin on renomedullary interstitial cells, *Lab. Invest.* **34**:522.

Lo Chang, T., and Sweeley, C. C., 1963, Characterization of lipids from canine adrenal glands, *Biochemistry* **2**:592.

Morrison, A. B., and Schneeberger-Keeley, E. E., 1969, The phagocytic role of renal medullary interstitial cells and the effect of potassium deficiency on this function, *Nephron* **6**:584.

Muirhead, E. E., Leach, B. E., Byers, L. W., Brooks, B., Daniels, E. G., and Hinman, J. W., 1971, Antihypertensive neutral renomedullary lipids (ANRL), in: *Kidney Hormones* (J. W. Fisher, ed.), Academic Press, London, p. 485.

Nissen, H. M., 1967, On the lipid droplets in renal interstitial cells I. A histochemical study, *Z. Zellforsch. Mikrosk. Anat.* **83**:76.

Nissen, H. M., 1968*a*, On lipid droplets in renal interstitial cells II. A histological study on the number of droplets in salt depletion and acute salt repletion, *Z. Zellforsch. Mikrosk. Anat.* **85**:483.

Nissen, H. M., 1968*b*, On lipid droplets in renal interstitial cells III. A histological study on the number of droplets during hydration and dehydration, *Z. Zellforsch. Mikrosk. Anat.* **92**:52.

Nissen, H. M., and Bojesen, I., 1969, On lipid droplets in renal interstitial cells IV. Isolation and identification, *Z. Zellforsch. Mikrosk. Anat.* **97**:274.

Oshima, M., and Carpenter, M. P., 1968, The lipid composition of the prepubertal and adult rat testis, *Biochim. Biophys. Acta* **152**:479.

Osvaldo-Decima, L., 1973, Ultrastructure of the lower nephron, in: *Handbook of Physiology*, Section 8: *Renal Physiology* (J. Orloff and R. W. Berliner, eds.), American Physiological Society, Washington, D. C., pp. 81–102.

Peterson, J. A., and Rubin, H., 1970, The exchange of phospholipids between cultured chick embryo fibroblasts as observed by autoradiography, *Exp. Cell Res.* **60**:383.

Sbarra, A. S., Shirley, W., Baumstock, J. S., 1963, Effect of osmolality on phagocytosis, *J. Bacteriol.* **85**:306.

Sen, S., Smeby, R. R., and Bumpus, F. M., 1967, Isolation of a phospholipid renin inhibitor from kidney, *Biochemistry* **6**:1572.

Stoffel, W., and Ach, K. L., 1964, Der Stoffwechsel der ungesättigten Fettsäuren II. Eigenschaften des kettenverlängernden Enzyms zur Frage der Biohydrogenierung der ungesättigten Fettsäuren, *Z. Physiol. Chem.* **377**:123.

Stoffel, W., Ecker, W., Assad, H., and Sprecher, H., 1970, Enzymatic studies on the mechanism of the retroconversion of C_{22}-polyenoic fatty acids to their C_{20}-homologues, *Hoppe-Seylers Z. Physiol. Chem.* **351**:1545.

Szokol, M., and Soltész, M. B., 1973, Histochemical study on the oxidative enzymes of the interstitial cells of the renal medulla in rats, *Acta Histochem.* **46**:120.

Takayasu, K., Okuda, K., and Yoshikawa, I., 1970, Fatty acid composition of human and rat adrenal lipids: Occurence of w-6 docosatrienoic acid in human adrenal cholesterol ester, *Lipids* **5**:743.

Tsai, P. Y., and Geyer, R. P., 1978, Effect of exogenous fatty acids on the retention of phospholipid acyl groups by mouse L. fibroblasts, *Biochim. Biophys. Acta* **528**:344.

Whereat, A. F., 1971, Fatty acid biosynthesis in aorta and heart, in: *Advances in Lipid Research 9* (R. Paoletti and D. Kritchevsky, eds.), Academic Press, New York and London, pp. 119–159.

Yatsu, F. M., and Moss, S., 1970, Brain fatty acid elongation and multiple sclerosis, *Nature* **227**:1132.

Zilversmit, D. B., 1969, Chylomicrons, in: *Structural and Functional Aspects of Lipoproteins in Living Systems* (E. Tria and A. M. Scame, eds.), Academic Press, London and New York, p. 346.

Zusman, R. M., and Keiser, H. R., 1977, Prostaglandin biosynthesis by rabbit renomedullary interstitial cells in tissue culture: Stimulation by angiotensin II, bradykinin and arginine vasopressin, *J. Clin. Invest.* **60**:215.

CHAPTER 7

Alterations in the Renal Medullary and Papillary Interstitial Cells in Experimental and Spontaneous (Essential) Hypertension

ANIL K. MANDAL and JOHN A. NORDQUIST

1. INTRODUCTION

It is reasonably well established that renal medulla and papilla of animals (rat, dog, rabbit) contain vasodepressor or antihypertensive substances that consistently reduce blood pressure in hypertensive animals (Muirhead, 1976). Much indirect evidence points toward the presence of similar vasodepressor substance(s) in human kidneys (Muehrcke *et al.*, 1970; Prezyna *et al.*, 1973; Mandal *et al.*, 1979). This hypothesis is further supported by the finding of large amounts of prostaglandins in human renal papilla (Vance *et al.*, 1973). However, the question of where in the papilla the vasodepressor substances are synthesized and/or stored has yet to be completely resolved. Within the papilla exist many interstitial cells that appear to be secretory, since they contain dilated endoplasmic reticulum, ribosomes, and conspicuous granules. These renal papillary interstitial cells (RIC) are considered by many to be the most probable site for the formation of vasodepressor substance(s). Furthermore, the location of the RIC, juxtaposed as they are between the tubules and the peritubular capillaries, strongly supports this proposed function.

ANIL K. MANDAL • Department of Medicine, Veterans Administration Medical Center and University of Oklahoma College of Medicine, Oklahoma City, Oklahoma 73104. JOHN A. NORDQUIST • Renal Electron Microscopy Laboratory, Veterans Administration Medical Center, Oklahoma City, Oklahoma 73104.

The RIC are present in decreasing frequency from the inner to the outer aspect of the kidney. Thus, the RIC are abundant in the papilla, far less abundant in the medulla, and rarely, if ever, observed in the cortex. The number of RIC, however, varies from species to species; it is far greater in rat, for instance, than in dog or man. The RIC populations among different types of rats appear to be similar. The striking anatomic appearance of the RIC in rat has stimulated investigators to study their functional characteristics, especially in relation to hypertension.

2. EXPERIMENTAL HYPERTENSIONS

Since the RIC as a whole, or their granular contents, were considered to be the source of vasodepressor or antihypertensive substance(s), several studies were initiated in recent years to observe the effect of induced hypertension on the RIC and their granular contents.

Rat kidneys were often selected for study due to the presence of a solitary papilla, which provides a representative sample of RIC and granularity.

2.1. Salt–Doca Hypertension (Muehrcke *et al.*, 1969)

Eighty Sprague–Dawley male rats weighing 125–175 g and housed in individual cages were divided into eight groups (A through H) consisting of 10 rats in each group. All animals were fed Purina Rat Chow *ad libitum*. Groups A and E served as controls. The rats from Groups E through H had undergone unilateral nephrectomy. Group B rats were given 4% NaCl solution to drink; Group C rats received subcutaneous injections of 3 mg desoxycorticosterone trimethylacetate (DOCA) daily, except Sunday; Group D rats had 4% NaCl solution to drink, and received subcutaneous injections of 3 mg DOCA daily, except Sunday. The rats of Groups F, G, and H had treatments identical to those described for Groups B, C, and D, respectively.

Observations were made on the general appearance of the animals together with body weight and blood pressure. Systolic blood pressures were recorded, using a small-animal blood pressure cuff–transducer on quiescent rats, several times during the observation period and also on the day of sacrifice. At two-week intervals, 2 animals from each group were anesthetized with ether; the abdomen was then incised and the kidneys were removed. Both kidneys were cut open transversely. From one kidney, a wedge section from the cortex to the papilla was fixed in Helly's solution for light microscopy (LM). From another kidney, the papillary apex (tip) was fixed in ice-cold 2% glutaraldehyde for electron microscopy (EM). [For

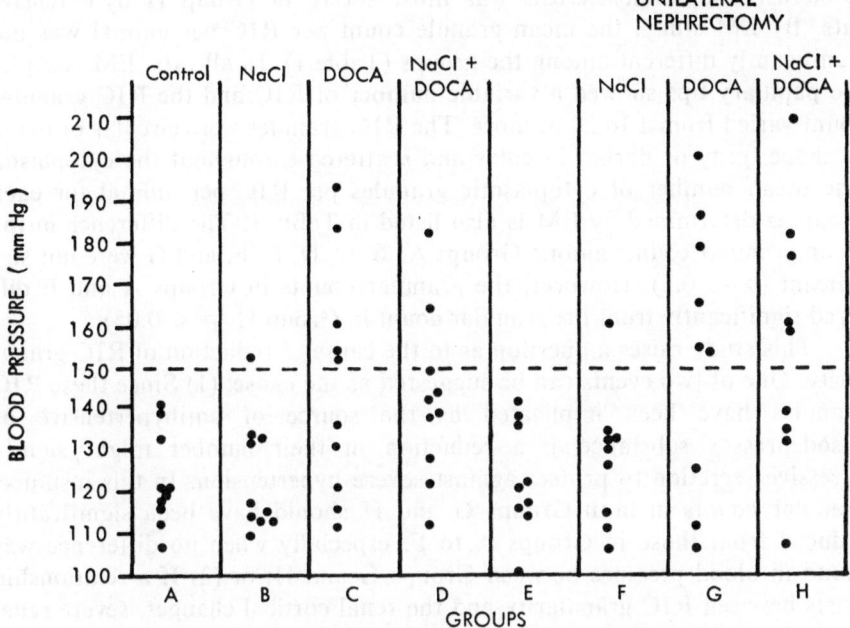

FIGURE 1. Scattergram of systolic blood pressures in rats at the time of sacrifice. The uni-lateral nephrectomized rats given DOCA (Group G) and both DOCA and saline solution (Group H) had a higher incidence of hypertension than the rats in Groups C and D. [Reproduced from Muehrcke *et al.* (1969) by the kind permission of the editor.]

details of the techniques mentioned throughout this chapter for the fixation of tissue, and the sectioning and staining of the sections for LM and EM studies, see Chapter 2 of Mandal (1979).] Granular counts were done in 100 RIC from methylene blue–azure II-stained 0.5-μm sections. Thin sections were studied using an RCA EMU 3H electron microscope. At least 100–200 RIC were photographed. Fifty whole RIC were selected randomly for quantitation of their granular contents.

Observations were made on all rats during a period of 33–100 days. Blood pressure measurements at the time of sacrifice are shown in Fig. 1. All rats in Group A remained normotensive; one rat in Group B had hypertension; five of nine rats (55%) in Group C had hypertension; two rats in Group D had hypertension; all rats in Group E were normotensive; one rat in Group F had hypertension; eight of nine rats (88%) in Group G had hypertension; and five of nine (55%) in Group H had hypertension.* Histopathologically, while the kidneys appeared normal in Group A rats, they exhibited varying degrees of abnormalities in rats from Group C through Group H. The abnormalities consisted of glomerulosclerosis and arterio-

* One rat in each of Groups C, G, and H died.

152 ANIL K. MANDAL and JOHN A. NORDQUIST

losclerosis. Arteriolosclerosis was most severe in Group H hypertensive rats. By LM study, the mean granule count per RIC per animal was not significantly different among the groups (Table 1). In all rats, EM study of the papillary tips showed a variable number of RIC and the RIC granular count varied from 1 to 20 or more. The RIC granules were circular or ovoid in shape, gray or darker in color and scattered throughout the cytoplasm. The mean number of cytoplasmic granules per RIC per animal for each group as determined by EM is also listed in Table 1. The difference in the mean granular counts among Groups A, B, C, D, E, F, and G were not significant ($p < 0.2$). However, the granular counts in Groups A and E differed significantly from the granular count in Group H ($p < 0.05$).

This study raises a question as to the cause of reduction of RIC granularity. One of two events can be suggested as the cause: (1) Since these RIC granules have been implicated as the source of antihypertensive or vasodepressor substance(s), a reduction in their number might signify excessive secretion to protect against severe hypertension. In this instance, granular counts in both Groups G and H should have been significantly reduced from those in Groups A to F, especially when no difference was found in blood pressure between Groups G and H; or (2) If a relationship exists between RIC granularity and the renal cortical changes, severe renal cortical derangements accompanying hypertension can be associated with reduction of RIC granularity. Group G did not demonstrate renal cortical changes as severe as those seen in Group H. It is possible then that the decreased RIC granularity in Group H is secondary to advanced glomerular and vascular disease.

TABLE 1

Mean Counts of Cytoplasmic Granularity in Rat Renal Medullary Interstitial Cells[a]

Experimental group	Light microscopy mean count of cytoplasmic granularity per interstitial cell per animal	Electron microscopy mean count of osmiophilic granularity per interstitial cell per animal
A	6.4 ± 0.82	8.8 ± 1.2*
B	6.4 ± 2.5	7.9 ± 1.1
C	4.8 ± 1.11	9.5 ± 0.9
D	5.6 ± 2.57	6.7 ± 1.0
E	9.3 ± 3.8	8.2 ± 1.2*
F	5.8 ± 1.3	9.4 ± 1.6
G	4.7 ± 1.22	6.5 ± 1.8
H	5.0 ± 1.73	5.6 ± 0.8*

[a] Reproduced from Muehrcke et al. (1969) by the kind permission of the editor of the *Journal of Laboratory and Clinical Medicine*.
* Groups A and E vs. Group H, $p < 0.05$.

Although half of the animals in Group C developed hypertension, the renal parenchymal changes were comparatively mild and the mean RIC granularity was not different from that of the control group. It was concluded from this study that the decreased granularity of the renal medullary or papillary interstitial cells in rats appeared secondary to advanced glomerular and vasular diseases and the consequent decrease in medullary blood flow.

2.2. "Postsalt" Hypertension (Tobian *et al.*, 1969)

Hypertension was induced in 21 male weanling rats by feeding them a dry diet containing 8% NaCl and tap water *ad libitum* for 7 weeks or more and by unilateral kidney removal sometime during the treatment period. Thereafter all rats sustained hypertension even on normal diets for 3 months. After three months, these rats were sacrificed and their kidneys were removed. Small portions from the centers of the papillae were fixed in 2% osmium tetroxide, dehydrated in alcoholic solution and embedded in Epon. Sections of 0.5 μm thickness were cut and stained with methylene blue and azure II and the RIC granules were counted using LM. In addition, determinations of sodium and urea concentrations in the papilla were made. The hypertensive rats had significant reductions of RIC granularity compared to that in normotensive control rats (79 vs. 136 per 100 square counts; $p < 0.001$). The granule counts correlated well with sodium and urea concentrations of the papilla in both hypertensive and normotensive rats. The papilla concentrations of sodium and urea in the hypertensive rats were significantly lower than those in the normotensive control rats and, because papillary granular counts are commensurate with sodium and urea gradients of the papilla, the granular reductions in hypertensive rats can be considered secondary to functional changes in the papilla or hypertension.

2.3. Goldblatt Hypertension (Ishii and Tobian, 1969)

In this experiment, 38 rats were made hypertensive by constriction of the unilateral renal artery. The contralateral kidney remained untouched. The normotensive control rats had a sham operation on the unilateral renal artery. The technique for the study of RIC granularity was essentially the same as that described for the postsalt hypertension study. The granular counts in the paired kidneys in both hypertensive and normotensive rats are shown in Table 2. It will be found that the average granular count for the untouched kidneys in the hypertensive rat was significantly lower than that for the untouched kidneys of normotensive control rats. The average granule count for the clipped kidneys in the hypertensive rats also was significantly lower than that for the sham-operated kidneys in the normoten-

TABLE 2

Counts of Interstitial Cell Granules in Rats with Goldblatt Hypertension and in Normotensive Control Rats[a,b]

Group	Right kidneys ("untouched" kidneys)	Left kidneys ("clipped" or sham-operated kidneys)
Hypertensive rats ($n = 38$)	99 ± 5.6	115 ± 4.9
Normotensive rats ($n = 19$)	133 ± 3.6	136 ± 5.7
p Value[c]	0.001	0.02

[a] Reproduced from Ishii and Tobian (1969) by the kind permission of Dr. L. Tobian.

[b] Granule counts per 100 tissue squares are shown as a mean $\pm$ SEM. Each tissue square represents 711.1 2 square units on the surface of the cut section.

[c] p Values show the significance of the difference between the hypertensive and normotensive groups, using Student's t test.

sive control rats. Since the granular mass in both untouched and clipped kidneys of the hypertensive rats was significantly decreased from that in the normotensive control rats, this decrease can be attributed to hypertension. This finding is further supported by the evidence of nephrosclerosis in the untouched kidneys and elevated blood urea nitrogen in the hypertensive rats.

Because the number of papillary granules decreased consistently in all types of experimentally induced hypertension, it becomes apparent that the granular reduction is secondary to hypertension. The probabilities of a relationship between granular alterations and hypertension will be discussed later in this chapter. For the moment, it seems reasonable to conclude that quantitative or qualitative changes in RIC granular morphology may be a reflection of the functional derangement of the papilla resulting from hypertension and/or arteriologlomerular changes.

2.4.   Spontaneous Hypertension (Spontaneously Hypertensive Rat)

2.4.1.   *Ultrastructural Analysis of Renal Papillary Interstitial Cell (Mandal et al., 1974)*

The RIC in eight spontaneously hypertensive rats (SHR) were studied using electron microscopy for quantitation of the granular counts. The results were compared with those in six age- and sex-matched normotensive Wistar rats (NR).

Immediately after direct arterial pressures were recorded under light ether anesthesia, the rats were killed and their kidneys removed. The papilla was dissected from each kidney and cut into two horizontal halves from base to tip. Each half was then cut into three pieces representing basal, tip, and midpapillary areas. Each piece was then fixed in 4% glutaraldehyde. Only one kidney from each rat was studied. The uniform areas of maximum cellularity from methylene blue–azure II-stained 0.5-μm sections were selected for further study by EM. In general, this area represented the core of the papilla rather than the periphery and was from the tip or middle third of the sectioned papilla rather than the basal third. Thin sections (300–400 Å) were studied with an RCA EMU 3G electron microscope. EM study was not done if a patchy distribution of RIC was observed in the so-called thick sections by LM.

At least 50 whole RIC from each rat were studied at random. The cytoplasmic granules of the RIC were quantitatively analyzed according to the following criteria: average number of granules per RIC (counting only those cells with granules), number of RIC with more than 10 granules per cell (hypergranular cells), and number of agranular cells, including cytoplasmic processes (cells completely devoid of granules). All SHR were hypertensive; their average mean arterial pressure of 159 mm Hg was significantly ($p < 0.001$) higher than the average mean arterial pressure of 114 mm Hg in NR.

Using EM, each RIC was evaluated with respect to size, shape, cytoplasmic constituents (including granularity), and cytoplasmic processes. Other than the reduced granularity in the SHR, there was no appreciable difference in the cellular morphology between groups. The average number of granules per RIC in SHR ranged from 2.1 to 7.7; the granularity of the NR ranged from 5.0 to 8.4 ($p < 0.05$). Furthermore, the NR had more hypergranular RIC than did the SHR ($p < 0.05$) (Table 3).

This study demonstrated that the SHR has a significantly greater number of agranular RIC, a lesser number of RIC with excess granularity, and a lesser average number of granules per RIC. One may speculate that the reduced RIC granularity may result from genetic factors in these SHR; however, this explanation seems unlikely since the hypogranularity was also observed in rats with experimentally induced hypertension. It therefore seems likely that the reduced granularity in these disparate types of hypertension may be a result, rather than a cause, of the elevated arterial pressure.

TABLE 3

Analysis of Renal Papillary Interstitial Cell Granularity[a,b]

Index	Normal Wistar	Spontaneously hypertensive
Average number of granules per cell	7.1 ± 0.49	4.6 ± 0.68*
Percentage of hypergranular cells	16.7 ± 4.7	6.2 ± 2.4*
Percentage of agranular cells	7.9 ± 2.6	30.0 ± 7.2*

[a] Reproduced from Mandal et al. (1974) by the kind permission of the editor.
[b] Values are means ± SEM.
* $p < 0.05$.

2.4.2. Morphological Study of the Renal Papillary Granule: Analysis in the Interstitial Cell and in the Interstitium (Mandal et al., 1975)

Renal papillae from 24 male rats, 14 NR and 10 SHR, averaging 20 weeks of age, were studied. All rats weighed 200–250 g and were fed on standard Purina Rat Chow. In 16 rats (8 NR and 8 SHR), direct arterial pressures were recorded under light ether anesthesia, after which their kidneys were removed. The entire papillae were immediately dissected from the kidneys, cut into 0.5- to 1-mm pieces, and fixed in iced 4% glutaraldehyde. In four rats (2 NR and 2 SHR), the left kidney was perfused with 6% glutaraldehyde prior to removal according to the technique reported by Osvaldo and Latta (1966). All four kidneys became uniformly blanched and rock hard after glutaraldehyde perfusion. After removal of the kidneys, their papillae were scooped out and cut into 0.5- to 1-mm pieces and then fixed further in iced 6% glutaraldehyde. In order to evaluate the durabiltiy of these granules, eight papillae from four NR kidneys were homogenized in a Potter–Elvehjem homogenizer and then centrifuged at 6000 rpm for 30 min. The sediment was fixed, processed, and embedded in a way similar to that for intact tissues. The ultrathin sections were stained with: (1) uranyl acetate and lead citrate (UA + LC); (2) freshly prepared 2% aqueous solution of phosphotungstic acid (PTA) in highly acid (pH 1.4–2.2), neutral (pH 6.8), and highly alkaline (pH 10–12) media for 10 min; and (3) 1% periodic acid and diluted silver methenamine (2 parts silver to 8 parts water) (PASM). The granular morphology was studied and the following features were noted: appearance, shape, size, presence or absence of membrane, and other morphologic alterations. In four NR and four SHR, the total number of intracellular and extracellular granules was quantified to determine the difference in the total and differential types of granularity between the two groups. All the blocks from each renal papilla in four NR and four SHR were studied. In order to identify the specificity of PTA for protein material, human serum albumin was similarly treated with PTA (pH 6.8) for 2 min and then studied electron microscopically.

Twenty-four-hour urinary collections were made from four NR and four SHR while the animals were housed in metabolic cages. The urine was filtered and the filtrate was then centrifuged. Smears were made from both the sediment and the supernatant and examined by LM after staining with toluidine blue and methylene blue and azure II. The sediment and the supernatant were stained with PTA and examined by EM. The total and differential counts of the renal papillary granules in NR and SHR are shown in Table 4.

Characteristics of Granules in Intact Papillae. In UA + LC-stained sections, three types of granules were observed in all rats: layered, homo-

TABLE 4

Differential Count of Total Renal Papillary Granules (per Papilla per Rat) in Four Normotensive and Four Spontaneously Hypertensive Rats[a,b]

Group	Total number of granules	Layered granules	Homogeneously dark granules	Gray granules
Normotensive Wistar rats	3881	2259	1589	32.5
	(822)	(1223)	(1044)	(22)
Spontaneously hypertensive rats	2659	1736	374	550.0
	(642)	(680)	(213)	(59.5)
p Values	0.10	0.10	0.10	0.001

[a] Reproduced from Mandal *et al.* (1975) by the kind permission of the editor.
[b] Values are means (± SEM).

geneously dark, and gray (Figs. 2–4*). The layered granules comprised 58% and 65% of the total granularity in the NR and SHR, respectively (Table 4); they were characterized by a large central core of deep electron-dense (dark) material surrounded by a thick rim of less electron-dense (gray) material. The outer border was smooth and dark in a large proportion of these granules (triple-layered) but fuzzy or irregular in a smaller number (double-layered). The homogeneously dark granules demonstrated no layering and a less distinct outer border, comprising 41% and 14% of the total granularity in the NR and SHR, respectively (Table 4). The gray granules demonstrated an irregular or crenated border. They constituted 0.84% of the total granularity in NR but 21% in SHR ($p < 0.001$) (Table 4). In PTA-stained sections, the interstitial cell membrane and its cytoplasmic constituents (other than granules) were poorly visible. In a neutral medium, the granules generally appeared homogeneously dark but without any contrast. However, in an acid medium (pH 1.4–2.2) the granules were electron dense and exhibited some layering, which was never as conspicuous as when stained with UA + LC. After PASM staining, almost all the granules in NR and most granules in SHR were found to consist of a network of heavy silver deposits, appearing as dark beads. The SHR had a greater number of granules with a network of fine silver deposits (Fig. 5).

All intracellular granules varied in size between 0.76 and 1.24 μm in NR and between 0.71 and 1.13 μm in SHR. In some SHR, large intracellular granules were often encountered, which ranged in size from 0.3 to 5.7 μm with an average size of 2 μm (Fig. 6). The layered granules were almost always spherical but a variety of other shapes were also observed. The gray granules were mostly irregular. The layered granules frequently demonstrated an interwoven network pattern, a budding appearance, a

* Figures 2–13 appear on an insert following page 160.

peripheral fusion, and an interconnection through the central dark part. Also frequently observed were elongation and margination of the granules toward the cellular membrane (Fig. 7a,b). In some, ballooning of a portion of the cellular membrane overlying a granule, fusion of the cellular and granular membranes (Fig. 7a), extrusion of a granule from the cell (Fig. 7b), and free granules overlying craters of the cellular membranes were also noted. All these findings seemed to indicate the liberation of intracellular granules into the free interstitium. Mitochondria were observed adhering to the intracellular granules and not infrequently enveloping them with their membranes (Fig. 8).

A variable number of granules were found extracellularly in all intact papillae. These granules were surrounded by neither cytoplasmic constituents nor cellular membranes and were located adjacent to the IC (Figs. 2, 9a), along the tubular and capillary basement membranes, or inside the tubular and capillary lumina (Fig. 9b). The layered granules comprised 60% and 57% of the total free granularity in NR and SHR, respectively. The remaining granules of both groups were, for the most part, homogeneously dark. No free gray granules were seen in NR but they were occasionally observed in SHR. With the exception of size, ultrastructural characteristics of the free granules were identical with those of the granules found intracellularly. The free granules appeared slightly larger in size. Their sizes varied between 0.9 and 1.7 μm in NR and between 1.0 and 1.9 μm in SHR. However, the difference in average size between intracellular granules and free granules was not significant.

In the homogenized papillae, granules were mostly layered, rarely homogeneously dark, and never gray (Fig. 10). Ultrastructurally, the granules were identical to those in the intact papillae. Albumin appeared (PTA stain) as homogeneously dark spherical droplets, although they were much smaller than any of the papillary granules.

LM of the urinary specimens revealed dark clumps of granules in SHR only. The granules were similar to those observed in renal papillary sections by LM. EM revealed many layered granules with irregular borders in all four SHR; these were seen only occasionally in one NR (Fig. 11).

3. VALUE OF ELECTRON MICROSCOPY IN DEFINING THE CHEMICAL NATURE OF PAPILLARY INTERSTITIAL GRANULES

The various ultrastructural appearances of the granules, e.g., layered, homogeneously dark, and gray, suggest possible lipid, protein, and glycoprotein chemical moieties in these granules. The binding of osmium to lipid, especially unsaturated fatty acids, renders them dark and may explain the positive visualization of unstained granules as well as their variable appearances in highly contrasting UA + LC-stained sections. Thus, from the studies mentioned previously, it appears that the layered granules may be composed of unsaturated (central electron-dense core) and saturated (outer less-electron-dense rim) fatty acids. Following the same logic, the homogeneously dark granules may be composed of only unsaturated fatty acids, and the gray ones may contain only saturated fatty acids.

Reports of studies on isolated lipid droplets having ultrastructural features similar to those in the intact papillae and with chemical compositions consisting of triglycerides; unsaturated fatty acids; long-chain saturated fatty acids, including arachidonic acid; and cholesterol ester (Änggård et al., 1972; Nissen and Bojesen, 1969) offer supportive evidence for these ultrastructural assessments. Identical electron-dense granules inside the RIC grown in tissue culture and the identification of neutral and acidic lipids in the cellular extract further reinforce the concept of a lipoid nature for the RIC granules. Although most evidence implicates lipids as the major granular constituent, it is difficult to exclude the presence of some protein and glycoprotein due to the intense staining observed with acidic PTA and PASM, respectively (Glauert, 1965; Hayat, 1970). The identification of small amounts of protein in the isolated lipid droplets from homogenized renal papillae (Bohman and Maunsbach, 1972) tends to support this latter ultrastructural conclusion.

4. RELATIONSHIP OF RENAL PAPILLARY INTERSTITIAL GRANULES TO ESSENTIAL (SPONTANEOUS) HYPERTENSION

Notwithstanding some disagreements among investigators, it can be stated with fairness and reasonable certainty that the renal papillary granules interact in the physiopathological mechanism of hypertension. Almost all investigators found reduced granularity in both rats with experimentally induced hypertension and spontaneously hypertensive rats (Ishii and Tobian, 1969; Tobian et al., 1969; Muehrcke et al., 1969; Mandal et al., 1974, 1975; Jurukova and Somova, 1976). However, the mechanism of reduction of the granularity in hypertensive states is still unclear. It is largely assumed that the granular reduction is secondary to hypertension. At a glance, this seems right, but it is difficult to explain how hypertension reduces the papillary interstitial cellular granularity. A variety of observations and conjectures have been made in this regard.

Papillary ischemia has been suggested as a cause of changes in the papillary interstitium. While Ganguli et al. (1977) found significant decrease in renal papillary plasma flow in SHR, Solez et al. (1976) showed renal papillary plasma flow to be higher in nonhydronephrotic SHR than in hydronephrotic SHR. These two observations would seem contradictory.

Limas and Limas (1977) found that SHR had increased granule counts with mild to moderate degrees of renal arteriolar sclerosis but decreased granularity with severe and extensive vascular lesions. We have not studied, and neither is there any published report on, the status of the papillary IC granularity of old SHR (>52 weeks), which uniformly demonstrate severe arteriologlomerular lesions. Surely, interstitial cellular granularity was reduced in salt–DOCA hypertensive rats that demonstrated extensive cortical lesions. Although there is a good probability that arteriolo- glomerular lesions resulting from hypertension may induce papillary ischemia and consequent granular reduction, more convincing data are necessary to confirm this preliminary observation.

It has been hypothesized that the SHR secrete more antihypertensive material(s) in an effort to reduce arterial pressure (Tobian and Azar, 1971). Thus, if the granules are the source of vasodepressor substances, a reduced granularity even in young SHR may be attributed to this adaptive mechanism. To generate support for this hypothesis an experiment was initiated, which did demonstrate that the hypertensive rat renal papilla secretes significantly more prostaglandins than does the normotensive rat renal papilla (Tobian and Azar, 1971).

5. RELATIONSHIP OF INTERSTITIAL CELLULAR GRANULES TO RENOMEDULLARY VASODEPRESSOR SUBSTANCES

Two major types of vasodepressor substances have been isolated from renomedullary extracts: (1) the antihypertensive neutral renomedullary lipid (ANRL) of Muirhead, and (2) acidic lipid or prostaglandins. The papillary granules, by virtue of their lipoid characteristics, and their abundance both inside RIC and in extracellular locations, would seem to be a major source of neutral lipid.

Likewise, these granular lipids appear to be an important source of prostaglandin synthesis. This hypothesis is supported by experiments *in vivo* and *in vitro* on lipogenesis (see Chapter 6) and by observations of granular alterations following indomethacin treatment (see Chapter 5). Although the morphologic observations are not so much in agreement regarding the decrease or increase in the number of granules, there is a better concordance as far as the size of the granules is concerened. This may mean that indome- thacin, by inhibiting prostaglandin synthesis, makes the granules adynamic, and they may then imbibe water and undergo enlargement. However, there are studies that argue against the granules as a possible source of prosta- glandins. Änggård et al. (1972) analyzed subcellular fractions of the

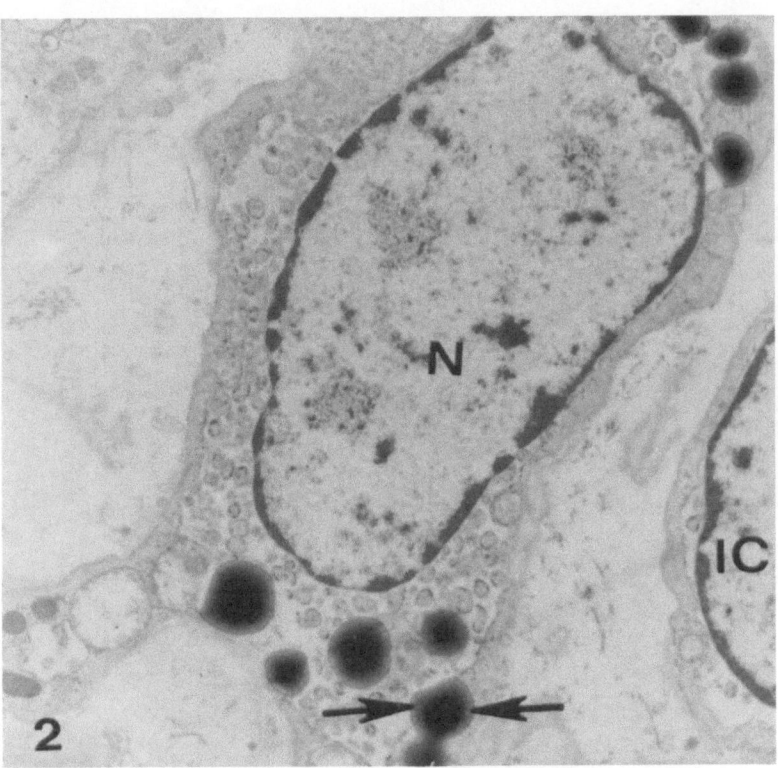

FIGURE 2. An interstitial cell shows a large nucleus (N) occupying three fourths of the cell surface area and several conspicuous layered granules. The central electron-dense material and the thick peripheral rim of lighter material give these granules a very conspicuous appearance. One of the granules (arrows) has marginated toward the cell membrane. note part of an adjacent interstitial cell (IC). From a spontaneously hypertensive rat (UA + LC ×8000).

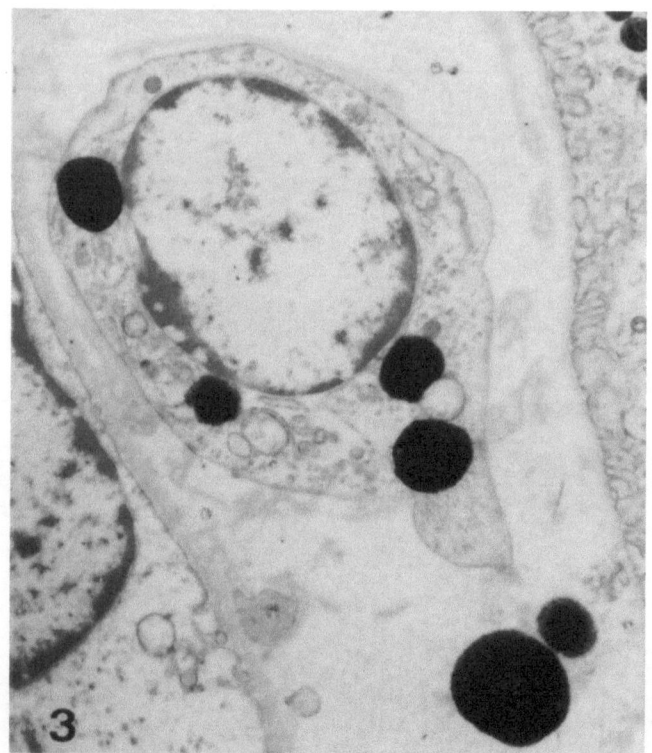

FIGURE 3. This interstitial cell contains homogeneously dark granules. Note free granules identical to those intracellularly, and located adjacent to the cell. The cell membrane reveals no disruptive changes. From a normotensive Wistar rat (UA + LC ×8000).

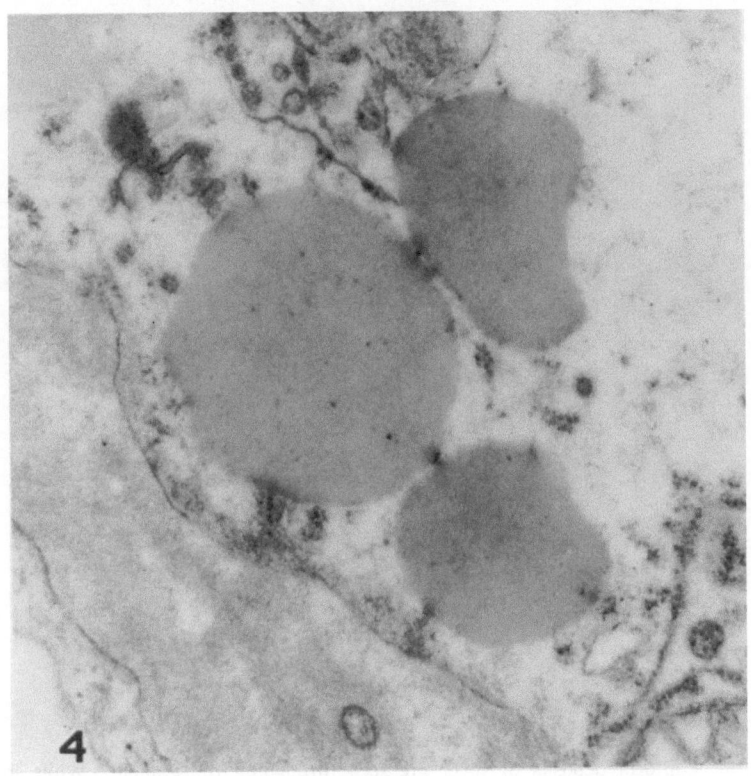

FIGURE 4. Gray granules within an interstitial cell reveal irregular crenated margins. From a spontaneously hypertensive rat (UA + LC ×26,000).

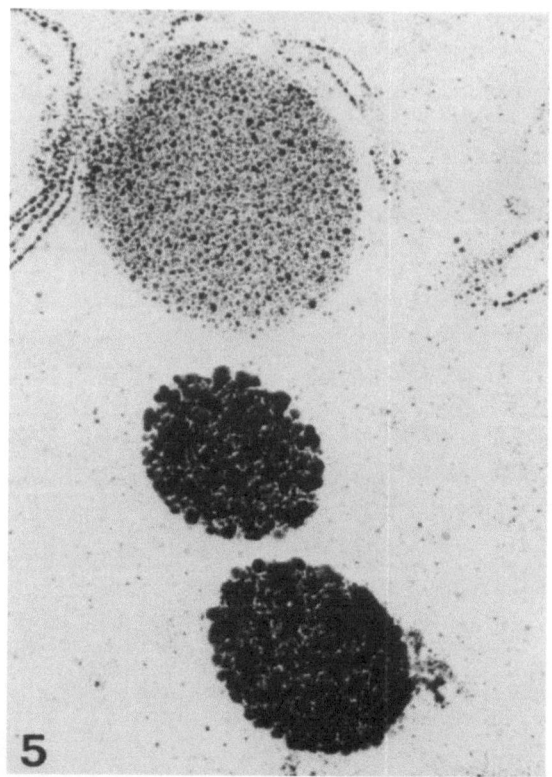

FIGURE 5. Uniform deposits of silver are seen throughout the granules. While in some granules the deposits are fine (largest granule at the top), large beads of silver are seen in other granules (smaller granules at the bottom). From a normotensive Wistar rat (PASM ×26,000).

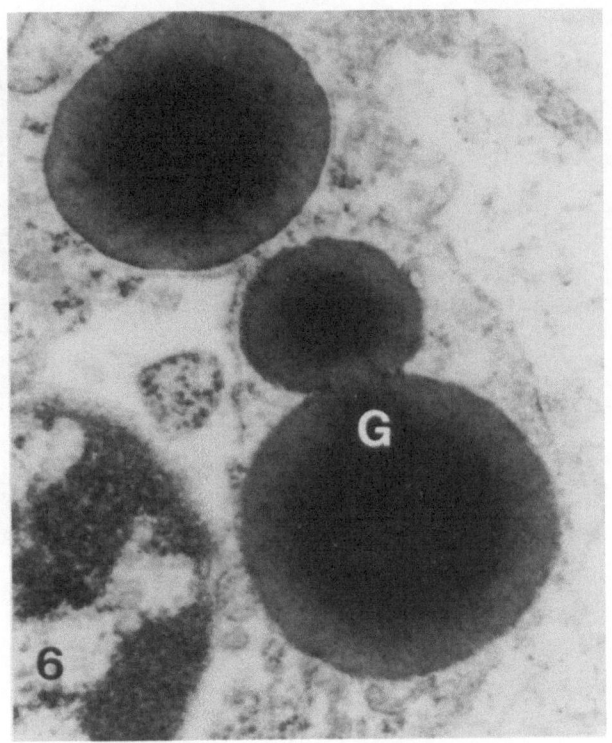

FIGURE 6. Very large granules within the interstitital cell. Note budding appearance of a granule (G). From a normotensive Wistar rat (UA + LC ×26,000).

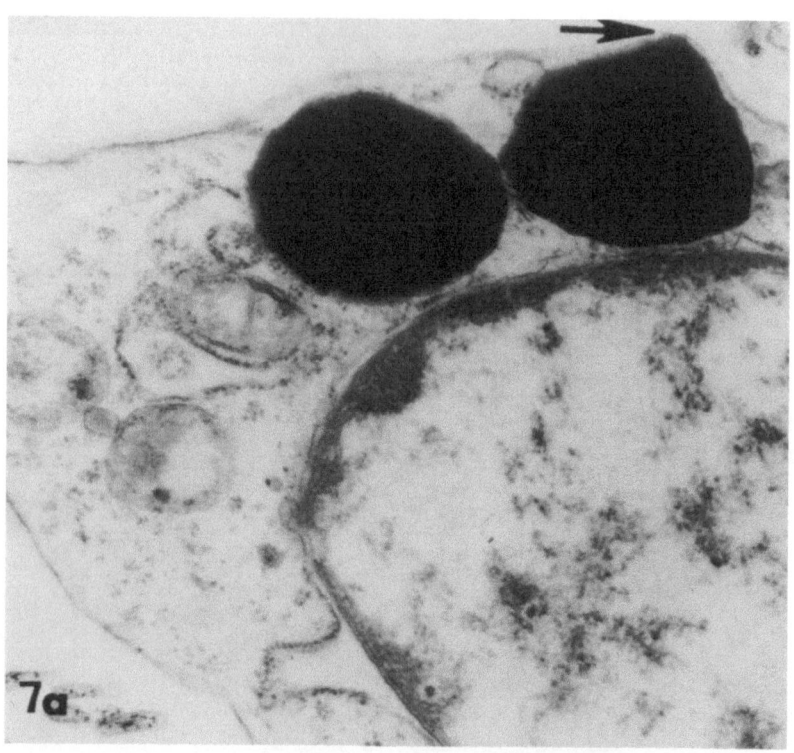

FIGURE 7. Possible mechanisms of extrusion of intracellular granules into the interstitium. (a) Ballooning of the cellular membrane over a granule (arrow) (UA + LC ×26,000), (b) Breach

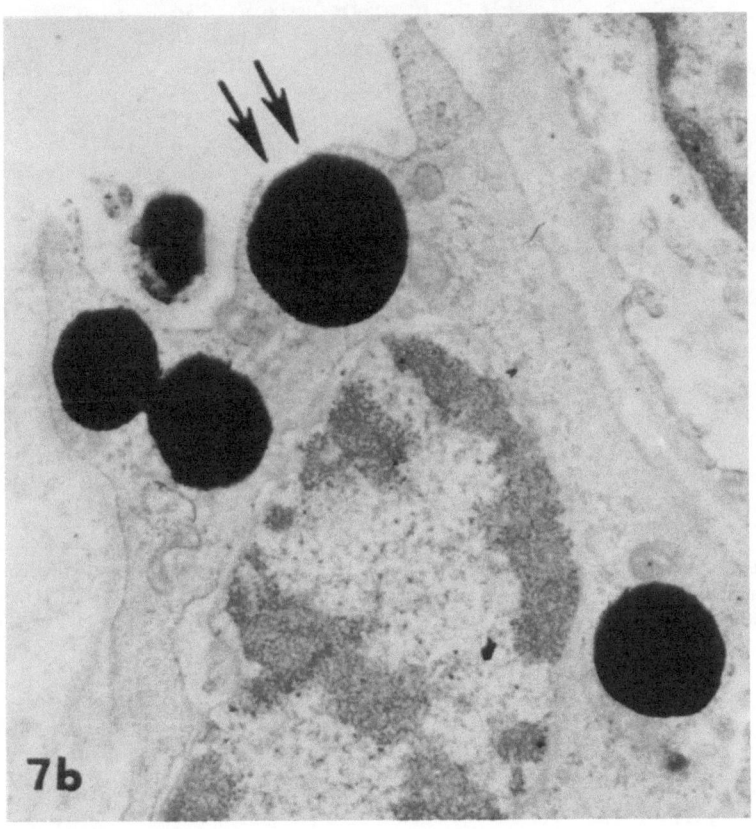

of the cellular membrane over a granule (double arrows) (UA + LC ×17,000). Both from a normotensive Wistar rat.

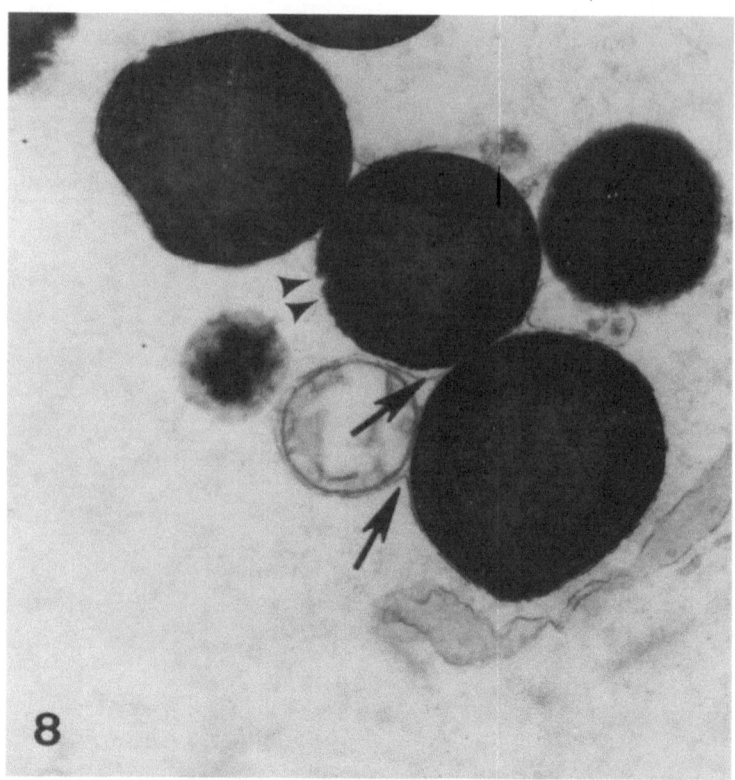

FIGURE 8. A mitochondrial membrane is seen encircling granules (arrows). Breach of the granular membrane (arrowheads) is also seen. From a normotensive Wistar rat (UA + LC ×27,000).

FIGURE 9. Free granules in a variety of extracellular locations: (a) In the free interstitium (arrows) in the neighborhood of an interstitial cell (UA + LC ×8000). (b) In a row along the basement membrane (BM) of a capillary loop (CP) (UA + LC ×15,000). Both from a normotensive Wistar rat.

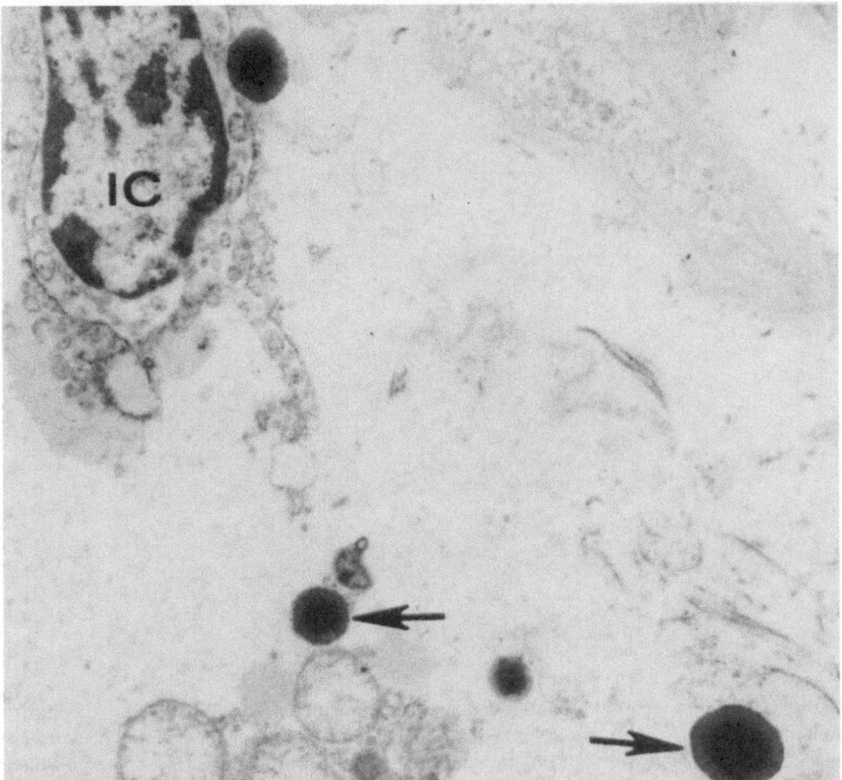

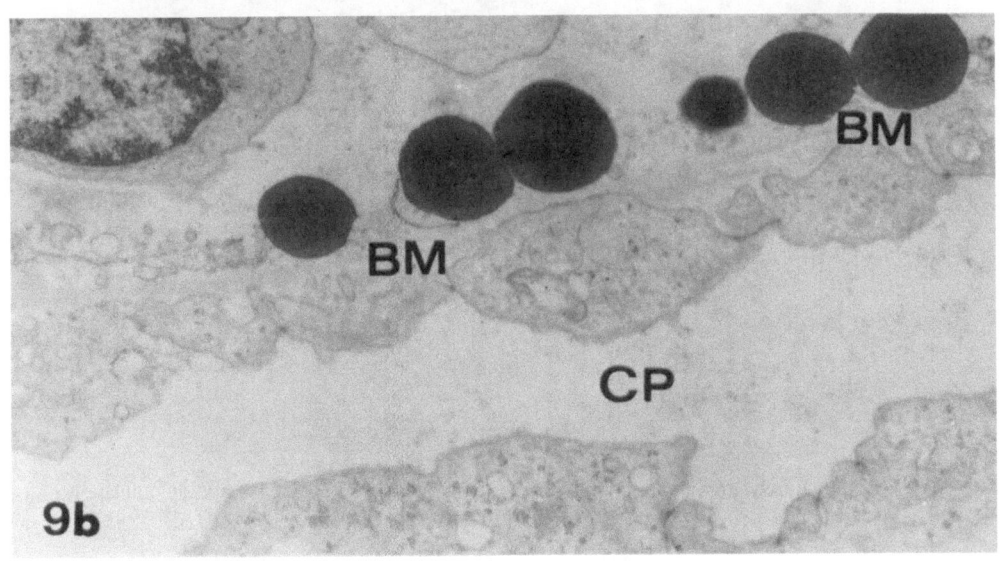

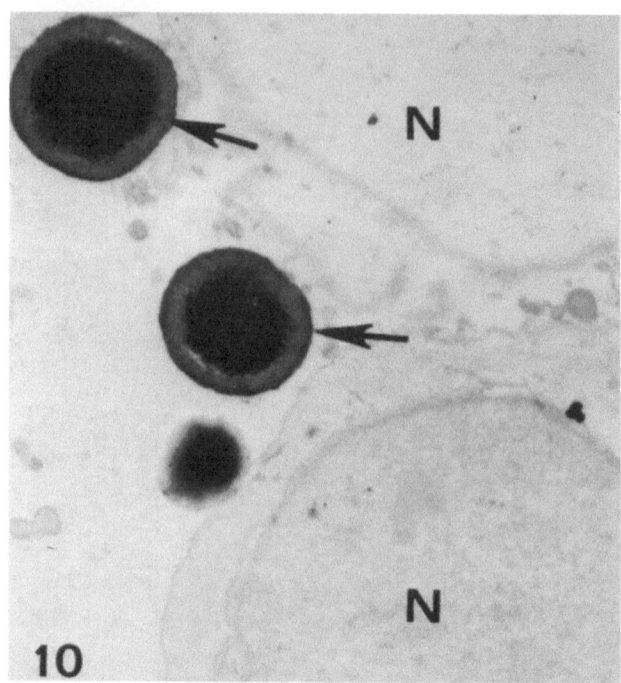

FIGURE 10. Homogenized renal papillae from normotensive Wistar rat demonstrate remnants of cell nuclei (N) and other cellular constituents like mitochondria, but also preservation of granules. The layering of the granules (arrows) into a central electron-dense portion and a peripheral thick rim of lighter material is obvious (UA + LC ×18,000).

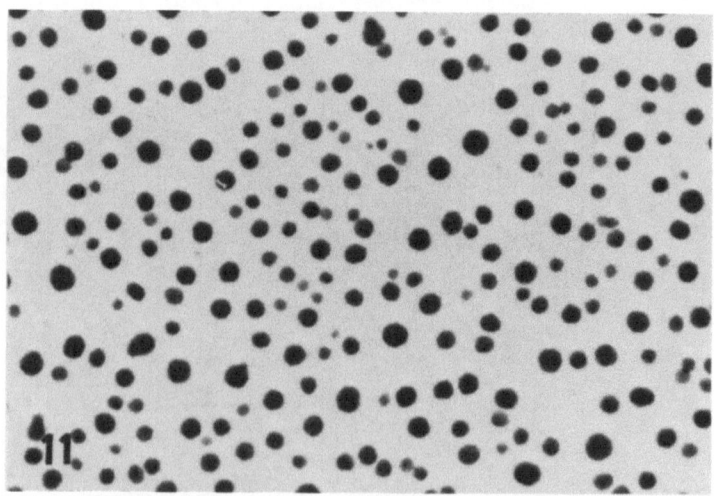

FIGURE 11. Purely granular materials in the 24-hr urinary sediment from a spontaneously hypertensive rat (PTA ×3000).

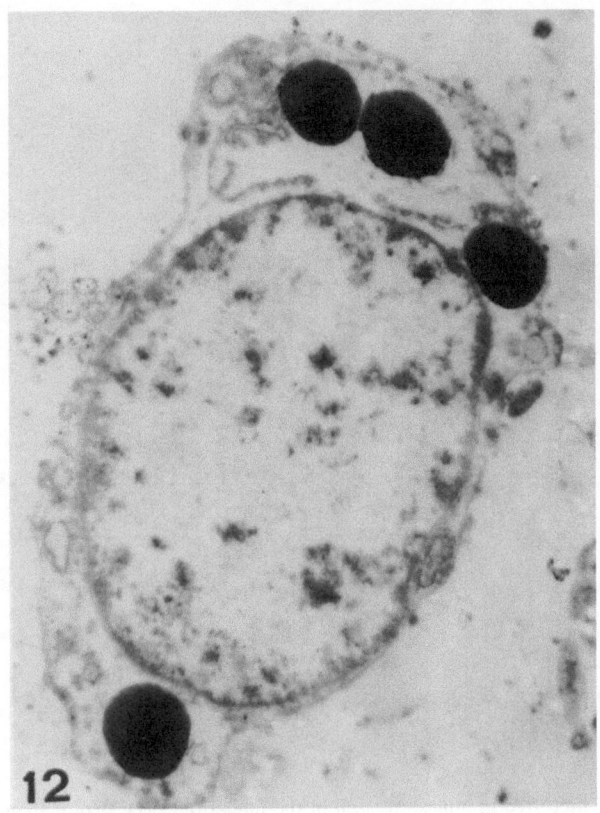

FIGURE 12. Layered granules in a papillary interstitial cell from a normal human kidney. The layering is not as prominent as it is in the rat renal papillary granule (UA + LC ×9000).

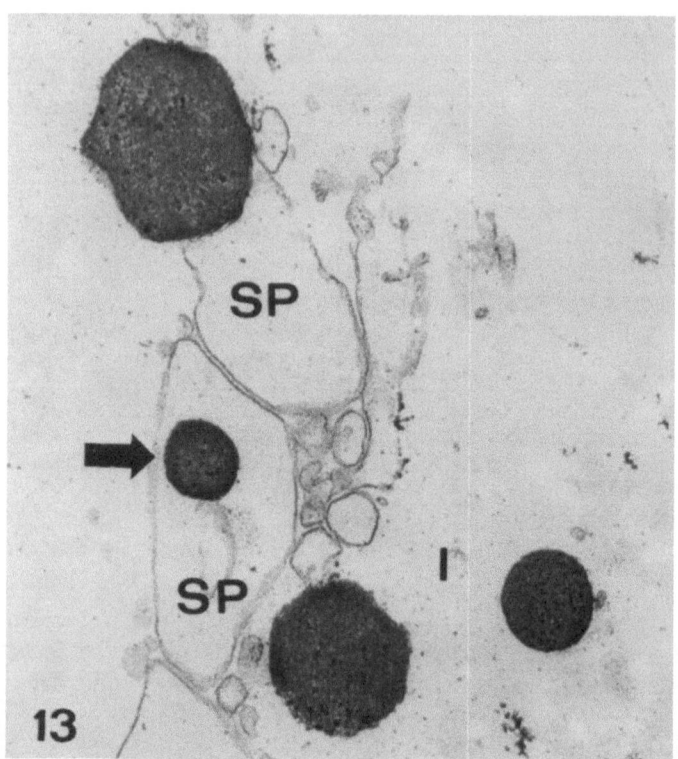

FIGURE 13. Three free granules are seen in the interstitium (I); two of them are apposed to the stellate processes (SP). Note an identical granule within the SP (arrow). From a normal human kidney (PASM ×17000).

homogenates from rabbit renal papilla for prostaglandins, prostaglandin precursor acids, prostaglandin synthetase, and 15-hydroxy prostaglandin dehydrogenase. The subcellular fractions consisted of lipid droplets, supernatant, microsomes, and mitochondria, verified by EM. While most of the prostaglandins were found in the supernatant, only a low concentration of arachidonic acid was measured in the lipid droplets.

These conflicting reports make it harder to determine the contribution of RIC granules in the production of renal vasodepressor substance(s). Nonetheless, the evidence is strong in favor of RIC as the major source of renal vasodepressor substance(s).

If we implicate the papillary interstitial granules in the pathogenesis of spontaneous or essential hypertension, an important question must be answered to confirm this role. The question concerns the functional integrity of the granules, i.e., are these granules merely located in the papilla and functionless or are they functional in producing certain substances. Ultrastructural studies have contributed significantly in defining the functional characteristics of the papillary granules. The different types of granules, their extracellular location, and their appearance in the urine are some of the notable features in that have characterized the dynamic functional aspects of the granules.

Three types of granules (layered, homogenously dark, and gray) have been described. It is unknown whether these variable types are normally present intracellularly or whether they appear *in situ* by chemical transformation. Chemical transformation is a possibility because of the observation of mitochondria in close proximity to the layered or homogeneously dark granules, but never in proximity to the gray granules. Since mitochondrial membrane has lipolytic enzymes, this juxtaposition suggests that layered and homogeneously dark, but not gray, granules are subjected to enzymatic action. In addition, gray granules, being devoid of membranes and of irregular shape, may represent the "chemical end product" of the other two granular types. In this case, a significantly greater number of gray granules in SHR may be accounted for by the increased release of lipid material (which may be the ANRL of Muirhead).

The secretory nature of the RIC can be attributed mainly to the large number of granules contained within them, but this proposed function is also supported by the presence of numerous free granules unassociated with cytoplasm or other cellular constituents throughout the interstitium. Our failure to find any difference in the ultrastructural characteristics between the free granules and those found intracellularly lends further support. The rare finding of disruption or fuzziness of RIC membrane and the frequent appearance of agranular cells with intact cellular membrane further justifies our notion that these free granules are intracellular granules that may have been extruded through an intact cellular membrane. The release of intracellular granules into the extracellular space appears to take place via a membrane fusion mechanism (Lagunoff, 1973). Therefore, gray granules having no membrane are unable to fuse with the cellular membrane and this may explain their absence or rare occurrence within free interstitium.

Still remaining unexplained is the disposition of the free granules. Their location throughout the interstitium and inside the lumina of capillaries and tubules seems to indicate their pathways into the bloodstream and urine, respectively. The presence of granules inside the capillary lumina may imply the release of granules or granular material(s) through the circulatory pathway. This would be consistent with Muirhead's hypothesis of the endocrine-type antihypertensive functions of the renal medulla.

Another speculation concerns the function of the RIC granules in modulating renin secretion. Since indomethacin blocks prostaglandin synthesis and lowers plasma renin activity, it can be assumed that indomethacin also exerts an inhibitory effect on juxtaglomerular cell (JGC) granularity. It is unknown whether or not decrease in renin production is the result of inhibition of prostaglandin synthesis. The latter is a distinct possibility because Weber et al. (1976) failed to increase plasma renin activity after renal ischemia in rats and rabbits pretreated with indomethacin. Simultaneous quantitative analysis of RIC granularity and JGC granularity, along with measurements of renin and prostaglandin levels in rats pretreated with indomethacin could confirm the relationship between RIC granularity and JGC granularity.

6. SIGNIFICANCE OF THE STUDIES OF THE RENAL PAPILLARY INTERSTITIAL CELLS IN RAT

Although abundant data have been accumulated concerning the vasodepressor (antihypertensive) function of the renal papillary interstitial cells and granules in rat, the evidence is weak in support of a similar function for the human kidneys. However, it is now established that the human renal papilla possesses interstitial cells and granules identical to those found in rat.

The authors studied papillae of five kidneys from four cadaver donors whose hearts were still beating, using EM. The kidneys were made available for EM study after they were found unsuitable for transplantation owing to low antigen match. All papillae had RIC, stellate processes, and intracellular and free granules. As in rat, three types of granules have been observed, namely (in order of frequency) homogeneously dark, gray, and layered; the free granules were identical to the granules within the RIC

(Figs. 12–13). These granules resemble those found in the rat renal papilla (Mandal *et al.*, 1979).

The ultrastructural resemblances between the rat and human renal papillary granules suggest that human papillary interstitial granules, like those of the rat, may be the source of renal vasodepressor substance(s). This notion can be both supported and challenged by several contradictory observations. In support: (1) Vance *et al.* (1973) found a high concentration of prostaglandins in the human renal papilla. (2) Muehrcke *et al.* (1970) found significant reduction of RIC granularity in the kidneys of malignant hypertensive patients compared to those in normotensive subjects. (3) Renal medullary fibroma in man is found to be composed of renomedullary IC. These RIC and their granules resemble those in the normal human renal papilla as well as in rat renal papilla (Lerman *et al.*, 1972). (4) Large amounts of prostaglandins were found in the renomedullary body (tumor) (Prezyna *et al.*, 1973). These observations are opposed by the study of Stuart *et al.* (1976). They found no difference in blood pressures and heart weights in of patients with and without renal medullary fibroma (interstitial cell tumor). Further opposition is provided by the observations of Martin and Tiltman (1976). They found renomedullary IC tumors in 16% of 223 cases (autopsies); however, no correlation was found between these tumors and the presence or absence of hypertension. Thus, these last two observations tend to nullify the idea that renomedullary nodule (tumor) composed of renomedullary IC represents a response to hypertension.

7. OBSTACLES TO HUMAN STUDY

Although it has been established that the renal papillae in normal human subjects contain interstitial cells and granules similar to those in normotensive and hypertensive rats, their interaction in the physiopathological mechanism of essential hypertension is completely unknown. There also remains uncertainty about the means of obtaining information regarding the status of RIC granules in the defensive mechanism against essential hypertension. The reasons for the uncertainty include: (1) the difficulty of performing renal biopsies, or any renal biopsies, in hypertensive patients or their asymptomatic family members; (2) the fact that percutaneous or open biopsies for the diagnosis of renal disease are simply inadequate for this purpose; and (3) the finding that autopsy materials are suboptimum for EM, particularly for cellular and granular studies. Notwithstanding these difficulties, good information can be derived from studies of donor kidneys that are not transplanted and studies of nephrectomy specimens from hypertensive patients.

REFERENCES

Änggård, E., Bohman, S.-O., Griffin, J. E., Larsson, C., and Maunsbach, A. B., 1972, Subcellular localization of the prostaglandin system in the rabbit renal papilla, *Acta. Physiol. Scand.* **84**:231.

Bohman, S.-O., and Maunsbach, A. B., 1972, Ultrastructural and biochemical properties of subcellular fractions from rat renal medulla, *J. Ultrastruct. Res.* **38**:225.

Ganguli, M., Tobian, L., O'Donnel, M., and Azar, S., 1977, Plasma flow and the sodium concentration in renal papilla in young and adult Kyoto hypertensive rats (SHR), *Fed. Proc.* **36**:531.

Glauert, A. M., 1965, Section staining, cytology, autoradiography, and immunochemistry for biological specimens, in: *Techniques for Electron Microscopy* (D. Kay, ed.), F. A. Davis, Philadelphia, p. 254.

Hayat, M. A., 1970, *Principles and Techniques of Electron Microscopy: Biological Applications*, Van Nostrand Reinhold, New York, p. 241.

Ishii, M. and Tobian, L., 1969, Interstitial cell granules in renal papilla and the solute composition of renal tissue in rats with Goldblatt hypertension, *J. Lab. Clin. Med.* **74**:47.

Jurukova, Z., and Somova, L., 1976, On the cytoplasmic granularity of renomedullary interstitial cells in experimental hypertension, *Acta Biol. Med. Ger.* **35**:1213.

Lagunoff, D., 1973, Membrane fusion during mast cell secretion, *J. Cell Biol.* **57**:252.

Lerman, R. J., Pitcock, J. A., Stephenson, P., and Muirhead, E. E., 1972, Renomedullary interstitial cell tumor, *Human Pathol.* **3**:559.

Limas, C. J., and Limas, C., 1977, Prostaglandin metabolism in the kidneys of spontaneously hypertensive rats, *Am. J. Physiol.* **233**:H87.

Mandal, A. K., 1979, *Electron Microscopy of the Kidney in Renal Disease and Hypertension: A Clinicopathological Approach*, Plenum Medical, New York, p. 279.

Mandal, A. K., Frohlich, E. D., Chrysant, K., Pfeffer, M. A., Yunice, A. A., and Nordquist, J. A., 1974, Ultrastructural analysis of renal papillary interstitial cell of spontaneously hypertensive rats, *J. Lab. Clin. Med.* **83**:256.

Mandal, A. K., Frohlich, E. D., Chrysant, K., Nordquist, J. A., Pfeffer, M., and Clifford, M., 1975, A morphological study of the renal papillary granule: Analysis in the interstitial cell and in the interstitium, *J. Lab. Clin. Med.* **85**:120.

Mandal, A. K., Nordquist, J. A., Thigpen, M. W., and James, T. M., 1979, Electron microscopy studies of papillary interstitial granules in normal human kidneys, *Ann. Clin. Lab. Sci.* **9**:37.

Martin, M. R., and Tiltman, A. J., 1976, Incidence of renomedullary interstitial cell tumors and correlation with hypertension, *S. Afr. Med. J.* **50**:2099.

Muehrcke, E. C., Mandal, A. K., Epstein, M., and Volini, F. I., 1969, Cytoplasmic granularity of renal medullary interstitial cells in experimental hypertension, *J. Lab. Clin. Med.* **73**:299.

Muehrcke, R. C., Mandal, A. K., and Volini, F. I., 1970, Renal interstitial cells: Prostaglandins and hypertension, *Circ. Res.* **27**(Suppl. 1):109.

Muirhead, E. E., 1976, Renomedullary antihypertensive endocrine function. *Acta. Biol. Med. Ger.* **35**:1181.

Nissen, H. M., and Bojesen, I., 1969, On lipid droplets in renal interstitial cells IV. Isolation and identification, *Z. Zellforsch. Mikrosk. Anat.* **97**:274.

Osvaldo, L., and Latta, H., 1966, The thin limbs of the loop of Henle, *J. Ultrastruct. Res.* **15**:144.

Prezyna, A., Attalah, A., Vance, K., Schoolman, M., and Lee, J., 1973, The renomedullary interstitial cell origin associated with high prostaglandin content, *Prostaglandins* **3**:669.

Solez, K., D'Agostini, R. J., Buono, R. A., Vernon, N., Wang, A. L., Finer, P. M., and
    Heptinstall, R. H., 1976, The renal medulla and mechanisms of hypertension in the spon-
    taneously hypertensive rat, *Am. J. Pathol.* **85**:555.
Stuart, R., Salyer, W. R., Salyer, D. C., and Heptinstall, R. H., 1976, Renomedullary inter-
    stitial cell lesions and hypertension, *Hum. Pathol.* **7**:327.
Tobian, L., and Azar, S., 1971, Antihypertensive and other functions of the renal papilla,
    Trans. Assoc. Am. Physicians **8**:281.
Tobian, L., Ishii, M., and Duke, M., 1969, Relationship of cytoplasmic granules in renal
    papillary interstitial cells to "post-salt" hypertension, *J. Lab. Clin. Med.* **73**:309.
Vance, V. K., Attallah, A. A., Prezyna, A., and Lee, J. B., 1973, Human renal prostaglandins,
    Prostaglandins **3**:647.
Weber, P. C., Larsson, C., Hamberg, M., Anggard, E., Corey, E. J., and Samuelsson, B.,
    1976, Effects of stimulation and inhibition of the renal prostaglandin synthetase system on
    renin release in vivo and in vitro, *Clin. Sci. Mol. Med.* **51**(Suppl. 3):271.

CHAPTER **8**

Regulation of Plasma Flow and Other Functions of the Renal Papilla in Hypertension

MUKUL C. GANGULI

1. STUDIES OF PLASMA FLOW TO THE RENAL PAPILLA IN EXPERIMENTAL AND SPONTANEOUS HYPERTENSION

1.1. Introduction

Following the demonstration of a countercurrent multiplier system within the renal medulla as a mechanism for urinary concentration, a great deal of attention has been focused on the importance of the medullary circulation in the concentrating process and on the factors affecting this part of the renal circulation (Hargitay and Kuhn, 1951; Wirz *et al.*, 1951).

Blood entering the renal medullary tissue via the vasa recta is derived from the postglomerular circulation of the juxtamedullary nephrons. The anatomical arrangement of these vasa rectae in bundles is highly suited for countercurrent exchange. It has been pointed out that changes in medullary blood flow may influence the medullary concentration of solutes, particularly sodium and urea, and, thereby, the osmolal concentration of urine (Berliner *et al.*, 1958; Thurau *et al.*, 1960a).

Using a photoelectric technique, Thurau *et al.* (1960a) demonstrated that medullary blood flow is increased more than cortical blood flow during osmotic diuresis in the dog. They also noted about a 70% increase in medullary blood flow during water diuresis. Using the Lilienfield method in rats, we have found a 61% and 33% increase of papillary plasma flow during osmotic and water diuresis, respectively. In addition, several workers

MUKUL C. GANGULI • Hypertension Section, Department of Internal Medicine, University of Minnesota Hospital and School of Medicine, Minneapolis, Minnesota 55455.

have reported a marked reduction of both sodium and urea content in the rat renal medulla during osmotic and water diuresis (Atherton *et al.*, 1968*a,b*; Bray, 1960; Saikia, 1965).

Conversely, in a nondiuretic state, a significantly reduced papillary sodium concentration has been noted in four forms of experimental hypertension in rats (Tobian *et al.*, 1969; Ishii and Tobian, 1969; Tobian and Ishii, 1969; Ganguli and Tobian, 1978). By virtue of this finding, one could theorize that the high arterial pressure produced a high plasma flow in the papilla, which could conceivably wash out some of the countercurrent solute gradient in these medullas. However, it is not yet certain whether or not hypertensive rats have a high rate of plasma flow in the papilla. If inner medullary plasma flow is not "autoregulated," then the elevated arterial pressure of chronic hypertension could produce a very high rate of papillary plasma flow in this region.

There is an abundance of evidence that the blood flow to the kidney as a whole is ordinarily autoregulated with great accuracy (Thurau, 1964; Ochwadt, 1956; Waugh, 1964; Hinshaw, 1964; Arendshorst *et al.*, 1975; Heller and Horacek, 1977; Stern *et al.*, 1979). In chronic hypertensive rats (Goldblatt hypertension and Dahl and Kyoto spontaneous hypertension), total renal blood flow is similar to that observed in normotensive control animals, suggesting the presence of autoregulation, even in the hypertensive kidney (Girndt and Ochwadt, 1969; Ben-Ishay *et al.*, 1967; Nishiyama *et al.*, 1976; Arendshorst and Beierwaltes, 1979).

The pressure–flow relationship of the renal medullary circulation, however, has been studied by a few investigators, but the results are conflicting. Precise measurements of medullary blood flow may still be lacking because of methodological difficulties. All techniques employed so far are indirect, based on the measurement of indicator transit time or volume of distribution.

Using a photoelectric technique, Kramer *et al.* (1960) found that the inner medullary blood flow was linearly related to perfusion pressure, while the cortical blood flow exhibited good autoregulation. Miyamato and Gordon (1970) noted that, following a sudden rise in perfusion pressure, the medullary blood flow increased while cortical and total renal blood flow remained unchanged. Girndt and Ochwadt (1969) concluded that, in chronic rat hypertension, autoregulation of blood flow to the renal medulla is not maintained. Indeed, medullary blood flow was greatly elevated in the contralateral kidney when compared with the clamped kidney, while total renal blood flow did not change significantly.

On the other hand, an equally well-developed autoregulation of both cortical and medullary blood flow has been described in dogs by Aukland (1966) and Loyning (1971). Whereas these authors measured the local clearance of hydrogen gas from different areas of the kidney, Wolgast

(1968) and Grangsjo and Wolgast (1972), used an indicator dilution technique to measure the transit time of labeled red cells with small needle-shaped beta-sensitive detectors. Recently, Stern *et al.* (1979), using a laser–Doppler spectroscopy method, indicated that the blood flow in the papillary vasa recta is autoregulated as a function of blood pressure in the same manner as are total and cortical blood flow.

With this background, we will report our results of the studies of plasma flow to the renal papilla in three forms of experimental rat hypertension—postsalt, Goldblatt, and deoxycorticosterone (DOCA) hypertension—and in two models of genetic hypertension—Dahl and Kyoto rats with spontaneous hypertension.

1.2. Methods

Since no one major artery supplies the renal medulla, direct measurement of medullary flow is not feasible. As mentioned earlier, all techniques employed so far are indirect, involving the use of tracers or indicators. The radioactive albumin uptake method developed by Lilienfield *et al.* (1961) seemed to be a satisfactory means of measuring papillary flow. Hence, the method used to measure the plasma flow in the renal papilla of the rat was essentially similar to that of Lilienfield *et al.* with slight modifications made by Ganguli and Tobian (1974) and Solez *et al.* (1974).

The principles underlying the Lilienfield method can be described as follows: The renal papilla contains a large amount of exchangeable albumin (Lilienfield *et al.*, 1958), with the highest concentrations found in vasa recta blood at the tip of the papilla. This strongly suggests that much, if not all, of the exchangeable albumin is intravascular (Thurau *et al.*, 1960*b*). The anatomical arrangement of the vasa rectae in the papilla makes it possible that blood entering these capillaries displaces the blood already present with relatively little mixing. Because of the small amount of mixing, the slow flow rate, and the greater length of the blood vessels in the renal papilla, considerable time must elapse between the entrance of blood into the papilla and its exit. As measured photoelectrically, the average transit time of circulating albumin in the renal papilla of dogs has been found to be in the range of 1–2 min (Kramer *et al.*, 1960). If no significant washout of incoming radioactive albumin occurs within the first 20 or 30 sec, the accumulation rate of radioactivity in this region during this time can be taken as a measure of the rate at which plasma is flowing into the papilla. However, in order to convert radioactive counts into volume of plasma flow, one needs to know the average plasma concentration of radioactive albumin during the interval that the radioactive plasma is flowing into the papilla. This information was obtained by continuously sampling arterial blood throughout the infusion period. During this time interval, blood from the carotid artery was slowly collected at approximately the same rate of withdrawal as fluid containing radioactive albumin entering the right atrium. Hence, no change in arterial pressure occurred during the procedure.

After an interval of 24 sec, the kidney pedicle was instantaneously ligated and the collection of blood from the carotid artery terminated. Since linear accumulation of radioactive albumin in the papilla of the adult rat (300–350 g) lasts 36 sec (Fig. 1), an accumulation time of 24 sec is well within the linear period and should provide an accurate index of plasma flow to the papilla. In dogs, the radioactive counts in the papilla increase almost linearly for about 60 sec after the start of infusion. In young rats (100–115 g), however, papillary uptake of labeled albumin reaches a plateau after only 21 sec of infusion.

Following ligation of the renal pedicle, the kidney was removed and the renal papilla was carefully dissected out and placed in an airtight preweighed bottle to obtain the wet weight of the papilla. Then the radioactivity of the papilla was ascertained in a gamma scintillation counter. The samples of blood from the carotid artery were similarly weighed and counted. Tissue radioactivity is expressed as counts per minute

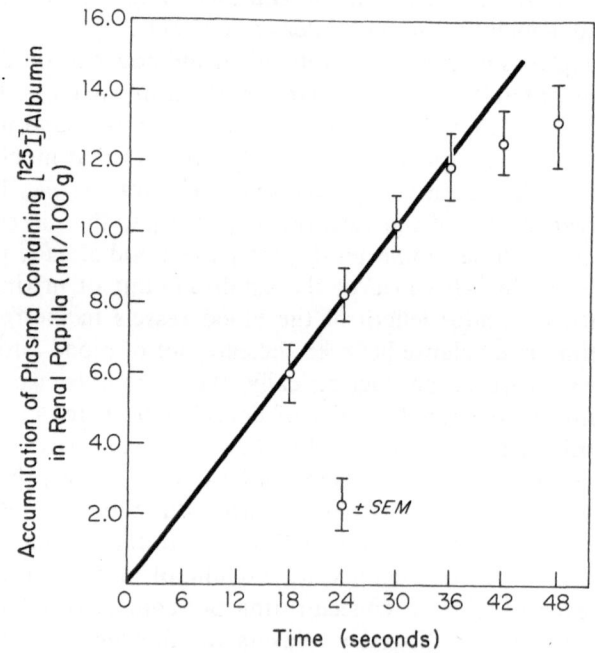

FIGURE 1.   Mean accumulation of plasma containing [^{125}I]albumin at various time intervals following the start of [^{125}I]albumin infusion.

TABLE 1

Blood Pressure and Renal Papillary Plasma Flow in Three Forms of Experimental Rat Hypertension[a]

Group	Number of rats	Blood pressure (mm Hg)	Papillary plasma flow (ml/100 g papilla per min)
Postsalt hypertension			
Normotensive control rats	51	124	41.9
Postsalt hypertensive rats	66	195[b]	35.6[c]
Goldblatt hypertension			
Control kidneys	12	140	23.4
Contralateral kidneys	13	174[b]	20.4[c]
Clipped kidneys	11	174[b]	17.6[b]
DOCA hypertension			
Control rats	17	141	21.8
DOCA rats	13	175[b]	18.8[c]

[a] Part of the data from Ganguli and Tobian (1974), by permission of the American Physiological Society.
[b] Significantly different from the corresponding control: $p < 0.001$.
[c] Significantly different from the corresponding control: $p < 0.01$.

per gram of tissue. Blood radioactivity is expressed as counts per minute per milliliter of plasma after making corrections for the hematocrit. The radioactive counts per gram of papilla divided by counts per milliliter of plasma give an estimate of the volume of plasma accumulating in a gram of papilla during 24 sec of elapsed time. This value should represent papillary plasma flow.

1.3. Results

Postsalt Hypertension. Hypertension was induced by placing male weanling Holtzman rats on chow containing 8% NaCl. Another group of weanling rats fed with chow containing 0.3% NaCl served as controls. After 4 months, the rats in both experimental and control groups were given food containing 0.6% NaCl. Beginning 3 weeks thereafter, blood pressure was measured by the microphonic method weekly for 3 consecutive weeks and the average of these pressures was considered the "true" blood pressure. Rats of the experimental group with blood pressure over 180 mm Hg (range 180–230) constituted the hypertensives, while rats of the control group with blood pressure under 135 mm Hg (range 110–135) were used as normotensives.

While 51 normotensive rats had average papillary plasma flows of 41.9 ml/100 g papilla per minute, 66 hypertensive rats averaged 35.6 ml/100 g papilla per min (Table 1). Thus, the hypertensive group had a 15% lower plasma flow than the normotensive group ($p < 0.01$).

Goldblatt Hypertension. Hypertension was produced in male Sprague–Dawley rats weighing 170–200 g by unilateral renal artery constriction with a silver clip (0.013 in.). The opposite kidney was left untouched. Blood pressure was recorded by the microphonic method immediately prior to renal artery clipping as well as 4 and 5 weeks after clipping.

Papillary plasma flow was measured in the left kidney at the sixth week (Table 1). The plasma flow to the renal papilla averaged 23.4 ml/100 g papilla per min in control rats. The "untouched" contralateral kidney of hypertensive rats averaged 20.4 ml/100 g papilla per min, which was 13% less than that in control rats. The difference was significant ($p < 0.01$). The plasma flow in the clipped kidney of hypertensive rats averaged 17.6 ml/100 g papilla per min, which was 25% lower compared to that of control rats ($p < 0.001$). The clipped kidney also had a 14% lower plasma flow than the untouched contralateral kidney ($p < 0.02$).

DOCA Hypertension. DOCA hypertension was produced in male Sprague–Dawley rats weighing between 170–200 g by giving desoxycorticosterone pivalate, 125 mg, subcutaneously at 0 and at 3 weeks. In addition, the rats received 1% NaCl in their drinking water. Papillary plasma flow was measured 5 weeks after the first administration of DOCA (Table 1). The papillary plasma flow in DOCA rats was significantly reduced from that in control rats (18.8 ml vs. 21.8 ml/100 g papilla per min) ($p < 0.01$).

Dahl Hypertension. Two strains of rats have been developed by Dahl *et al.* (1962). One group, the salt-sensitive (S) strain, invariably becomes hypertensive when fed a NaCl diet (8% NaCl in dry chow). The other group, the salt-resistant (R) strain, never becomes hypertensive when fed an 8% NaCl diet. The S strain is so named because it is Sensitive to salt hypertension. The R strain denotes Resistant to salt hypertension.

Female rats of R and S strains about 16 weeks of age and weighing 235–285 g were studied. They were divided equally into groups, according to duration of feeding schedule, amount of NaCl fed, and type of rat (Table 2). The two levels of dietary NaCl, 0.3% and 8.0%, were considered as either "normal" or "high-salt," respectively. All rats had received 0.3% NaCl chow since weaning. After that, high-salt feeding was carried out in both R and S rats for both 1- and 4-week periods. Concomitant feeding of a diet with 0.3% NaCl was carried out in other R and S rats. The papillary plasma flow was then measured in a round-robin fashion among groups I through IV and among groups V through VIII.

When eating a normal diet containing 0.3% NaCl, both R rats and S rats have fairly normal blood pressures, averaging 129 and 144 mm Hg, respectively. The S rats were considered to have borderline hypertension

TABLE 2
Blood Pressure and Renal Papillary Plasma Flow in Two Dahl Rat Strains[a]

Group	Type of rat[b]	Number of rats	Percent NaCl in diet	Blood pressure (mm Hg)	Papillary plasma flow (ml/100 g papilla per min)
One-week feeding					
I	R	13	0.3	130	25.6
II	S	10	0.3	145[c]	20.4[c]
III	R	12	8.0	128	33.8
IV	S	9	8.0	152[d]	24.8[c]
Four-week feeding					
V	R	9	0.3	127	25.7
VI	S	8	0.3	142[c]	17.7[d]
VII	R	9	8.0	127	29.5
VIII	S	7	8.0	162[d]	20.0[d]

[a] From Ganguli et al. (1976), by permission of the American Heart Association, Inc.
[b] R, hypertension-resistant rats; S, hypertension-sensitive rats.
[c] Significantly different from the preceding mean: $p < 0.005$.
[d] Significantly different from the preceding mean: $p < 0.001$.

because their mean blood pressure was about 15 mm Hg higher than that of R rats ($p < 0.005$). These borderline hypertensive S rats (groups II and VI) had a mean papillary plasma flow of 19.2 ml/100 g papilla per min, which was 25% lower than the 25.6 ml/100 g papilla per min plasma flow ($p < 0.001$) of the normotensive R rats (groups I and V). When both S and R rats were challenged with a high (8%) NaCl diet for 1 week, however, a contrast between change in blood pressure and papillary flow was found in these two strains of rats. The R rats showed no increase in blood pressure (128 mm Hg). In the S rats, blood pressure increased significantly (152 mm Hg) ($p < 0.001$). The R rats also had a significantly higher papillary plasma flow than the S rats (33.8 ml vs. 24.8 ml/100 g papilla per min, respectively) ($p < 0.005$). When the same comparison was made after 4 weeks of high-salt feeding, R rats still demonstrated normal blood pressure (127 mm Hg). The blood pressure of the S rats increased to 162 mm Hg. The papillary plasma flow of both R and S rats decreased further but the difference was still significant. R rats had a flow rate of 29.5 ml/100 g papilla per min, whereas S rats showed 20.0 ml/100 g papilla per min ($p < 0.001$).

In addition, the effect of varying salt intake within the same strain was compared. When R rats were challenged with a high (8%) NaCl diet for 1 week, the papillary plasma flow increased from 25.6 ml/100 g papilla per min on 0.3% NaCl to 33.8 ml/100 g papilla per min on 8% NaCl with a 32% net increase ($p < 0.001$). Similarly, S rats, fed 8% NaCl, also showed an increase in papillary plasma flow from 20.4 to 24.8 ml/100 g papilla per min with a 22% increase ($p < 0.05$). When they were fed a high (8%) salt diet for 4 weeks, R rats showed a significant increase in papillary plasma flow from 25.7 ml/100 g papilla per min to 29.5 ml/100 g papilla per min with a 15% rise ($p < 0.025$) in contrast to a nonsignificant increase of papillary plasma flow from 17.7 to 20.0 ml/100 g papilla per min in S rats.

Kyoto Spontaneous Hypertension. When plasma flow to the renal papilla was measured in Dahl rats on a low-sodium diet, the papillary plasma flow in the hypertension-prone rats was found to be 25% lower than that in the hypertension-resistant strain, even though both strains had levels of blood pressure within the normal range. It was of interest to determine whether or not the same type of relationship was present in the Kyoto spontaneously hypertensive rat during various stages of development of hypertension. These rats were compared with Kyoto normotensive control rats of the same age. All rats were fed chow with 0.3% NaCl and tap water *ad libitum.* This amount of dietary sodium is considered normal. Table 3 gives the blood pressure and renal papillary plasma flow of Kyoto nor-motensive rats (WKY) and Kyoto hypertensive rats (SHR) in three dif-ferent age groups. At 6 weeks of age, when the Kyoto hypertensive rat is in a phase of rapidly rising blood pressure, WKY rats had a mean papillary plasma flow of 44.7 ml/100 g papilla per min, while SHR rats had a mean papillary plasma flow of 41.0 ml/100 g papilla per min, which is 8% less than that in the normotensive controls ($p < 0.06$). At this age, the hyperten-sive rats had a mean blood pressure of 154 mm Hg, which is significantly higher than the 108 mm Hg in controls ($p < 0.001$). At 9 weeks of age, Kyoto hypertensive rats had reached a mean blood pressure of 177 mm Hg, compared to 117 in the control group ($p < 0.001$). Papillary plasma flow

TABLE 3

Blood Pressure and Renal Papillary Plasma Flow in Two Strains of Kyoto Rats

Age group	Type of rat[a]	Number of rats	Body weight (g)	Blood pressure (mm Hg)	Papillary plasma flow (ml/100 g papilla per min)
6 weeks	WKY	24	130	108	44.7
	SHR	24	133	154[b]	41.0
9 weeks	WKY	24	210	117	36.8
	SHR	30	208	177[b]	32.7[c]
17 weeks	WKY	24	327	118	33.2
	SHR	26	326	182[b]	29.5[b]

[a] WKY, Kyoto normotensive rats; SHR, Kyoto hypertensive rats.
[b] Significantly different from the preceding mean: $p < 0.001$.
[c] Significantly different from the preceding mean: $p < 0.005$.

averaged 36.8 ml/100 g papilla per min in the normotensive group, compared to 32.7 ml/100 g papilla per min in the hypertensive group, an 11% reduction of flow in the hypertensive group ($p < 0.005$). At 17 weeks of age, the Kyoto hypertensive rats had a slight increase in blood pressure over that at 9 weeks of age but the papillary plasma flow did not change.

1.4. Discussion

All our findings indicate that the renal papillae in hypertensive rats do not exhibit an increase of plasma flow in the presence of elevated inflow pressure to the kidneys. Thus, it may be stated that the hypertensive papillae autoregulate their plasma flow in different types of longstanding hypertension. In fact, the hypertensive papillae have a plasma flow actually lower than normotensive kidneys despite the high inflow pressure. In view of this reduced plasma flow, the low sodium and urea levels found in hypertensive papillae (Tobian et al., 1969; Ishii and Tobian, 1969; Ganguli and Tobian, 1978; Ganguli et al., 1977a) are evidently not due to a washout effect arising from a rapid plasma flow.

It is not clear just why the hypertensive renal papillae have lower plasma flow than the normotensive renal papillae. An increased vascular resistance per total papilla must be present and the rise in resistance is proportionately greater than the rise in arterial pressure. There are three types of vasculatures containing smooth muscle cells involved in the supply of blood to the papilla. These include the afferent and efferent arterioles of the juxtamedullary glomeruli as well as the descending limbs of the vasa rectae (Moffat, 1967). Any or all of these three areas could have an increased narrowing of the lumen resulting from either a nonmyogenic structural narrowing of the vascular channels or an increased contraction of the vascular smooth muscle. In addition, evidence obtained in the rat suggests that appropriate adjustments in preglomerular vascular resistance occur in response to changes in perfusion pressure within the autoregulatory range (Gomez, 1951; Lowenstein et al., 1970; Azar et al., 1976; Arendshorst and Beierwaltes, 1979). Another interesting theory for renal autoregulation outlined by Thurau (Thurau and Schneerman, 1965; Thurau et al., 1967) postulates that the sodium concentration (or load) at the macula densa should determine the release of renin from the juxtamedullary apparatus, thereby determining the preglomerular resistance. As the renin concentration in juxtaglomerular apparatus of the juxtamedullary glomeruli (Bing and Wiberg, 1958; Peart, 1959) is low, there should be no well-developed autoregulation of the blood flow to the medulla, but this is in disagreement with the findings. This disparity is further substantiated by the low sodium concentration in the papilla in all kinds of rat hypertension. Furthermore, Tobian et al. (1974b) noted that isolated kidneys from hypertensive rats released significantly lesser amounts of renin at all levels of inflow pressure. After consideration of different mechanisms, Stein (1976) believes that myogenic theory most reasonably accounts for the renal autoregulation phenomenon.

Papillary plasma flow significantly increases in normotensive R rats and in ordinary Sprague–Dawley rats when they are challenged with a high NaCl intake. This increase in papillary plasma flow may enhance the well-known natriuretic action of the collecting duct and thereby expedite the excretion of a large sodium load (Stein *et al.*, 1975; Sonnenberg, 1974; Diezi *et al.*, 1973). When the S rat was challenged with a high NaCl intake, there was only a limited rise in papillary plasma flow, which was strikingly lower than that of the R rat after 4 weeks on the same high NaCl intake (Table 2). This reduced papillary flow could result in a lower rate of Na^+ excretion in hypertensive rats. Leaving such speculations aside, it has been demonstrated that isolated S kidneys do indeed have an intrinsic limitation of natriuresis at any of three tested inflow pressures (Tobian *et al.*, 1978*a*), as in kidneys of postsalt hypertension and Kyoto spontaneous hypertension (Tobian *et al.*, 1974*b*). However, the sodium output markedly increases with increments of inflow pressure. Hence, the disproportionate vasoconstriction of vessels in hypertensive papillae possibly is another way to increase Na^+ excretion through a mechanism of pressure natriuresis (Selkurt, 1951). This shift in the pressure natriuresis curve would indicate that these hypertensive kidneys need a high arterial pressure for adequate sodium excretion. Hypertension thus tends to be maintained by a "resetting" of the pressure natriuresis curve. Nishiyama *et al.* (1976) noted that blood flow was normal in most vascular beds in the Kyoto hypertensive rat when measured as flow per unit weight of tissue. In the various vascular beds in hypertension, the high arterial inflow pressure is just balanced by elevated vascular resistance, so the tissue blood flow remains normal. The resistance of vessels supplying the hypertensive papilla, however, appears to be disproportionately greater than the vascular resistance of any other vessels in the body.

Thus, the pattern of a decreased papillary plasma flow is common to these five types of hypertension. It is plausible that this low papillary plasma flow is a genuine, repeating hallmark for all types of experimental and genetic rat hypertension.

2. RELATIONSHIP BETWEEN RENOMEDULLARY INTERSTITIAL CELL GRANULES, SODIUM, AND PROSTAGLANDINS IN NORMOTENSIVE AND HYPERTENSIVE RATS

2.1. Introduction

The renal medulla thus far can be implicated in a variety of ways in the pathogenesis of hypertension. For instance, interstitial cells are found to be abundantly located in the inner medulla and papilla. They are unique in that they have many cytoplasmic granules filled with lipid material, suggesting that these cells have some secretory function. The lipid granules *per se* do not contain much prostaglandin (PG); however, granules are very rich in arachidonic acid and thus could be considered as a storehouse of precursor material for PG synthesis (Comai *et al.*, 1975), particularly PGE_2, a powerful vasoactive and natriuretic agent. In the kidney, 90% of the PGE_2 is synthesized in the renal medulla (Van Dorp, 1971), not only by the interstitial cells, but also by cells of collecting ducts (Muirhead *et al.*, 1972; Zanszen and Nugteren, 1971). These renomedullary collecting ducts are also important regulators of ultimate sodium excretion. Since hypertension is affected by sodium balance in the body, the collecting ducts of the medulla could conceivably have an important connection to hypertension. Lastly, the renal papilla contains very high concentrations of sodium and urea as a result of countercurrent systems operating within this region of the kidney. Here we will report the interrelationships between renomedullary interstitial cells, prostaglandins, and sodium in hypertension, during prostaglandin synthesis inhibition and during high NaCl intake.

2.2. Results

2.2.1. *Sodium, Prostaglandin E_2, and Interstitial Cell Granules in Hypertension*

In postsalt hypertensive rats, the sodium concentration in the papilla averaged 95 mEq/kg of wet papilla, a 33% reduction ($p < 0.001$) compared to that (141 mEq/kg of wet papilla) of normotensive control rats (Table 4).

TABLE 4
Interstitial Cell Granule Count and Sodium Concentration of Renal Papilla[a]

Group	Number of rats	Blood pressure (mm Hg)	Average granule count (no./100 squares)	Papillary sodium (mEq/kg wet weight)
Postsalt hypertension				
Normotensive control rats	10	124	136	141
Postsalt hypertensive rats	21	178[b]	79[b]	95[b]
Goldblatt hypertension				
Control kidneys	38	120	135	136
Clipped kidneys	38	189[b]	115[c]	122
Contralateral kidneys	38	189[b]	99[b]	107[d]

[a] From Tobian (1972), by permission.
[b] Significantly different from the corresponding control: $p < 0.001$.
[c] Significantly different from the corresponding control: $p < 0.02$.
[d] Significantly different from the corresponding control: $p < 0.01$.

In the hypertensive group the PGE_2 concentration of the whole kidney averaged 217 ng/100 g of dry solids, a 36% decrease ($p < 0.05$) compared to PGE_2 content (340 ng/100 g of dry solids) in the normotensive control group.

Sodium concentration of the renal papilla was measured in 30 Kyoto hypertensive rats (SHR) and 24 Kyoto normotensive rats (WKY), both 10 weeks of age. The average papillary sodium concentrations in WKY and SHR were 198 mEq and 170 mEq/kg of papillary water, respectively (Table 5). The papillary sodium concentration was significantly reduced ($p < 0.001$) in hypertensive papillae. PGE_2 concentrations of quick-frozen papillae from WKY and SHR are given in Table 5. Papillary PGE_2 was 3.4 times higher in SHR (63.5 ng/100 mg of dry papilla) than in normotensive WKY (18.7 ng/100 mg of dry papilla).

It has also been reported (Tobian et al., 1969; Ishii and Tobian, 1969; Tobian, 1972) that papillary interstitial cell granularity is significantly reduced in postsalt hypertensive rat kidneys, in both clipped and contra-lateral kidneys of Goldblatt hypertensive rats (Table 4), and in SHR kidneys compared to age-matched normotensive WKY rats (Mandal et al., 1974). This is commensurate with reduced papillary sodium, but is apparently incompatible with elevated PGE_2 found in the SHR renal papilla.

2.2.2. Effect of Prostaglandin Synthesis Inhibition on Interstitial Cell Granules and Sodium

The effect of inhibition of prostaglandin synthesis (using indomethacin) on the granularity of renomedullary interstitial cells and papillary sodium

TABLE 5
Sodium and Prostaglandin Concentrations in the Renal Papilla

Group	Sodium (mEq/kg H_2O)	PGE_2 (ng/100 mg dry, fat-free solids)
WKY	198	18.7
SHR	170[a]	63.5[b]
Control rats	185	76.9
Indomethacin rats	358[a]	<0.5[b]
Rats on normal-NaCl (0.3%) diet for 2 weeks	171	76.9
Rats on high-NaCl (8%) diet for 2 weeks	224[a]	38.9[c]

[a] Significantly different from the preceding mean: $p < 0.001$.
[b] Significantly different from the preceding mean: $p < 0.01$.
[c] Significantly different from the preceding mean: $p < 0.04$.

concentration has been studied. Comai *et al.* (1974) noted that indomethacin administration (2.5 and 5 mg/kg intravenously for 3 days, in rabbits) increased the number of interstitial cell lipid droplets from 2.19 in controls to 6.73 and 11.58, respectively, in indomethacin-treated animals ($p < 0.01$). The response to indomethacin was found to be dose-dependent.

Thirty minutes after intravenous administration of indomethacin (10 mg/kg), papillary sodium concentration averaged 358 mEq/kg H_2O, which is significantly higher ($p < 0.001$) than the 185 mEq/kg H_2O in control rats given only diluent. In addition, a 97% reduction of papillary PGE_2 concentration in indomethacin-treated rats compared to that in control rats was noted (Table 5).

2.2.3. *Papillary Prostaglandin E_2 and Sodium during High NaCl Intake*

It has been reported that infusion of either PGE_2 or PGA_2 intravenously or into the renal artery usually causes a marked natriuresis and water diuresis. Thus, it is very logical to conceive that medullary PGE_2 may act as a local natriuretic hormone (Johnston *et al.*, 1967; Vander, 1968; Lee, 1972; Martinez-Maldonado *et al.*, 1972).

PGE_2 and sodium concentration in the renal papilla were measured in normal Sprague–Dawley rats fed either a normal or high-NaCl diet (Table 5). While 60 rats on a normal-NaCl (0.3%) diet for 2 weeks had an average PGE_2 concentration of 76.9 ng/100 mg of dry papilla, an equal number of rats on a high-NaCl (8%) diet for 2 weeks had an average PGE_2 concentration of 38.9 ng/100 mg of dry papilla. Thus, the rats on the high-NaCl diet had a 50% reduction in papillary PGE_2 concentration ($p < 0.04$). These results are quite similar to those of an earlier study (Tobian *et al.*, 1974a) in which PGE_2 level in the whole quick-frozen kidney was significantly reduced (40%) after 2 weeks on a high-salt diet. In 20 rats fed a normal-NaCl (0.3%) diet, the sodium concentration in the renal papilla averaged 171 mEq/kg papillary H_2O. In 20 other rats fed a high-NaCl (8%) diet for 2 weeks, the papillary sodium concentration averaged 224 mEq/kg papillary H_2O, a 31% increase ($p < 0.001$).

2.3. Discussion

The evidence indicates a significant reduction in the granularity of renal papillary interstitial cells in postsalt, Goldblatt, DOCA, and Kyoto spontaneous hypertension. Along with decreased granularity of these interstitial cells there is, *vis à vis*, a reduced concentration of renal papillary sodium. This suggests a possible relationship between a deranged function of the renal papilla and hypertension. The low sodium concentration in the papilla was first thought to result from increased papillary blood flow producing a so-called "washout" effect. However, when papillary plasma flow was measured in rats with postsalt, Goldblatt, DOCA, and Kyoto spontaneous hypertension, it was found to be significantly lower than that of the normotensive control rats. Thus, the low sodium level in the papilla of hypertensive rats apparently is not due to a "washout" phenomenon.

It was also postulated that the decreased number of interstitial cell granules in the papilla of the hypertensive rat might be a manifestation of "sickness" or degeneration of the interstitial cells. Such a situation would be analogous to the atrophic beta cell in the pancreatic islets of subjects with severe juvenile diabetes. Although postsalt hypertensive rats were found to have a lower concentration of intrarenal PGE_2 in situ, determination of PGE_2 release by incubating renal papillae for two hours in modified Kreb's solution showed that the hypertensive papillae actually released 52% more PGE_2 than the normotensive papillae. In addition, a maximum fall in blood pressure was noted when hypertensive rats received implanted fragments of "hypertensive" renal papillae (Tobian and Azar, 1971). Hence, it can be stated that these "hypertensive" papillae are capable of making and releasing PGE_2 and are therefore not comparable to the atrophied pancreatic beta cells seen in juvenile diabetes.

Total intrarenal PGE_2 concentration was not different between SHR and WKY rats (Tobian and O'Donnell, 1976). However, when PGE_2 concentration was measured in quick-frozen renal papillae it was 3–4 times higher in the SHR. On the other hand, Dunn et al. (1976), using radioimmunoassay, found no difference in medullary PGE_2 between control and SHR; however, they did observe a substantially greater activity in vitro of prostaglandin synthetase, i.e., increased synthetic rate of PGE_2 in renomedullary microsomes isolated from the hypertensive rats. Sirois and Gagnon (1974), using Goldblatt and SHR models of hypertension, have observed a decreased release of PGE_2-like material from the renal papillae obtained from the hypertensive animals. Two other groups have also reported a reduction in renal PGE_2 synthesis in renal models of hypertension (Leary et al., 1974; Pugsley et al., 1975).

In papillae of SHR, then, changes in interstitial cell granularity parallel changes in sodium concentration. Papillary PGE_2 concentration, however, changes in the opposite direction, i.e., a rise in papillary PGE_2 accompanies the reduction in papillary sodium and interstitial cell granularity. It has been noted that reduction of prostaglandins by indomethacin leads to a heightened papillary sodium concentration. Hence, in hypertensive rats, it can be hypothesized that the opposite phenomenon is occurring, i.e., a rise in papillary PGE_2 is causing a reduction of papillary sodium. Decreased granularity in hypertensive papillae may be a measure of depleted lipid precursors of PGE_2 production and therefore increased in situ medullary PGE_2 and increased PGE_2 synthetic ability.

This general interrelationship between papillary interstitial cell granularity, sodium concentration, and PGE_2 levels has also been found in two normotensive situations. Use of either indomethacin or meclofenamate, two prostaglandin synthesis inhibitors, demonstrates a profound reduction in renal prostaglandin levels, as well as a striking increase in papillary sodium concentrations (Ganguli et al., 1977b). Again, interstitial cell granularity changes in the same direction as sodium concentration, as increased granularity of interstitial cells is observed after 3 days of indomethacin administration (Comai et al., 1975).

After inhibition of prostaglandin synthesis, countercurrent multiplication of sodium chloride appears to function supernormally while average medullary concentration of urea is unaffected. It is conceivable that reducing prostaglandin synthesis with indomethacin could cause the ascending limb to increase its rate of chloride pumping or decrease its rate of sodium and chloride "back leak." This would bring about an increased concentration of chloride and sodium in the papilla. An alternative hypothesis could relate to the collecting tubule, which is reported to synthesize prostaglandins. The collecting tubular epithelium actively transports sodium and some back leak of sodium also occurs. Stokes and Kokko (1977) noted that PGE_2 inhibits net sodium transport in isolated collecting tubules. Thus, it is possible that reducing prostaglandin levels with indomethacin either greatly enhances the rate of pumping or greatly reduces the sodium back leak in the collecting tubule. Such types of alterations of collecting duct function could induce a large increase in sodium concentration within the papilla.

Another instance of this general interrelationship is seen during high NaCl intake, which is associated with an increased concentration of papillary sodium together with a decreased concentration of papillary PGE_2. Regarding interstitial cell granularity, Muehrcke et al. (1969) found no change while Azar et al. (1971) noted a decrease in granularity under a high-NaCl regime. It seems that a change in interstitial cell granularity in stressed normotensive situations is equivocal, unlike the hypertensive state. This bears out the statement of Muehrcke et al. (1969) that cytoplasmic granularity of papillary interstitial cells of normal animals is relatively constant but decreases when the animals develop sustained hypertension associated with morphological vascular abnormalities in the kidney. Hence, decreased granularity appears to be a secondary phenomenon. According to Tobian et al. (1978b), with a high NaCl intake, the rat requires a physiological adaptation that permits the urinary excretion of a very large amount of NaCl, while at the same time conserving body water through the excretion of a highly concentrated urine. The sharply increased concentration of sodium in the renal papilla would provide an enhanced driving force for osmotic reabsorption of water from the collecting tubules. Moreover, the reduction in the level of PGE_2 in the papilla could conceivably enhance the

TABLE 6

Relationship of Papillary Interstitial Cell Granules, Sodium, and PGE_2[a]

	Interstitial cell granules	Sodium	PGE_2
Postsalt hypertension	↓	↓	—
Goldblatt hypertension	↓	↓	—
DOCA hypertension	↓	↓	—
Kyoto spontaneous hypertension	↓	↓	↑
PG synthesis inhibition	↑	↑	↓
High-NaCl diet	→	↑	↓

[a] ↑, Increase; ↓, decrease; →, no change; —, not measured.

action of antidiuretic hormone on the collecting tubular cells, permitting maximum osmotic movement of water from collecting tubular fluid to the renomedullary interstitium. Thus, both the reduction in papillary PGE_2 level and the increase in papillary sodium would encourage the elaboration of a more hyperosmotic urine.

2.4. Summary

In summary, it would appear that decreased granularity of papillary interstitial cells is common to these four types of hypertension. In addition, there is, *vis à vis*, a reduced concentration of papillary sodium. On the other hand, an elevated PGE_2 was seen in the SHR renal papilla, i.e., a rise in papillary PGE_2 accompanies the reduction of papillary sodium. The same general interrelationship has also been noted in two normotensive situations. Reduction of PGE_2 by indomethacin accompanied both an increase in papillary sodium concentration and interstitial cell granularity. In addition, reduced papillary PGE_2 resulting from a high salt intake was associated with a concomitant increase in sodium concentration of the renal papilla. These findings so far provide strong suggestions that PGE_2 does have a great deal of influence on the handling of sodium and chloride in the renal papilla.

A summary of the interrelationship of interstitial cells, sodium, and PGE_2 is presented in Table 6.

REFERENCES

Arendshorst, W. J., and Beierwaltes, W. H. 1979, Renal and nephron hemodynamics in spontaneously hypertensive rats, *Am. J. Physiol.* **236**:F246.

Arendshorst, W. J., Finn, W. F., and Gottschalk, C. W., 1975, Autoregulation of blood flow in the rat kidney, *Am. J. Physiol.* **228**:127.

Atherton, J. C., Hai, M. A., and Thomas, S., 1968a, The time course of changes in renal tissue composition during mannitol diuresis in the rat, *J. Physiol.* **197**:411.

Atherton, J. C., Hai, M. A., and Thomas, S., 1968b, The time course of changes in renal tissue composition during water diuresis in the rat, *J. Physiol.* **197**:429.

Aukland, K., 1966, Study of renal circulation with inert gas; measurements in tissue, *Proceedings of the 3rd International Congress on Nephrology* (J. S. Handler, ed.), Karger, Basel, pp. 188–200.

Azar, S., Tobian, L., and Ishii, M., 1971, Effect of varying levels of dietary Na on sodium in papilla and on the number of papillary interstitial cell granules, *Fed. Proc. Fed. Am. Soc. Exp. Biol.* **30**:609 (abstr).

Azar, S., Johnson, M. A., Bruno, L., and Tobian, L., 1976, Single nephron dynamics in the Kyoto hypertensive and normotensive rat, Proc. Int. Symp. Spontaneously Hypertensive Rat, 2nd, Newport Beach, CA, DHEW Publication No. (NIH) 77-1179, U.S. Government Printing Office, Washington, D.C.

Ben-Ishay, D., Knudsen, K. D., and Dahl, L. K., 1967, Renal function studies in the early stage of salt hypertension in rats, *Proc. Soc. Exp. Biol. Med.* **125**:575.

Berliner, R. W., Levinsky, N. G., Davidson, D. G., and Eden, M., 1958, Dilution and concentration of the urine and the action of antidiuretic hormone, *Am. J. Med.* **24**:730.

Bing, J., and Wiberg, B., 1958, Localization of renin in the kidney, *Acta. Pathol. Microbiol. Scand.* **44**:138.

Bray, G. A., 1960, Freezing point depression of rat kidney slices during water diuresis and antidiuresis, *Am. J. Physiol.* **199**:1211.

Comai, K., Prose, P., Farber, S. J., and Paulsrud, J. R., 1974, Correlation of renal medullary prostaglandin content and renal interstitial cell lipid droplets, *Prostaglandins* **6**:375.

Comai, K., Farber, S. J., and Paulsrud, J. R., 1975, Analyses of renal medullary lipid droplets from normal, hydronephrotic, and indomethacin treated rabbits, *Lipids* **10**:555.

Dahl, L. K., Heine, M., and Tassinari, L., 1962, Effect of chronic salt ingestion; evidence that genetic factors play an important role in susceptibility to experimental hypertension, *J. Exp. Med.* **115**:1173.

Diezi, J., Michoud, P., Aceves, J., and Giebisch, G., 1973, Micropuncture study of electrolyte transport across papillary collecting duct of the rat, *Am. J. Physiol.* **224**:623.

Dunn, M. J., Howe, D., and Harrison, M., 1976, Renal prostaglandin synthesis in the spontaneously hypertensive rat, *J. Clin. Invest.* **58**:862.

Ganguli, M., and Tobian, L., 1974, Does the kidney autoregulate papillary plasma flow in chronic postsalt hypertension? *Am. J. Physiol.* **226**:330.

Ganguli, M., and Tobian, L., 1978, Renal papillary plasma flow in Goldblatt and DOCA hypertension, *Circulation* **58**:II-212 (abstr).

Ganguli, M., Tobian, L., and Dahl, L., 1976, Low renal papillary plasma flow in both Dahl and Kyoto rats with spontaneous hypertension, *Circ. Res.* **39**:337.

Ganguli, M., Tobian, L., O'Donnell, M., and Azar, S., 1977a, Plasma flow and the sodium concentration in renal papilla in young and adult Kyoto hypertensive rats (SHR rats), *Fed. Proc. Fed. Am. Soc. Exp. Biol.* **36**:531 (abstr).

Ganguli, M., Tobian, L., Azar, S., and O'Donnell, M., 1977b, Evidence that prostaglandin synthesis inhibitors increase the concentration of sodium and chloride in rat renal papilla, *Circ. Res.* **40**(Suppl. I):135.

Girndt, J., and Ochwadt, B., 1969, Durchblutung des Nierenmarks, Gesamtnierendurchblutung und cortico-medulläre Gradienten beim experimentellen renalen Hochdruck der Ratte, *Pflügers Arch.* **313**:30.

Gomez, D. M., 1951, Evaluation of renal resistance with special reference to changes in essential hypertension, *J. Clin. Invest.* **30**:1143.

Grangsjo, G., and Wolgast, M., 1972, The pressure–flow relationship in renal cortical and medullary circulation, *Acta Physiol. Scand.* **85**:228.

Hargitay, B., and Kuhn, W., 1951, Das Multiplikationsprinzip als Grundlage der Harnkonzentrierung in der Niere, *Z. Elektrochem.* **55**:539.

Heller, J., and Horacek, V., 1977, Autoregulation of renal blood flow in the rat, *Pflügers Arch.* **370**:81.

Hinshaw, L. B., 1964, Mechanism of renal autoregulation: Role of tissue pressure and description of multifactor hypothesis, *Circ. Res.* **14**–**15**(Suppl. I):120.

Ishii, M., and Tobian, L., 1969, Interstitial cell granules in renal papilla and the solute composition of renal tissue in rats with Goldblatt hypertension, *J. Lab. Clin. Med.* **74**:47.

Johnston, H. H., Herzog, J. P., and Lauler, D. P., 1967, Effect of prostaglandin E_1 on renal hemodynamics, sodium and water excretion, *Am. J. Physiol.* **213**:939.

Kramer, K., Thurau, D., Deetjen, P., 1960, Hämodynamik des Nierenmarks. Capilläre Passagezeit, Blutvolumen, Durchblutung, Gewebshematokrit und O_2-Verbrauch des Nierenmarks in situ, *Arch. Ges. Physiol.* **270**:251.

Leary, W. P., Ledingham, J. G., and Vane, J. R., 1974, Impaired prostaglandin release from the kidneys of salt-loaded and hypertensive rats, *Prostaglandins* **7**:425.

Lee, J. B., 1972, Natriuretic "hormone" and the renal prostaglandins, *Prostaglandins* **1**:55.

Lilienfield, L. S., Rose, J. C., and Lassen, N. A., 1958, Diverse distribution of red cells and albumin in the dog kidney, *Circ. Res.* **6**:810.

Lilienfield, L. S., Maganzini, H. G., and Bauer, M. H., 1961, Blood flow in the renal medulla, *Circ. Res.* **9**:614.

Lowenstein, J., Beranbaum, E. R., Chasis, H., and Baldwin, D. S., 1970, Intrarenal pressure and exaggerated natriuresis in essential hypertension, *Clin. Sci.* **38**:359.

Loyning, E. W., 1971, Effect of reduced perfusion pressure on intrarenal distribution of blood flow in dogs, *Acta Physiol. Scand.* **83**:191.

Mandal, A. K., Frohlich, E. D., Chrysant, K., Pfeffer, M. A., Yunice, A., and Nordquist, J. A., 1974, Ultrastructural analysis of renal papillary interstitial cell of spontaneously hypertensive rats, *J. Lab. Clin. Med.* **83**:256.

Martinez-Maldonado, M., Tsaparas, N., Eknoyan, G., and Suki, W. N., 1972, Renal actions of prostaglandins: Comparison with acetylcholine and volume expansion, *Am. J. Physiol.* **222**:1147.

Miyamoto, J., and Gordon, S., 1970, The cortical and medullary blood flows of the isolated dog's kidney, *Jpn. J. Physiol.* **20**:584.

Moffat, D. B., 1967, The fine structure of the blood vessels of the renal medulla with particular reference to the control of medullary circulation, *J. Ultrastruct. Res.* **19**:532.

Muehrcke, R. C., Mandal, A. K., Epstein, M., and Volini, F. I., 1969, Cytoplasmic granularity of the renal medullary interstitial cells in experimental hypertension, *J. Lab. Clin. Med.* **73**:299.

Muirhead, E. E., Germain, G., Leach, B. E., Pitcock, J. A., Stephenson, P., Brooks, B., Brosius, W. L., Daniels, E. G., and Hinman, J. W., 1972, Production of renomedullary prostaglandins by renomedullary interstitial cells grown in tissue culture, *Circ. Res.* **31**(Suppl. II):161.

Nishiyama, K., Nishiyama, A., and Frohlich, E. D., 1976, Regional blood flow in normotensive and spontaneously hypertensive rats, *Am. J. Physiol.* **230**:691.

Ochwadt, B., 1956, Zur selbstseuerung des Nierenkreislaufes, *Pflügers Arch. Ges. Physiol.* **262**:207.

Peart, W. S., 1959, Renin and hypertension, *Ergebn. Physiol.* **50**:409.

Pugsley, D. J., Beilin, L. J., and Peto, R., 1975, Renal prostaglandin synthesis in the Goldblatt hypertensive rat, *Circ. Res.* **36**—**37**(Suppl. I):81.

Saikia, T. C., 1965, Composition of the renal cortex and medulla of rats during water diuresis and antidiuresis, *Q. J. Exp. Physiol.* **50**:146.

Selkurt, E. E., 1951, Effects of pulse pressure and mean arterial pressure modifications on renal hemodynamics and electrolyte and water excretion, *Circulation* **4**:541.

Sirois, P., and Gagnon, D. J., 1974, Release of renomedullary prostaglandins in normal and hypertensive rats, *Experientia* **30**:1418.

Solez, K., Kramer, E. C., Fox, J. A., and Heptinstall, R. H., 1974, Medullary plasma flow and intravascular leukocyte accumulation in acute renal failure, *Kidney Int.* **6**:24.

Sonnenberg, H., 1974, Medullary collecting duct function in antidiuretic and in salt or water diuretic rats, *Am. J. Physiol.* **226**:501.

Stein, J. H., 1976, The renal circulation, in: *The Kidney* (B. M. Brenner and F. C. Rector, eds.), Saunders, Philadelphia, p. 234.

Stein, J. H., Kirschenbaum, M. A., Bay, W. H., Osgood, R. W., Ferris, T. F., 1975, Role of the collecting duct in the regulation of sodium balance, *Circ. Res.* **36–37**(Suppl I):119.

Stern, M. D., Bowen, P. D., Parma, R., Osgood, R. W., Bowman, R. L., and Stein, J. H., 1979, Measurement of renal cortical and medullary blood flow by laser–doppler spectroscopy in the rat, *Am. J. Physiol.* **236**:F80.

Stokes, J. B., and Kokko, J. P., 1977, Inhibition of sodium transport by prostaglandin E_2 across the isolated, perfused rabbit collecting tubule, *J. Clin. Invest.* **59**:1099.

Thurau, K., 1964, Renal hemodynamics, *Am. J. Med.* **36**:698.

Thurau, K., and Schneermann, J., 1965, Die Natriumkonzentration and den Makula densa Zellen als regulierender Faktor für das Glomerulusfiltrat, *Klin. Wochenschr.* **43**:410.

Thurau, K., Deetjen, P., and Kramer, K., 1960a, Hämodynamik des Nierenmarks. II. Mitteilung. Wechselbeziehung zwischen vascularem und tubularem Gegenstromsystem bei arteriellen Drucksteigerungen, Wasserdiurese und osmotischer Diurese, *Pflügers Arch. Ges. Physiol.* **270**:270.

Thurau, K., Sugiura, T., and Lilienfield, L. S., 1960b, Micropuncture of renal vasa recta in hydropenic hamsters, *Clin. Res.* **8**:383.

Thurau, K., Schneermann, J., Nagl, J., Horster, W., and Wahl, M., 1967, Composition of tubular fluid in the macula densa segment as a factor regulating the function of the juxtaglomerular apparatus, *Circ. Res.* **20–21**(Suppl. II):79.

Tobian, L., 1972, A viewpoint concerning the enigma of hypertension, *Am. J. Med.* **52**:595.

Tobian, L., and Azar, S., 1971, Antihypertensive and other functions of the renal papilla, *Trans. Assoc. Am. Physicians* **84**:281.

Tobian, L., and Ishii, M., 1969, Interstitial cell granules and solutes in renal papilla in post-Goldblatt hypertension, *Am. J. Physiol.* **217**:1699.

Tobian, L., and O'Donnell, M., 1976, Renal prostaglandins in relation to sodium regulation and hypertension, *Fed. Proc. Fed. Am. Soc. Exp. Biol.* **35**:2388.

Tobian, L., Ishii, M., Duke, M., 1969, Relationship of cytoplasmic granules in renal papillary interstitial cells to "post-salt" hypertension, *J. Lab. Clin. Med.* **73**:309.

Tobian, L., O'Donnell, M., Smith, P., 1974a, Intrarenal prostaglandin levels during normal and high sodium intake, *Circ. Res.* **34–35**(Suppl. I):83.

Tobian, L., Johnson, M. A., Lange, J., Magraw, S., 1974b, Effect of varying perfusion pressure on the output of sodium and renin and the vascular resistance in kidneys of rats with "post-salt" hypertension and Kyoto spontaneous hypertension, *Circ. Res.* **36–37**(Suppl. I):162.

Tobian, L., Lange, J., Azar, S., Iwai, J., Koop, D., Coffee, K., and Johnson, M. A., 1978a, Reduction of natriuretic capacity and renin release in isolated, blood-perfused kidneys of Dahl hypertension-prone rats, *Circ. Res.* **43**(Suppl. I):92.

Tobian, L., O'Donnell, M., and Ganguli, M., 1978b, Relationship of prostaglandins and sodium in renal papilla in Kyoto hypertensive rats and during high sodium diets, *Trans. Assoc. Am. Physicians* **91**:204.

Vander, A. J., 1968, Direct effects of prostaglandin on renal function and renin release in anesthesized dog, *Am. J. Physiol.* **214**:218.

Van Dorp, D., 1971, Recent developments in the biosynthesis and analyses of prostaglandin, *Ann. N.Y. Acad. Sci.* **180**:181.

Waugh, W. H., 1964, Myogenic nature of autoregulation of renal flow in the absence of blood corpuscles, *Circ. Res.* **14–15**(Suppl. I):156.

Wirz, H., Hargitay, B., and Kuhn, W., 1951, Lokalisation des Konzentrierungsprozesses in der Niere durch direkte Kryoskopie, *Helv. Physiol. Pharmacol. Acta* **9**:196.

Wolgast, M., 1968, Studies on the regional blood flow with P^{32}-labelled red cells and small beta-sensitive semiconductor detectors, *Acta Physiol. Scand. Suppl.* **313**:1.

Zanszen, F. H. A., and Nugteren, D. H., 1971, Histochemical localization of prostaglandin synthetase, *Histochemie* **27**:159.

CHAPTER 9

Prostaglandin E$_2$ Biosynthesis by Renomedullary Interstitial Cells

In Vitro Studies and Pathophysiological Correlations

RANDALL MARK ZUSMAN

1. INTRODUCTION

In the past decade, there has been a virtual explosion in the number of publications dealing with the biochemistry and physiology of the prostaglandins. The recent discoveries of the thromboxanes (Hamberg *et al.*, 1975) and of prostacyclin (Moncada *et al.*, 1976) have added to the manifold studies of the metabolism of arachidonic acid (Fig. 1) to the prostaglandin (PG) endoperoxides PGG$_2$ and PGH$_2$ (Hamberg *et al.*, 1974) and the subsequent synthesis of thromboxane A$_2$ (TXA$_2$) via thromboxane synthetase, an enzyme specifically inhibitable by imidazole (Needleman *et al.*, 1976*a,b*, 1977*a,b*; of prostacyclin (PGI$_2$) via prostacyclin synthetase (Moncada *et al.*, 1976; Needleman *et al.*, 1977*a,b*), an enzyme inhibitable by 15-hydroperoxy arachidonic acid (Moncada and Vane, 1977; Needleman et al., 1978); and of PGE$_2$ and PGF$_{2\alpha}$ by isomerization and peroxidation (Karim, 1976*a,b*). The entire prostaglandin cascade is initiated by a cyclooxygenase that adds two molecules of oxygen to arachidonic acid, a 20-carbon polyunsaturated fatty acid (Lands *et al.*, 1974; Flower and Vane, 1974). This cyclooxygenase enzyme is inhibited by the nonsteroidal antiinflammatory agents, such as

RANDALL MARK ZUSMAN • Harvard Medical School, Boston, Massachusetts 02115, and Cardiac and Hypertension Units, Medical Services, Massachusetts General Hospital, Boston, Massachusetts 02114.

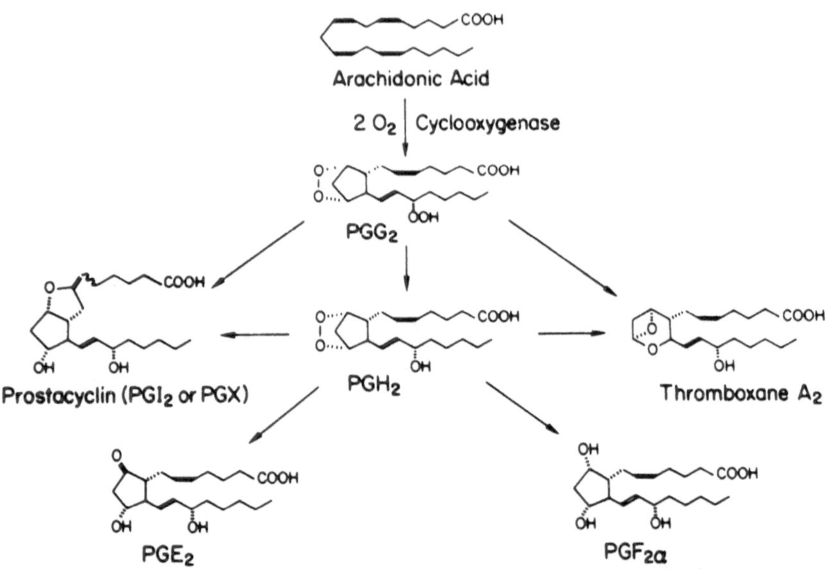

FIGURE 1. Pathways of arachidonic acid metabolism to prostaglandins E_2 and $F_{2\alpha}$, thromboxane A_2, and prostacyclin.

indomethacin, ibuprofen, meclofenamic acid, and naproxen, and is specifically acetylated by acetylsalicylic acid (aspirin) (Rome and Lands, 1975; Pong and Levine, 1976; Lands and Rome, 1976).

Although much progress has been made in understanding the chemistry of arachidonic acid metabolism, less is known about the regulation of prostaglandin synthesis at the cellular level. This relative deficiency in our knowledge is due to the numerous factors that have been shown to affect prostaglandin synthesis, and the many interlocking systems that characterize organ function *in vivo*. In no organ is this more apparent than the kidney (Dunn and Hood, 1977). Although the synthesis of prostaglandins by the kidney *in vivo* and by renal medullary slices *in vitro* has been shown to be sensitive to various physiological and pharmacological manipulations (Karim, 1976a,b; McGiff and Malik, 1976; Dunn and Hood, 1977), little is known about the factors that regulate prostaglandin syntbesis at the cellular level. Since arachidonic acid is not found as the free acid within cellular cytoplasm, but rather is esterified in phospholipids, triglycerides, and cholesterol esters (Lands and Rome, 1976), researchers have assumed that the rate-limiting step in renal prostaglandin synthesis is the rate of arachidonic acid release from these storage forms within the cell. The factors affecting deacylation of arachidonic acid remained largely unknown until the completion of recent studies.

A minimum of five cellular sites within the kidney are capable of prostaglandin synthesis. Using histochemical, anatomical, and/or immunological techniques, investigators have demonstrated that the mesangial cells of the glomerulus (Smith and Bell, 1978; Hassid *et al.*, 1979), the epithelial cells of Bowman's capsule (Smith and Bell, 1978), the endothelium of the renal vasculature (Smith and Bell, 1978), the interstitial cells of the medulla (Janszen and Nugteren, 1971; Bohman, 1977; Tobian and Azar, 1971; Muirhead *et al.*, 1972; Dunn *et al.*, 1976; Smith and Bell, 1978; Zusman and Keiser, 1977*a*), and the epithelial cells of the collecting ducts (Janszen and Nugteren, 1971; Smith and Bell, 1978) all metabolize arachidonic acid to PGE$_2$ or PGF$_{2\alpha}$, TXA$_2$, and/or prostacylcin. Yet because of the multiple sites of synthesis and the many intrarenal compensatory mechanisms that characterize the kidney, it has been difficult to isolate the factors that affect prostaglandin synthesis using organ studies *in vivo* or experiments involving tissue slices *in vitro*.

Although the kidney is capable of synthesizing TXA$_2$ (Morrison *et al.*, 1977) and prostacyclin (Needleman *et al.*, 1978), the major product of arachidonic acid metabolism in the kidney is PGE$_2$ (Crowshaw *et al.*, 1970; Frolich *et al.*, 1975; Dunn and Hood, 1977). The isolation of rabbit renomedullary interstitial cells in tissue culture using techniques of autologous implantation (Muirhead *et al.*, 1972; Zusman and Keiser, 1977*a*) has provided a model system for the study of the regulation of arachidonic acid metabolism and PGE$_2$ biosynthesis. This system allows for the precise regulation of the environment in which the cells are grown and provides an opportunity for the determination of the effects of physiological stimuli and pharmacological agents on PGE$_2$ biosynthesis by a uniform population of cells growing as a monolayer in tissue culture.

2. REGULATION OF ARACHIDONIC ACID METABOLISM BY RABBIT RENOMEDULLARY INTERSTITIAL CELLS IN TISSUE CULTURE

When grown in RPMI-1640 tissue culture medium, and studied in Krebs's bicarbonate buffer (pH 8.1, osmolarity 300 mOsm/liter) in an atmosphere of 95% air–5% carbon dioxide, rabbit renomedullary interstitial cells synthesize 1.8 ± 0.4 pmoles PGE$_2$/μg cellular protein per hr (mean $\pm$ SEM, $N = 24$) (Zusman and Keiser 1977*a,b*, 1980). When arachidonic acid is added to the tissue culture medium, PGE$_2$ synthesis can be increased to a maximum of 200 ± 12 pmoles PGE$_2$/μg cellular protein per hr ($N = 4$) at arachidonic acid concentrations equal to or in excess of 3.3 mM.

2.1. Prostaglandin E$_2$ Synthesis

2.1.1. *Effects of Sodium, Potassium, and Osmolality (Table 1)*

The renomedullary interstitial cells are found *in vivo* in a region of the kidney characterized by a widely divergent ionic composition and osmotic

TABLE 1

The Effects of Angiotensin II, Potassium-Free Media, Hyperosmolality, and Dexamethasone on Prostaglandin E_2 Synthesis, Arachidonic Acid Release, Phospholipase Activity, and the Arachidonic Acid Storage Pool in Rabbit Renomedullary Interstitial Cells in Tissue Culture[a]

Experimental conditions	Prostaglandin E_2 synthesis (pmoles PGE_2/μg protein per hr)	Radiolabeled materials released (fmoles/μg protein per hr)		Phospholipase activity (fmoles arachidonic acid released/μg protein per hr)	Arachidonic acid storage pool (pmoles/μg protein)	
		Arachidonic acid	PGE_2		Phospholipids	Triglycerides
Basal	1.8 ± 0.4	66 ± 5	9.8 ± 0.6	422 ± 13	17.17 ± 0.14	15.13 ± 0.39
Angiotensin II (2 nM)	27.1 ± 1.4*	3870 ± 140*	622 ± 63*	1641 ± 76*	14.14 ± 0.29*	15.14 ± 0.24
Potassium (0 mEq/liter)	3.2 ± 0.5*	120 ± 10*	18.2 ± 1.3*	395 ± 29	16.22 ± 0.18*	15.09 ± 0.23
Hyperosmolality (1200 mOsm/liter)	7.9 ± 0.7*	254 ± 18*	39.7 ± 2.5*	441 ± 31	15.83 ± 0.18*	14.75 ± 0.26
Dexamethasone (500 nM)	1.0 ± 0.2*	25 ± 3*	4.1 ± 0.9*	419 ± 18	17.54 ± 0.11*	14.70 ± 0.31

[a] Rabbit renomedullary interstitial cells were incubated for 1 hr in Krebs-bicarbonate buffer (pH 8.1, potassium concentration 3 mEq/liter, osmolality 300 mosmole/liter). PGE_2 synthesis was measured by radioimmunoassay (Zusman and Keiser, 1977a); arachidonic acid and PGE_2 release were measured after thin-layer chromatography of the incubation medium from cells incubated with radiolabeled arachidonic acid (Zusman and Keiser, 1977b); phospholipase activity was measured as the rate of release of arachidonic acid from a radiolabeled arachidonic-acid-containing phospholipid substrate (Zusman and Brown, 1979); the distribution of arachidonic acid in the cellular lipid storage pool was measured by thin-layer chromatographic separation of the lipids extracted from cells incubated with tritium-labeled arachidonic acid (Zusman and Brown, 1979). Each value represents the mean ± standard error of the mean ($N = 6$). An asterisk (*) indicates statistical significance ($p < 0.01$) compared to basal values.

tonicity as compared with the cellular environment of the remainder of the kidney or other organ systems. As a result of the countercurrent system of the loop of Henle, the renal papillary interstitium with which the interstitial cells are in equilibrium may have an osmolality of as high as 1200 mosmole/liter; furthermore, the interstitial cells are also in equilibrium with the urinary space when the epithelial surface of the collecting duct is under the influence of antidiuretic hormone. Because the ionic composition of the urine with repect to sodium and potassium can vary greatly in response to the dietary intake of these cations, the renomedullay interstitial cells may be exposed to marked swings in interstitial fluid cationic composition.

When the osmolality of the incubation medium in which the cells were grown was increased from 300 mosmole/liter (the osmolality of plasma) to 1200 mosmole/liter (the maximal osmolality of the renal papilla and the maximum concentration of rabbit urine during marked fluid depression), a progressive increase in the rate of PGE₂ synthesis was observed to a maximum of 7.9 ± 0.7 pmoles PGE₂/μg cellular protein per hr.

If the osmolality of the incubation buffer was held constant at 300 mOsm/liter but the sodium content was increased from zero to 100 mEq/liter PGE₂ synthesis was not affected. However, when potassium was removed from the buffer (normal potassium concentration is 3 mEq/liter), PGE₂ synthesis increased from 1.8 ± 0.4 to 3.2 ± 0.5 pmoles PGE₂/μg cellular protein per hr ($p < 0.01$, $N = 6$). The addition of potassium to the incubation medium so as to increase the extracellular potassium concentration from 2.0 to 7.0 mEq/liter resulted in a 7% inhibition of PGE₂ synthesis per mEq/liter increase in the potassium concentration.

2.1.2. *Effects of Angiotensin II, Bradykinin, and Arginine Vasopressin (Table 1)*

Experiments *in vitro* using the isolated perfused kidney or renal slices and studies of renal prostaglandin release *in vivo* have shown that the vasoactive peptides, angiotensin II and bradykinin, stimulate renal prostaglandin synthesis. Angiotensin II, 2 nM, increased PGE₂ synthesis from 1.8 ± 0.4 to 27.1 ± 1.4 pmoles PGE₂/μg cellular protein per hr ($N = 6$, $p < 0.001$). Maximal stimulation of PGE₂ synthesis, 36.8 pmoles PGE₂/μg protein per hr, was elicited by an angiotensin II concentration of 4 nM.

Bradykinin, a potent vasodilator in the kidney and natriuretic agent, increased PGE₂ synthesis to 6.5 ± 0.5 pmoles PGE₂/μg protein per hr at a concentration of 100 nM; half-maximal stimulation of PGE₂ synthesis occurred at a bradykinin concentration of 32 nM.

Arginine vasopressin, the mammalian antidiuretic hormone, stimulated PGE₂ synthesis to 5.8 ± 0.4 pmoles PGE₂/μg cellular protein per hr at a concentration of 1 μM; half-maximal stimulation of PGE₂ synthesis occurred at a vasopressin concentration of 380 nM.

When the renomedullary interstitial cells were incubated with mepacrine (100 μM), a phospholipase inhibitor, or indomethacin (100 μM), a cyclooxygenase inhibitor, angiotension II (2 nM)-stimulated PGE_2 synthesis fell from 27.1 $\pm$ 1.4 to 13.7 $\pm$ 1.4 (N = 6, p < 0.01) and 0.21 $\pm$ 0.03 (N = 6, p < 0.001), pmoles PGE_2/μg cellular protein per hr, respectively. Bradykinin- and arginine- vasopressin-stimulated PGE_2 synthesis were also inhibited by mepacrine and indomethacin. The effects of mepacrine and indomethacin on polypeptide-stimulated PGE_2 synthesis suggest that these peptides stimulated phospholipase-mediated arachidonic acid release with a resultant increase in the concentration of free arachidonic acid that can be metabolized to PGE_2.

2.1.3. *Effects of Adrenal Steroid Hormones*

Adrenal steroid hormones have been shown to inhibit PGE_2 synthesis in a number of organs and tissues (Lewis and Piper, 1975; Kantrowitz *et al.*, 1975; Tashjian *et al.*, 1975; Floman and Zor, 1976; Hong and Levine, 1976; Gryglewski, 1976; Chang *et al.*, 1977; Chandrabose *et al.*, 1978; Zusman *et al.*, 1978). After incubation of the cells for 18 hr with dexamethasone (500 nM), basal PGE_2 synthesis fell from 1.8 $\pm$ 0.4 to 1.0 $\pm$ 0.2 picomoles PGE_2/μg cellular protein per hr (N = 6, p < 0.01).

2.1.4. *Effect of Protein Synthesis Inhibition*

Pong, Hong, and Levine (1977) have reported that protein synthesis inhibitors decrease peptide-hormone-stimulated PGE_2 in BALB/3T3 fibroblasts in tissue culture. Preincubation of renomedullary interstitial cells with cycloheximide (35 μM) for 2 hr decreased angiotensin II-stimulated PGE_2 synthesis from 27.1 $\pm$ 1.4 to 8.6 $\pm$ 1.1 pmoles PGE_2/μg cellular protein per hr (N = 6, p < 0.001). Cycloheximide also inhibited bradykinin- and vasopressin-stimulated PGE_2 synthesis, but had no effect on basal PGE_2 synthesis or on the effects of arachidonic acid, potassium, hyperosmolality, or corticosteroids on PGE_2 synthesis by the renomedullary interstitial cell in tissue culture.

2.2. Regulation of Arachidonic Acid Release (Tables 1 and 2)

Although experiments performed with the phospholipase inhibitor mepacrine and the cyclooxygenase inhibitor indomethacin suggest that angiotensin II-stimulated PGE_2 synthesis is due to an increase in the rate of arachidonic acid release, measurements of the rate of PGE_2 synthesis are not conclusive. It is possible, however, to label the arachidonic acid storage pool of the cells with radiolabeled (tritium-containing) arachidonic acid.

TABLE 2

The Effects of Cycloheximide, Mepacrine, and Indomethacin on Angiotensin II-Stimulated PGE$_2$ Synthesis, Arachidonic Acid Release, Phospholipase Activity, and the Arachidonic Acid Storage Pool in Rabbit Renomedullary Interstitial Cells in Tissue Culture[a]

Experimental conditions	Prostaglandin E$_2$ synthesis (pmoles PGE$_2$/μg protein per hr)	Radiolabeled materials released (fmoles/μg protein per hr)		Phospholipase activity (fmoles arachidonic acid released/μg protein per hr)	Arachidonic acid storage pool (pmoles/μg protein)	
		Arachidonic acid	PGE$_2$		Phospholipids	Triglycerides
Angiotensin II (2 nM)	27.1 ± 1.4	3870 ± 140	622 ± 63	1641 ± 76	14.14 ± 0.29	15.14 ± 0.24
+ cycloheximide (35 μM)	8.6 ± 1.1*	1307 ± 45*	211 ± 23*	974 ± 37*	15.79 ± 0.19*	14.87 ± 0.29
+ mepacrine (100 μM)	13.7 ± 1.4*	1880 ± 170*	209 ± 18*	806 ± 66*	16.18 ± 0.25*	14.94 ± 0.38
+ indomethacin (100 μM)	0.21 ± 0.03*	4090 ± 190	1.8 ± 0.1*	1601 ± 57	14.77 ± 0.60	14.98 ± 0.27

[a] Prostaglandin E$_2$ synthesis, arachidonic acid release, phospholipase activity, and the distribution of arachidonic acid in the cellular storage pool were measured as described in the footnote to Table 1. The cells were preincubated with cycloheximide, mepacrine, or indomethacin for a minimum of 2 hr prior to incubation with angiotensin II. Each value represents the mean ± standard error of the mean ($N = 6$). An asterisk (*) indicates statistical significance ($p < 0.01$) compared to the value obtained after incubation with angiotensin II alone.

Thin-layer chromatographic analysis of the radiolabeled materials released from these cells under different experimental conditions (Zusman and Keiser, 1977b) provides information regarding the rate of arachidonic acid release as well as the simultaneous rate of conversion of arachidonic acid to PGE_2. With these techniques, an increase in PGE_2 synthesis due to an increase in cyclooxygenase activity can be distinguished from an increase in PGE_2 synthesis secondary to an increase in the rate of arachidonic acid release. The latter would result in an increase in the precursor concentration in the cellular cytoplasm, whereas the former would result in an increase in the rate of conversion of arachidonic acid to PGE_2.

Angiotensin II (2 nM) stimulated tritium-labeled arachidonic acid release from 66 ± 5 to 3870 ± 140 fmoles [^{3}H]arachidonic acid/μg cellular protein per hr ($N = 6$, $p < 0.001$) and [^{3}H]-PGE_2 release from 9.8 ± 0.6 to 622 ± 63 fmoles [^{3}H]-PGE_2/μg cellular protein per hr ($N = 6$, $p < 0.001$). Mepacrine (100 μM) decreased angiotensin II-stimulated tritium-labeled arachidonic acid and PGE_2 release to 1880 ± 170 and 209 ± 18 fmoles/μg cellular protein per hr ($N = 6$, $p < 0.01$), respectively. Indomethacin (100 μM) decreased angiotensin II-stimulated, tritium-labeled PGE_2 release to 1.8 ± 0.1 ($N = 6$, $p < 0.001$), but had no effect on [^{3}H]arachidonic acid release, which was 4090 ± 190 fmoles [^{3}H]arachidonic acid/μg cellular protein per hr ($N = 6$). Cycloheximide (35 μM) decreased angiotensin II-stimulated tritium-labeled arachidonic acid and PGE_2 release to 1307 ± 45 and 211 ± 23 fmoles/μg cellular protein per hr ($N = 6$, $p < 0.01$), respectively.

An increase in the osmolality of the incubation medium from 300 to 1200 mOsm/liter resulted in an increase in the rate of tritium-labeled arachidonic acid and PGE_2 release to 254 ± 18 and 39.7 ± 2.5 fmoles/μg cellular protein per hr ($N = 6$, $p < 0.001$), respectively. An increase in the rate of PGE_2 synthesis has been observed in rat renal papillae *in vitro* exposed to hypertonic solutions (Danon *et al.*, 1978). In these experiments, a fall in the specific activity of PGE_2 synthesized from [^{14}C]arachidonic acid was observed in papillae incubated in hypertonic medium as compared to PGE_2 synthesis by papillae incubated in isotonic media; these results were interpreted as being consistent with an increase in the availability of endogenous arachidonic acid in tissue incubated in hypertonic solutions. The results of the experiments in rabbit renomedullary interstitial cells confirm that the mechanism of stimulation of PGE_2 synthesis by hypertonic media is an increase in the rate of arachidonic acid release from the endogenous arachidonic acid storage pool.

Removal of potassium from the incubation medium resulted in an increase in the rate of tritium-labeled arachidonic acid and PGE_2 release to 120 ± 10 and 18.2 ± 1.3 fmoles/μg cellular protein per hr ($N = 6$, $p < 0.01$), respectively, in comparison to arachidonic acid and PGE_2 release by cells incubated in tissue culture medium containing 3 mEq/liter potassium. Dexamethasone (500 nM) decreased tritium-labeled arachidonic acid and PGE₂ release to 23 ± 3 and 4.1 ± 0.9 fmoles/μg cellular protein per hr ($N = 6, p < 0.01$), respectively. Unlike the effect of protein synthesis inhibition on angiotensin II-stimulated arachidonic acid release, cycloheximide did not influence the effects of hyperosmolality, dexamethasone, or potassium-free buffer on arachidonic acid release and PGE₂ synthesis.

Neither angiotensin II, mepacrine, cycloheximide, potassium, hyperosmolality, nor dexamethasone affected the rate of conversion of arachidonic acid to PGE₂; the ratio of PGE₂ released to arachidonic acid released was 0.152 ± 0.008 ($N = 7$). Thus, these studies suggest that the cyclooxygenase activity of the cells remains constant and is not the rate-limiting factor in the regulation of PGE₂ synthesis under normal conditions. When the cells are exposed to persistently elevated concentrations of arachidonic acid, in excess of 1.6 mM, a progressive loss of cyclooxygenase activity occurs (Zusman and Keiser, 1980). This arachidonic acid-mediated deactivation of the cyclooxygenase is due to the generation of oxidizing free radicals during the synthesis of the prostaglandin endoperoxides (Egan et al., 1976).

2.3. Regulation of Phospholipase Activity (Tables 1 and 2)

Although the experiments in rabbit renomedullary interstitial cells in tissue culture described above (Zusman and Keiser, 1977a,b, 1980) as well as studies in the lung (Vargaftig and Hai, 1972) and in methylcholanthrene-transformed BALB/3T3 fibroblasts in tissue culture (Hong and Levine, 1976; Pong and Levine, 1976; Pong et al., 1977) suggest that polypeptide-hormone-stimulated PGE₂ synthesis is due to an increase in phospholipase-mediated arachidonic acid release, direct measurement of phospholipase activity has not been reported. After incubation of renomedullary interstitial cells with tritium-labeled arachidonic acid, the radiolabeled phospholipids can be extracted from the cells and purified by thin-layer chromatography (Ramwell and Daniels, 1969). Using these endogenously synthesized phospholipids as the substrates for a phospholipase assay, it is possible to measure phospholipase activity in a sonicate of the cells in tissue culture (Zusman and Brown, 1979, 1980).

Basal phospholipase activity was 422 ± 13 fmoles tritium-labeled arachidonic acid released/μg cellular protein per hr. The addition of angiotensin II (2 nM) increased phospholipase activity to 1641 ± 76 fmoles [³H]arachidonic acid released/μg cellular protein per hr. Cycloheximide (35 μM) and mepacrine (100 μM) decreased angiotensin-II-stimulated phospholipase activity to 974 ± 37 and 806 ± 66 fmoles [³H]arachidoinc acid released/μg cellular protein per hr ($N = 6, p < 0.001$), respectively.

Indomethacin (100 μM) had no effect on angiotensin II-stimulated phospholipase activity.

Phospholipase activity in cells incubated in potassium-free buffer, in hyperosmolar (1200 mOsm/liter) buffer, or with dexamethasone (500 nM) was 395 $\pm$ 29, 441 $\pm$ 31, and 419 $\pm$ 18 fmoles [^{3}H]arachidonic acid released/μM cellular protein per hr (N = 6), respectively; none of these values differ significantly from phospholipase activity measured under basal conditions (potassium concentration 3 mEq/liter, osmolality 300 mOsm/liter).

2.4. The Phospholipid–Triglyceride Arachidonic Acid Storage Pool

When incubated for 24 hr with tritium-labeled arachidonic acid, rabbit renomedullary interstitial cells incorporate 56% of the label into phospholipids, 43% into triglycerides, and 1% into cholesterol esters (Zusman and Keiser, 1977b; Zusman and Brown, 1979).

After incubation with angiotensin II (2 nM), the tritium-labeled arachidonic-acid-containing phospholipid concentration of the cells fell from 17.17 $\pm$ 0.14 to 14.14 $\pm$ 0.29 pmoles [^{3}H]arachidonic acid/μg cellular protein (N = 6, p < 0.001). After incubation with angiotensin II (2 nM) and cycloheximide (35 μM) or mepacrine (100 μM), the tritium-labeled arachidonic-acid-containing phospholipid concentration fell to 15.79 $\pm$ 0.19 and 16.18 $\pm$ 0.25 pmoles [^{3}H]arachidonic acid/μg cellular protein, respectively. These values are significantly lower than the concentration observed in the cells under basal conditions (N = 6, p < 0.01) and greater than the concentration after incubation with angiotensin II alone (p < 0.01). After incubation with angiotensin II and indomethacin (100 μM), the arachidonic-acid-containing phospholipid concentration was 14.77 $\pm$ 0.60 pmoles [^{3}H]arachidonic acid/μg cellular protein; this value was significantly lower (N = 6, p < 0.01) than the concentration under basal conditions, but not different from the concentration observed after incubation with angiotensin II alone.

Incubation of the cells in potassium-free buffer or under conditions of hyperosmolality (1200 mosmole/liter) resulted in a fall in the arachidonic-acid-containing phospholipid concentration to 16.22 $\pm$ 0.18 and 15.83 $\pm$ 0.18 pmoles [^{3}H]arachidonic acid/μg cellular protein (N = 6, p < 0.01), respectively. Incubation of the cells with dexamethasone (500 nM) resulted in an increase in the concentration of arachidonic-acid-containing phospholipids to 17.54 $\pm$ 0.11 pmoles [^{3}H]arachidonic acid/μg cellular protein (N = 6, p < 0.01) (Zusman and Brown, 1979).

The arachidonic-acid-containing triglyceride concentration of the rabbit renomedullary interstitial cells in tissue culture was 15.13 $\pm$ 0.39 pmoles

[^{3}H]arachidonic acid/μg cellular protein, and was unaffected by angiotensin II, hyperosmolality, dexamethasone, or incubation in potassium-free buffer (Zusman and Brown, 1979).

2.5. Summary

The rabbit renomedullary interstitial cells in tissue culture are a model system for the study of the regulation of arachidonic acid metabolism and PGE$_2$ biosynthesis at the cellular level (Zusman and Keiser, 1977a). Polypeptide-hormone-stimulated PGE$_2$ synthesis, such as that which occurs after incubation of the cells with angiotension II, bradykinin, or arginine vasopressin, is due to an increase in cellular phospholipase activity and the resultant increase in the cytoplasmic concentration of arachidonic acid, the precursor of PGE$_2$ (Zusman and Keiser, 1977b; Zusman and Brown, 1979). The stimulation of phospholipase activity by these vasoactive peptides can be blocked by cycloheximide, an inhibitor of protein synthesis (Zusman and Keiser, 1980; Zusman and Brown, 1979). Incubation with the protein synthesis inhibitor for as little as 2 hr results in maximal inhibition of angiotensin II-stimulated PGE$_2$ synthesis and arachidonic acid release; the time course of this effect suggests that a "labile" protein is synthesized in response to polypeptide hormone–receptor interaction. Either this "labile" protein activates latent phospholipase by serving as a cofactor for the reaction or by cleaving a subunit from the enzyme molecule, or it is the phospholipase itself. Pong et al. (1977), in their studies of PGE$_2$ synthesis by the BALB/3T3 fibroblast in tissue culture, have also observed a dependence of peptide-hormone-stimulated PGE$_2$ synthesis on an intact mechanism for protein synthesis and have found a time course of action of cycloheximide similar to that observed in interstitial cells.

Hyperosmolality and incubation in potassium-free media cause an increase in arachidonic acid release and PGE$_2$ synthesis; dexamethasone causes a decrease. Unlike the effect of angiotensin II, the effects of hyperosmolality, potassium-free media, and dexamethasone are not affected by protein synthesis inhibition and are not associated with a change in cellular phospholipase activity (Zusman and Keiser, 1977a, 1980; Zusman and Brown, 1979). Like angiotensin II, however, hyperosmolality and potassium-free media decrease the concentration of arachidonic acid in the form of phospholipids in the cells, dexamethasone increases the concentration of arachidonic acid in the form of phospholipids. Neither angiotensin II, hyperosmolality, potassium-free media, nor dexamethasone affects the concentration of arachidonic acid in the form of triglycerides in the cells. This series of observations suggests that the changes in arachidonic acid release and PGE$_2$ synthesis that occur after incubation with dexamethasone or in hypertonic or potassium-free media are not due to changes in phospholipase activity, but result from changes in the availability of phospholipids in the cell membrane as substrates for phospholipase action.

3. PATHOPHYSIOLOGICAL CORRELATIONS

3.1. Role of Prostaglandin E_2 in the Regulation of Vasopressin-Stimulated Water Permeability

PGE$_2$ inhibits vasopressin-stimulated water permeability in the toad (*Bufo marinus*) urinary bladder *in vitro* (Orloff *et al.*, 1965; Lipson *et al.*, 1971; Lipson and Sharp, 1971; Ozer and Sharp, 1972; Flores and Sharp, 1972; Omachi *et al.*, 1974; Albert and Handler, 1974; Urakabe *et al.*, 1975; Zusman *et al.*, 1977a,b, 1978; Zusman, 1980) and in the isolated perfused rabbit collecting tubule (Grantham and Orloff, 1968). It has been concluded that endogenous PGE$_2$ synthesis modulates basal and vasopressin-stimulated adenylate cyclase activity (Zusman *et al.*, 1977a; Orloff and Zusman, 1978; Zusman, 1980) because (1) PGE$_2$ also inhibits the water permeability response to vasopressin and theophylline, but not to cyclic 3′,5′-adenosine monophosphate (Orloff *et al.*, 1965; Zusman *et al.*, 1977a; Orloff and Zusman, 1978); (2) inhibition of PGE$_2$ synthesis enhances vasopressin- and theophylline- but not AMP-stimulated water flow (Albert and Handler, 1974; Zusman *et al.*, 1977a); and (3) PGE$_2$ inhibits vasopressin-stimulated AMP accumulation in the epithelial cells of the toad urinary bladder (Omachi *et al.*, 1974). Laboratory proof of the inhibition of basal and vasopressin-sensitive adenylate cyclase activity by PGE$_2$, however, has been difficult to obtain (Handler and Orloff, 1973).

The demonstration of vasopressin-stimulated PGE$_2$ synthesis in rabbit renomedullary interstitial cells in tissue culture (Zusman and Keiser, 1977a,b) suggested that endogenous PGE$_2$ might modulate the water permeability response to vasopressin of the mammalian kidney. In the toad urinary bladder *in vitro*, a model for a vasopressin-sensitive epithelial membrane, it was shown that vasopressin, but not theophylline or cAMP, stimulates endogenous PGE$_2$ biosynthesis (Zusman *et al.*, 1977a) via an increase in the rate of release of arachidonic acid from the cellular arachidonic acid storage pool. Like the mechanism of peptide-stimulated PGE$_2$ synthesis in the renomedullary interstitial cell, vasopressin-stimulated PGE$_2$ synthesis in the toad urinary bladder can be inhibited by mepacrine, a phospholipase inhibitor, or indomethacin, a cyclooxygenase inhibitor. Furthermore, as in the renomedullary interstitial cell, vasopressin-stimulated PGE$_2$ synthesis can be inhibited by cycloheximide and by adrenal steroid hormones (Zusman *et al.*, 1978). Agents that inhibit endogenous vasopressin-stimulated PGE_2 synthesis enhance vasopressin-stimulated water permeability (Zusman *et al.*, 1977*a,b*, 1978; Zusman, 1980). Evidence for the stimulation of renal PGE_2, synthesis *in vivo* by vasopressin and for the role of PGE_2 in the modulation of water reabsorption has been obtained in the rat (Berl *et al.*, 1977; Lum *et al.*, 1977; Walker *et al.*, 1978; Dunn *et al.*, 1977, 1978; Bell and Mya, 1977), in the rabbit (Lifschitz and Stein, 1977), in the dog (Anderson *et al.*, 1975; Berl and Schrier, 1973) and in humans (Berl *et al.*, 1977; Zusman *et al.*, 1979). Furthermore, the inhibition of PGE_2 synthesis appears to play an important role in the hyponatremic syndromes that occur after chlorpropamide administration (Ardvino *et al.*, 1966; Moses *et al.*, 1973; Zusman *et al.*, 1977*b,c*) and after the simultaneous administration of adrenocorticotrophic hormone and indomethacin (Zusman *et al.*, 1979). The site of synthesis of the intrarenal PGE_2 that inhibits vasopressin-stimulated water flow is as yet unproven. It is possible that vasopressin stimulates PGE_2 release from the medullary interstitial cells and that this PGE_2, which enters the tubule of the nephron at the loop of Henle and also may diffuse through the interstitial fluid, decreases vasopressin-stimulated cyclic AMP accumulation in the epithelial cells of the collecting duct. It is possible also that the collecting duct epithelia, which are capable of prostaglandin synthesis (Janszen and Nugteren, 1971; Bohman, 1977; Smith and Bell, 1978) synthesize PGE_2 in response to vasopressin and regulate their own water permeability response to the peptide hormone. The ability of the collecting duct epithelial cells to synthesize PGE_2 in response to vasopressin has not yet been proven *in vivo* or *in vitro*, and further investigation of this question awaits the isolation of these cells in tissue culture.

3.2. Enhanced Renal Prostaglandin E_2 Synthesis in Bartter's Syndrome and Other Hypokalemic Disorders

Bartter's syndrome is a disorder characterized by hypokalemic alkalosis, hyperreninemia, hyperaldosteronism, normotension, and vascular insensitivity to angiotension II (Bartter *et al.*, 1962). Histologic examination of renal biopsy tissue from patients with Bartter' syndrome reveals hyperplasia of the juxtaglomerular apparatus, consistent with the increased rate of renin production. Because of evidence for the role of prostaglandins in the regulation of renin release, the possibility that Bartter's syndrome was due to an excess of prostaglandin synthesis was investigated. It was found that these patients have an increased rate of renal prostaglandin synthesis (Verberckmoes *et al.*, 1976; Fichman *et al.*, 1976; Gill *et al.*, 1976; Norby *et al.*, 1976). Furthermore, histologic examination of the medullary and papillary regions of the kidney revealed hyperplasia of the medullary interstitial cells (Verberckmoes *et al.*, 1976). These findings provide a clinical correlation of the increased PGE_2 synthesis by renomedullary interstitial cells in tissue culture when incubated in potassium-free buffer. Depletion of the intracellular potassium, as occurs in potassium wasting disorders, presumably increases prostaglandin synthesis via the mechanism demonstrated in the medullary interstitial cell *in vitro*. It has been shown recently that potassium-depleted normal dogs (Galvez *et al.*, 1977) or normal humans (Gill and Bartter, 1978), or hypokalemic humans with disorders other than Bartter's syndrome (Gullner *et al.*, 1979) also have increased renal PGE_2 synthesis. Thus, the elevations of renal prostaglandin biosynthesis and renin and aldosterone release, the vascular insensitivity to angiotension II, and the associated abnormalities of the kallikrein–kinin system in such patients (Vinci *et al.*, 1978) are secondary to potassium depletion *per se*, and are not a primary etiologic factor in this disease. Bartter's syndrome is now thought to result from an abnormality of chloride transport in the loop of Henle (Gill and Bartter, 1978). The inhibition of prostaglandin biosynthesis with cyclooxygenase inhibitors corrects toward normal the plasma aldosterone and renin activity, plasma and urinary bradykinin, urinary PGE_2, kinin and kallikrein excretion, and vascular insensitivity to angiotension II, but does not correct the abnormality of chloride transport (Gill *et al.*, 1976; Gill and Bartter, 1978; Vinci *et al.*, 1978).

3.3. Renomedullary Interstitial Cell Tumor and Its Relationship to Hypertension

Adenomatous hyperplasia of the renomedullary interstitial cell results in the formation of tumorlike nodules, formerly known as fibromas of the renal medulla (Reese and Winstanley, 1958; Lerman *et al.*, 1972; Preszyna *et al.*, 1973). These nodules (1) are less than 1 cm in diameter, (2) may be solitary or multiple within an individual kidney, (3) are unencapsulated but may compress or encompass the surrounding tubular structures, and (4) have a high prostaglandin content. Light microscopic examination of tissue stained with oil red 0 or sudan black, and electron microscopy after fixation with osmium tetroxide, confirmed the presence of lipid-laden granules within the cellular cytoplasm; these granules are characteristic of the interstitial cell *in situ* and in tissue culture. The presence or absence of these nodules of renomedullary interstitial cells has not correlated with abnormalities of blood pressure or renal function (Stuart *et al.*, 1976; Martin and Tiltman, 1976). It is likely that the nodules represent benign adenomatous hyperplasia of this "endocrinelike" cell without any resultant pathophysiological abnormalities. On the other hand, fibrosis of the renal medulla with destruction of the interstitial cells was associated with an increase in blood pressure in one series of patients; the authors of this report suggested that the loss of the antihypertensive activity of the interstitial cells leads to an increase in blood pressure (Haggitt *et al.*, 1971). The preliminary report has not been followed by publication of more conclusive data, and the relationship between renomedullary interstitial cell tumors, renomedullary fibrosis, and blood pressure regulation thus remains unconfirmed.

3.4. Relationship of Angiotensin II Binding to Prostaglandin E₂ Synthesis in the Renomedullary Interstitial Cell

Angiotensin II binds to rabbit renomedullary interstitial cells with the characteristics of an interaction with a membrane receptor protein. Binding studies have revealed that hormone–receptor interaction (1) is saturable; (2) is reversible; (3) is selective for angiotensin II analogues with physiological activity; (4) is inhibited by sar^{1}ala^8-angiotensin II, an antagonist of angiotensin activity *in vivo;* and (5) occurs at concentrations of the peptide that are found under normal physiological conditions (Brown *et al.*, 1979*a,b*, 1980). Similarly, the stimulation of phospholipase activity, arachidonic acid release, and PGE₂ synthesis occurs over an angiotensin II concentration range that is consistent with the K_D of the receptor, which has been measured as 3.1 nM (Zusman and Brown, 1979). These studies suggest that *in vivo* renomedullary interstitial cell function is affected by changes in plasma renin activity and angiotensin II concentration. It is possible that abnormalities of angiotensin binding and activation of the phospholipase may occur in experimental animals or in humans with abnormalities of blood pressure regulation.

4. CONCLUSIONS

The renomedullary interstitial cell is a highly specialized, endocrinelike cell capable of prostaglandin E₂ synthesis (Fig. 2). The vasoactive polypeptides angiotensin II, bradykinin, and arginine vasopressin stimulate phospholipase activity, arachidonic acid release, and PGE₂ synthesis via a mechanism that is dependent on protein synthesis. On the other hand, potassium, osmolality, and dexamethasone affect arachidonic acid release and PGE₂ synthesis through mechanisms that are independent of phospholipase activity and protein synthesis. Physiological studies in experimental animals, isolated tissues *in vitro*, and humans suggest that the interstitial cells play a role in the pathophysiology of hypokalemic disorders and vasopressin-stimulated water permeability of the renal collecting duct. The relationship of tumors of renomedullary interstitial cells to renal function or abnormalities of blood pressure regulation remains unknown. However, the rabbit renomedullary interstitial cell in tissue culture can be used as a model system for the study of the cellular regulation of arachidonic acid

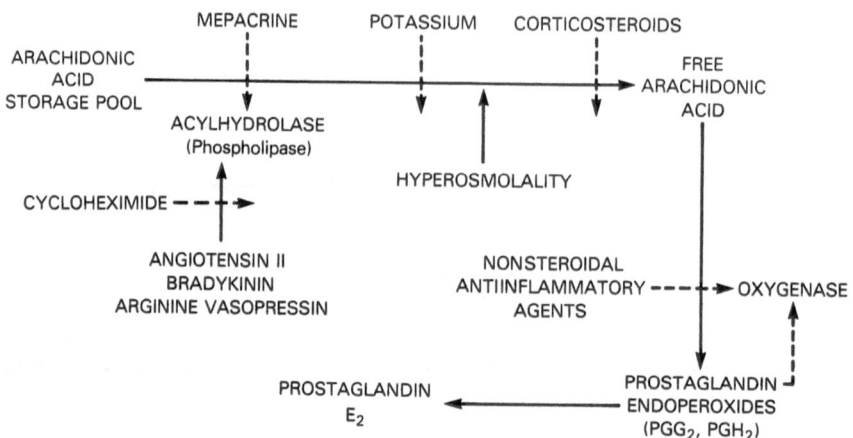

FIGURE 2. A schematic diagram summarizing the regulation of prostaglandin E_2 biosynthesis by rabbit renomedullary interstitial cells in tissue culture.

metabolism. The study of this system will provide information which may be applicable not only to renal prostaglandin biosynthesis but to the synthesis of prostaglandins, thromboxane A_2, and prostacyclin by platelets, vascular endothelium, renal glomeruli, and other tissues containing arachidonic acid cyclooxygenase.

REFERENCES

Albert, W. C., and Handler, J. S., 1974, Effect of PGE_1, indomethacin, and polyphloretin phosphate on toad bladder response to ADH, *Am. J. Physiol.* **226**:1382.

Anderson, R. S., Berl, T., McDonald, K. M., and Schrier, R. W., 1975, Evidence for an *in vivo* antagonism between vasopressin and prostaglandin in the mammalian kidney, *J. Clin. Invest.* **56**:420.

Ardvino, F., Ferraz, F. P. J., and Rodrigues, J., 1966, Antidiuretic action of chlorpropamide in idiopathic diabetes insipidus, *J. Clin. Endocrinol. Metab.* **26**:1325.

Bartter, F. C., Pronove, P., Gill, J. R., and McCardle, R. C., 1962, Hyperplasia of the juxtaglomerular complex with hyperaldosteronism and hypokalemic alkalosis, *Am. J. Med.* **33**:811.

Bell, C., and Mya, M. K. M., 1977, Release by vasopressin of E-type prostaglandins from the rat kidney, *Clin. Sci. Mol. Med.* **52**:103.

Berl, T., and Schrier, R. W., 1973, Mechanism of effect of prostaglandin E_1 on renal water excretion, *J. Clin. Invest.* **52**:463.

Berl, T., Raz, A., Wald, H., Horowitz, J., and Czackes, W., 1977, Prostaglandin synthesis inhibition and the action of vasopressin: Studies in man and rat, *Am. J. Physiol.* **232**:F529.

Bohman, S.-O., 1977, Demonstration of prostaglandin synthesis in collecting duct cells and other cell types of the rabbit renal medulla, *Prostaglandins* **14**:729.

Brown, C. A., Zusman, R. M., and Haber, E., 1979, Characterization of an angiotensin binding site in cultured rabbit renomedullary interstitial cells: Correlation of binding with prostaglandin synthesis, *Clin. Res.* **27**:501A.

Brown, C. A., Zusman, R. M. and Haber, E., 1979b, Correlation of prostaglandin biosynthesis with angiotensin binding to cultured rabbit renomedullary interstitial cells: Effects of potassium and protein synthesis inhibition, in: Proceedings of the International Conference on Prostaglandins, Washington, D.C., May 27–31, 1979, p. 14.

Brown, C. A., Zusman, R. M., and Haber, E., 1980, Characterization of an angiotensin binding site in cultured rabbit renomedullary interstitial cells: Correlation of binding with prostaglandin synthesis, *Trans. Am. Assoc. Phys.* **92**:169.

Chandrabose, K. A., Lapetina, E. G., Schmitges, C. J., Siegel, M. I., and Cuatrecasas, P., 1978, Action of corticosteroids in regulation of prostaglandin biosynthesis in cultured fibroblasts, *Proc. Natl. Acad. Sci. USA* **75**:214.

Chang, J., Lewis, G. P., and Piper, P. J., 1977, Inhibition by glucocorticoids of prostaglandin release from adipose tissue *in vitro*, *Br. J. Pharm.* **59**:425.

Crowshaw, K., McGiff, J. C., Strand, J. C., Lonigro, A. J., and Terragno, N. A., 1970, Prostaglandins in dog renal medulla, *J. Pharm. Pharmacol.* **22**:302.

Danon, A., Knapp, H. R., Oelz, O., and Oates, J. A., 1978, Stimulation of prostaglandin biosynthesis in the renal papilla by hypertonic mediums, *Am. J. Physiol.* **234**:F64.

Dunn, M. J., and Hood, V. L., 1977, Prostaglandins and the kidney, *Am. J. Physiol.* **233**:F169.

Dunn, M. J., Staley, R. S., and Harrison, M., 1976, Characterization of prostaglandin production in tissue culture of rat renal medullary cells, *Prostaglandins* **12**:37.

Dunn, M. J., Greeley, H. P., Horner, J., and Valtin, H., 1977, Renal excretion of prostaglandin E₂ and F₂α in Brattleboro homozygous diabetes insipidus rats, *Kidney Int.* **12**:555.

Dunn, M. J., Greeley, H. P., Valtin, H., Kinter, L. B., and Beewkes, R., 1978, Renal excretion of prostaglandins E₂ and F₂α in diabetes insipidus rats, *Am. J. Physiol.* **235**:E624.

Egan, R. W., Paxton, J., and Kuehl, F. A., 1976, Mechanism for irreversible self-deactivation of prostaglandin synthetase, *J. Biol. Chem.* **251**:7329.

Fichman, M. P., Telfer, N., Zia, P., Speckart, P., Golub, M. and Rude, R., 1976, Role of prostaglandins in the pathogenesis of Bartter's syndrome, *Am. J. Med.* **60**:785.

Floman, Y., and Zor, U., 1976, Mechanism of steroid action in inflammation: Inhibition of prostaglandin synthesis and release, *Prostaglandins* **12**:403.

Flores, A. G. A., and Sharp, G. W. G., 1972, Endogenous prostaglandins and osmotic water flow in the toad bladder, *Am. J. Physiol.* **223**:1392.

Flower, R. J., and Vane, J. R., 1974, Inhibition of prostaglandin biosynthesis, *Biochem. Pharmacol.* **23**:1439.

Frolich, J. C., Wilson, T. W., Sweetman, B. J., Siegal, M., Nies, A. S., Carr, K., Watson, J. T., and Oates, J. A., 1975, Urinary prostaglandins: Identification and origin, *J. Clin. Invest.* **55**:763.

Galvez, O. G., Bay, W., Roberts, B. W., and Ferris, T. F., 1977, The hemodynamic effects of potassium deficiency in the dog, *Circ. Res.* **40**(Suppl. I):1-11.

Gill, J. R., and Bartter, F. C., 1978, Evidence for a prostaglandin-independent defect in chloride reabsorption in the loop of Henle as a proximal cause of Bartter's syndrome, *Am. J. Med.* **65**:766.

Gill, J. R., Frolich, J. C., Bowden, R. E., Taylor, A. A., Keiser, H. R., Seyberth, H. W., Oates, J. A., and Bartter, F. C., 1976, Bartter's syndrome: A disorder characterized by high urinary prostaglandins and a dependence of hyperreninemia on prostaglandin synthesis, *Am. J. Med.* **61**:43.

Grantham, J. J., and Orloff, J., 1968, Effect of prostaglandin E₁ on the permeability response of the isolated collecting tubule to vasopressin, adenosine 3',5'-monophosphate and theophylline, *J. Clin. Invest.* **47**:1154.

Gryglewski, R. J., 1976, Steroid hormones, anti-inflammatory steroids, and prostaglandins, *Pharmacol. Res. Comm.* **8**:337.

Gullner, H.-G., Gill, J. R., Bartter, F. C., and Chan, J. C. M., 1979, A familial disorder with hypokalemic alkalosis, hyperreninemia, aldosteronism and high prostaglandins that is not Bartter's syndrome, *Clin. Res.* **27**:520A.

Haggitt, R. C., Pitcock, J. A., and Muirhead, E. E., 1971, Renal medullary fibrosis in hypertension, *Hum. Pathol.* **2**:587.

Hamberg, M., Svensson, J., and Samuelson, B., 1974, Prostaglandin endoperoxides: A new concept concerning the mode of action and release of prostaglandins, *Proc. Natl. Acad. Sci. USA* **71**:3824.

Hamberg, M., Svensson, J., and Samuelson, B., 1975, Thromboxanes: A new group of biologically active compounds derived from prostaglandin endoperoxides, *Proc. Natl. Acad. Sci. USA* **72**:2994.

Handler, J. S., and Orloff, J., 1973, The mechanism of action of antidiuretic hormone, in: *The Handbook of Physiology:* Section 8: *Renal Physiology* (J. Orloff and R. Berliner, eds.), American Physiological Society, Washington, D.C., pp. 791–814.

Hassid, A., Konieczkowski, M., and Dunn, M. J., 1979, Prostaglandin synthesis in isolated rat renal glomeruli, *Proc. Natl. Acad. Sci. USA* **76**:1155.

Hong, S. L., and Levine, L., 1976, Stimulation of prostaglandin synthesis by bradykinin and thrombin and their mechanisms of action on MC5-5 fibroblasts, *J. Biol. Chem.* **251**:5814.

Janszen, F. H. A., and Nugteren, D. H., 1971, Histochemical localization of prostaglandin synthetase, *Histochemie* **27**:159.

Kantrowitz, F., Robinson, D. R., McGuire, M. B., and Levine, L., 1975, Corticosteroids inhibit prostaglandin production by rheumatoid synovia, *Nature* **258**:737.

Karim, S. M. M. (ed.), 1976a, *Prostaglandins: Chemical and Biochemical Aspects*, University Park Press, Baltimore.

Karim, S. M. M. (ed.), 1976b, *Prostaglandins: Physiological, Pharmacological, and Pathological Aspects*, University Park Press, Baltimore.

Lands, W. E. M., and Rome, L. H., 1976, Inhibition of prostaglandin biosynthesis, in: *Prostaglandins: Chemical and Biochemical Aspects* (S. M. M. Karim, ed.), University Park Press, Baltimore, pp. 87–138.

Lands, W. E. M., leTellier, P. R., Rome, L., and Vanderhoek, J. Y., 1974, Regulation of prostaglandin synthesis, in: *Prostaglandin Synthetase Inhibitors* (H. J. Robinson and J. R. Vane, eds.), Raven Press, New York, pp. 1–7.

Lerman, R. J., Pitcock, J. A., Stephenson, P., and Muirhead, E. E., 1972, Renomedullary intersterstitial cell tumor (formerly fibroma of renal medulla), *Hum. Pathol.* **3**:559.

Lewis, G. P., and Piper, P. J., 1975, Inhibition of release of prostaglandins as an explanation of some of the actions of anti-inflammatory corticosteroids, *Nature* **254**:308.

Lifschitz, M. D. and Stein, J. H., 1977, Antidiuretic hormone stimulated renal prostaglandin E synthesis in the rabbit, *Clin. Res.* **25**:440A.

Lipson, L. C., and Sharp, G. W. G., 1971, Effect of prostaglandin E₁ on sodium transport and osmotic water flow in the toad bladder, *Am. J. Physiol.* **220**:1046.

Lipson, L., Hynie, S., and Sharp, G., 1971, Effect of prostaglandin E₁ on osmotic water flow and sodium transport in the toad bladder, *Ann. N.Y. Acad. Sci.* **180**:261.

Lum, H. M., Aisenberg, G. A., Dunn, M. J., Berl, T., Schrier, R. W., and McDonald, K. M., 1977, *In vivo* effect of indomethacin to potentiate the renal medullary cyclic AMP response to vasopressin, *J. Clin. Invest.* **58**:8.

McGiff, J. C., and Malik, K. U., 1976, Renal prostaglandins, in: *Prostaglandins: Physiological, Pharmacological, and Pathological Aspects* (S. M. M. Karim, ed.), University Park Press, Baltimore, pp. 201–246.

Martin, M. R., and Tiltman, A. J., 1976, Incidence of renomedullary interstitial cell tumors and correlation with hypertension, *S. Afr. Med. J.* **50**:2099.

Moncada, S., and Vane, J. R., 1977, The discovery of prostacyclin (PGX): A fresh insight into arachidonic acid metabolism, in: *Intersciences Prostaglandin Symposium*, Academic Press, New York, pp. 155–178.

Moncada, S., Gryglewski, R., Bunting, S., and Vane, J. R., 1976, An enzyme isolated from arteries transforms prostaglandin endoperoxides to an unstable substance that inhibits platelet aggregation, *Nature* **264**:633.

Morrison, A. R., Nishikawa, K., and Needleman, P., 1977, Unmasking of thromboxane A₂ synthesis by ureteral obstruction in the rabbit kidney, *Nature* **267**:259.

Moses, A. M., Numan, P., and Miller, M., 1973, Mechanism of chlorpropamide-induced antidiuresis in man: Evidence for release of ADH and enhancement of peripheral action, *Metab. Clin. Exp.* **22**:59.

Muirhead, E. E., Germain, G., Leach, B. E., Pitcock, J. A., Stephenson, P., Brooks, B., Brosius, W. L., Daniels, E. G., and Hinman, J. W., 1972, Production of renomedullary prostaglandins by renomedullary interstitial cells grown in tissue culture, *Circ. Res.* **30–31**(Suppl. II):11–161.

Needleman, P., Minkes, M., and Raz, A., 1976a, Thromboxanes: Selective biosynthesis and distinct biological properties, *Science* **193**:163.

Needleman, P., Moncada, S., Bunting, S., Vane, J. R., Hamberg, M., and Samuelsson, B., 1976b, Identification of an enzyme in platelet microsomes which generates thromboxane A₂ from prostaglandin endoperoxides, *Nature* **261**:558.

Needleman, P., Raz, A., Ferrendelli, J. A., and Minkes, M., 1977a, Application of imidazole as a selective inhibitor of thromboxane synthetase in human platelets, *Proc. Natl. Acad. Sci. USA* **74**:1716.

Needleman, P., Raz, A., Kulkaeni, S., Pure, E., Wyche, A., Denny, S. E., and Isakson, P. C., 1977b, Biological and chemical characterization of a unique endogenous vasodilator prostaglandin produced in isolated coronary artery and in intact perfused heart, in: *Interscience Symposium on Prostaglandins*, Academic Press, New York, pp. 199–215.

Needleman, P., Bronson, S. D., Wyche, A., Sivakoff, M., and Nicolaou, K. C., 1978, Cardiac and renal prostaglandin I₂: Biosynthesis and biological effects in isolated perfused rabbit tissues, *J. Clin. Invest.* **61**:839.

Norby, L., Flamenbaum, W., Lentz, R., and Ramwell, P. W., 1976, Prostaglandins and aspirin therapy in Bartter's syndrome, *Lancet* **2**:604.

Omachi, R. S., Robbie, D. E., Handler, J. S., and Orloff, J., 1974, Effect of ADH and other agents on cyclic AMP accumulation in toad bladder epithelium, *Am. J. Physiol.* **226**:1152.

Orloff, J., and Zusman, R., 1978, The role of prostaglandin E (PGE) in the modulation of the action of vasopressin on water flow in the urinary bladder of the toad and mammalian kidney, *J. Membr. Biol.* **40**:297.

Orloff, J., Handler, J. S., and Bergstrom, S., 1965, Effect of prostaglandin (PGE₁) on the permeability response of toad bladder to vasopressin, theophylline and adenosine 3′,5′-monophosphate, *Nature* **205**:397.

Ozer, A., and Sharp, G. W. G., 1972, Effect of prostaglandins and their inhibitors on osmotic water flow in the toad bladder, *Am. J. Physiol.* **222**:674.

Pong, S., and Levine, L., 1976, Prostaglandin synthetase systems of rabbit tissues and their inhibition by non-steroidal anti-inflammatory drugs, *J. Pharmacol. Exp. Ther.* **196**:226.

Pong, S., Hong, S. L., and Levine, L., 1977, Prostaglandin production by methycholanthrenetransformed mouse BALB/3T3: Requirement for protein synthesis, *J. Biol. Chem.* **252**:1408.

Preszyna, A., Attalah, A., Vance, V. K., Schoolman, M., and Lee, J. B., 1973, The renomedullary body: A newly recognized structure of renomedullary interstitial cell origin associated with high prostaglandin content, *Prostaglandins* **3**:669.

Ramwell, P. W., and Daniels, E. G., 1969, Chromatography of prostaglandins, in: *Lipid Chromatographic Analysis* (G. V. Marinetti, ed.), Marcel Dekker, New York, pp. 313–344.

Reese, A. J. M., and Winstanley, D. P., 1958, The small tumor-like lesions of the kidney, *Br. J. Cancer* **12**:507.

Rome, L. H., and Lands, W. E. M., 1975, Structural requirements for time dependent inhibition of prostaglandin biosynthesis by antiinflammatory drugs, *Proc. Natl. Acad. Sci. USA* **72**:4863.

Smith, W. L., and Bell, T. G., 1978, Immunohistochemical localization of the prostaglandin forming cyclo-oxygenase in renal cortex, *Am. J. Physiol.* **235**:F451.

Stuart, R., Salyer, W. R., Salyer, D. C., and Heptinstall, R. H., 1976, Renomedullary interstitial cell lesions and hypertension, *Hum. Pathol.* **7**:327.

Tashjian, A. H., Jr., Voelkel, E. F., McDonough, J., and Levin, L., 1975, Hydrocortisone inhibits prostaglandin production by mouse fibrosarcoma cells, *Nature* **258**:739.

Tobian, L., and Azar, S., 1971. Antihypertensive and other functions of the renal papilla, *Trans. Assoc. Am. Phys.* **84**:281.

Urakabe, S., Taksmitsu, Y., Shirai, D., Yuasa, S., Kimura, G., Orita, Y., and Abem H., 1975, Effect of different prostaglandins on the permeability of the toad urinary bladder, *Comp. Biochem. Physiol.* **52**:1.

Vargaftig, B. B., and Hai, N. D., 1972, Selective inhibition by mepacrine of the release of "rabbit aorta contracting substance" evoked by the administration of bradykinin, *J. Pharm. Pharmacol.* **24**:159.

Verbeckmoes, R., Van Damme, B., Clement, J., Amery, A. and Michielsen, P., 1976, Bartter's syndrome with hyperplasia of renomedullary cells. Successful treatment with indomethacin, *Kidney Int.* **9**:302.

Vinci, J. M., Gill, J. R., Bowden, R. E., Pisano, J. J., Izzo, J. L., Radfar, N., Taylor, A. A., Zusman, R. M., Bartter, F. C., and Keiser, H. R., 1978, Kallikrein–kinin system and its response to prostaglandin synthesis inhibition, *J. Clin. Invest.* **61**:1671.

Walker, L. A., Whorton, A. R., Siegel, M., France, R. and Frolich, J. C., 1978, Antidiuretic hormone increases renal prostaglandin synthesis in vivo, *Am. J. Physiol.* **235**:F180.

Zusman, R. M., 1980, Regulation of prostaglandin biosynthesis: Studies in the rabbit renomedullary interstitial cell and the toad urinary bladder in vitro, in: *Prostaglandins in Cardiovascular and Renal Physiology* (A. Scriabine, ed.), Spectrum Publications, pp. 93–121.

Zusman, R. M., and Brown, C. A., 1979, Role of phospholipase in the regulation of prostaglandin E$_2$ biosynthesis by rabbit renomedullary interstitial cells in tissue culture: Effects of angiotensin II, potassium, dexamethasone, hyperosmolality and inhibition of protein synthesis, in: Proceedings of the International Conference on Prostaglandins, Washington, D.C., May 27–31, 1979, p. 130.

Zusman, R. M., and Brown, C. A., 1980, Role of phospholipase in the regulation of prostaglandin E$_2$ biosynthesis by rabbit renomedullary interstitial cells in tissue culture: Effects of angiotensin II, potassium, dexamethane, hyperosmolality and inhibition of protein synthesis, in: *Advances in Prostaglandin and Thromboxane Research*, Vol. 6 (P. Ramwell, ed.), Raven Press, New York, p. 243.

Zusman, R. M., and Keiser, H. R., 1977a, Prostaglandin biosynthesis by rabbit renomedullary interstitial cells in tissue culture: Stimulation by angiotensin II, bradykinin and arginine vasopressin, *J. Clin. Invest.* **60**:215.

Zusman, R. M., and Keiser, H. R., 1977b, Prostaglandin E$_2$ biosynthesis by rabbit renomedullary interstitial cells in tissue culture: Mechanism of stimulation by angiotensin II,
bradykinin, and arginine vasopressin, *J. Biol. Chem.* **252**:2069.

Zusman, R. M., and Keiser, H. R., 1980, Regulation of prostaglandin E$_2$ biosynthesis by rabbit renomedullary interstitial cells in tissue culture: Effects of potassium, osmolality, corticosteroids, arachidonic acid, and protein synthesis inhibition, *Kidney Int.* **17**:277.

Zusman, R. M., Keiser, H. R. and Handler, J. S., 1977a, Vasopressin-stimulated prostaglandin E biosynthesis in the toad urinary bladder: Effect on water flow, *J. Clin. Invest.*
60:1339.

Zusman, R. M., Keiser, H. R., and Handler, J. S., 1977b, Inhibition of vasopressin-stimulated
prostaglandin E biosynthesis by chlorpropamide in the toad urinary bladder: Mechanism
of enhancement of vasopressin-stimulated water flow, *J. Clin. Invest.* **60**:1348.

Zusman, R. M., Keiser, H. R., and Handler, J. S., 1977c, A hypothesis for the molecular
mechanism of action of chlorpropamide in the treatment of diabetes mellitus and diabetes
insipidus, *Fed. Proc. Fed. Am. Soc. Exp. Biol.* **13**:2728.

Zusman, R. M., Keiser, H. R., and Handler, J. S., 1978, Effect of adrenal steroids on
vasopressin-stimulated PGE synthesis and water flow, *Am. J. Physiol.* **234**:F532.

Zusman, R. M., Vinci, J. M., Bowden, R. E., Horwitz, D., and Keiser, H. R., 1979, The effect
of indomethacin and adrenocorticotrophic hormone on renal function in man: An experimental model of inappropriate antidiuresis, *Kidney Int.* **15**:62.

CHAPTER 10

Influence of Renal Prostaglandins on Renin Release

PETER C. WEBER and WOLFGANG SIESS

1. INTRODUCTION

The key position of the kidney in the control of electrolyte balance and blood pressure is determined by a variety of local and systemic hormonal factors. The latter include the autonomic nervous system and cate-cholamines, the antidiuretic hormone (ADH), and adrenocortical hormones, and the former include the kinins, renin, and the prostaglandins (PGs), as well as other, as yet less well defined, endocrines of the kidney. Recent studies have led to new insights into the relationship between these hormonal systems and the regulation of renal blood flow, glomerular filtration rate, and the tubular handling of electrolytes. In discussing a functional relationship between PGs and the renin–angiotensin system, and the effects of PGs on electrolyte balance and blood pressure, it is necessary to consider their respective localizations within the kidney the factors causing their release, and their intrarenal and systemic actions.

2. THE RENIN–ANGIOTENSIN SYSTEM

2.1. The Juxtaglomerular Apparatus

Renin is synthesized and stored in the epitheloid cells of the juxtaglomerular apparatus (JGA) (Fig. 1), a structure adjacent to the glomeruli, which are localized exclusively in the kidney cortex. The granular cells of the JGA are highly differentiated vascular smooth muscle cells

PETER C. WEBER and WOLFGANG SIESS • Department of Internal Medicine, University Hospital, D-8000 Munich 2, West Germany.

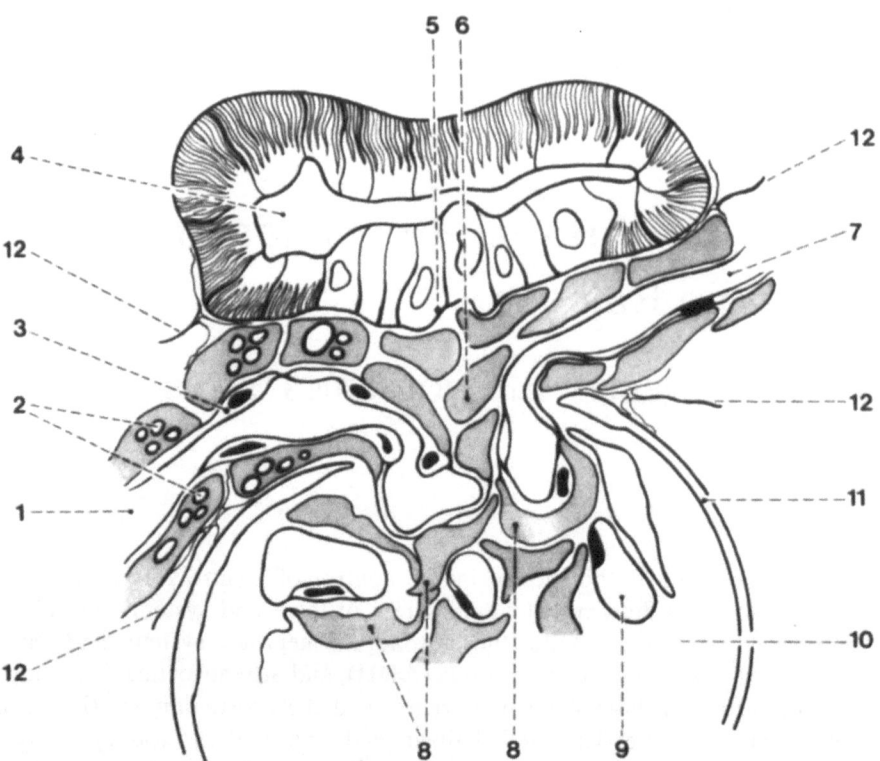

FIGURE 1. Schematic drawing of the structure of the juxtaglomerular apparatus and its relation to other elements of the glomerular vascular pole. (1) Afferent arteriole; (2) renin granules
in the myoepitheloid cells of the afferent arteriole; (3) endothelial cell of the arteriole; (4)
lumen of the distal tubule; (5) basal side of the macula densa cells; (6) Goormaghtigh cells; (7)
efferent arteriole; (8) mesangial cells of the glomerulus; (9) glomerular capillaries; (10)
glomerulus; (11) Bowman's capsule; (12) axons innervating vascular and distal tubular elements.

within the media of the afferent arteriole that contain both membrane-
bound granules and myofibrils. They are in close proximity to the endothelium of the arteriole on the one side and opposed to the macula densa (MD)
cells on the other side. The latter are specialized distal tubular cells found
where the distal tubule is close to the vascular pole of the glomerulus. Goormaghtigh cells are located in the area formed by the MD and the afferent
and efferent arteriole. Thereby, the JG cells have anatomical connections to
the glomerulus. There is a dense network of adrenergic nerve endings in the
JGA region (Barajas, 1970).

2.2. The Release of Renin

The physiological consequences of a release of the proteolytic enzyme renin from the granules of the JG cells are brought about by a series of reactions. From its substrate, angiotensinogen, renin cleaves the decapeptide prohormone angiotensin I (AI), and, from the reaction of AI with the converting enzyme (or kininase II), the active octapeptide hormone angiotensin II (AII) is generated. The major determinants of renin synthesis and/or release are extracellular volume, sympathetic nervous tone, and arterial blood pressure. These operate through activation of one or more of the three major mechanisms of renin release: the "baroreceptor," the adrenergic receptor, and the MD receptor (Reid *et al.*, 1978). The early findings of intrarenal formation of AII (Bailie *et al.*, 1971) and, more recently, the observation of tight junctions between preglomerular endothelial and JG cells (Forssman and Taugner, 1977), as well as the demonstration that most of the renin enters the circulation distal to the efferent arteriole (Morgan and Davis, 1975), imply that a major proportion of the renin–angiotensinogen reaction occurs in the interstitial compartment of the kidney. This may be of considerable importance for the intrarenal formation and action of AII.

3. THE RENAL PROSTAGLANDINS

3.1. Formation and Metabolism of Prostaglandins in the Kidney

The PG system constitutes a group of interrelated compounds that are generated by a multienzyme complex, the PG synthetase. By the action of phospholipase, arachidonic acid—the most abundant precursor of PGs—is cleaved from its esterified storage site of membrane phospholipids and is converted by the PG cyclooxygenase to the PG endoperoxides PGG_2 and PGH_2. These PG intermediates are the precursors of a spectrum of PGs characteristic for each tissue (Pace-Asciak and Rangaraj, 1977). The PG endoperoxides are further transformed by an isomerase to PGE_2 and its isomer, PGD_2. $PGF_{2\alpha}$ may be produced either from the PG endoperoxides by a reductase, or by the conversion of PGE_2, catalyzed by a PGE-9-ketoreductase (Lee and Levine, 1974). More recent studies of the metabolism of PGG_2 and PGH_2 led to the discovery of thromboxane (TX) A_2 (Hamberg *et al.*, 1975) and of prostacyclin or PGI_2 (Moncada *et al.*, 1976). While the formation of each of these PGs has been demonstrated in the kidney, PGA_2, previously thought to be representative of a circulating antihypertensive renal hormone (Lee *et al.*, 1965) probably originated from PGE_2 during sample work-up of renal tissue.

The metabolism and inactivation of the PGs occurs rapidly following their formation and there is no storage pool of PGs within tissues. The lipid droplets found within the interstitial cells in the renal medulla most probably represent PG precursor storage pools that may be influenced predominantly by chronic changes in lipid metabolism, due either to dietary intake or to chronic changes of kidney function (Nissen, 1968; Mandal *et al.*, 1967). The PG endoperoxides and TXA_2 are chemically very unstable. The classical PGs of the E, F, and D series are inactivated locally or by passage through the lungs by the PG dehydrogenase (Änggård and Larsson, 1971). In contrast, PGI_2 is only partly metabolized by the lungs and might be a circulating hormone (Gryglewski *et al.*, 1978).

3.2.   Regional and Cellular Localization of the Renal Prostaglandin System

The kidney has a high capacity to synthesize PGs. By immunohistochemical (Smith and Wilkin, 1977; Smith and Bell, 1978) and biochemical (Crowshaw, 1973; Larsson and Änggård, 1973; Whorton *et al.*, 1978) analyses, it has been demonstrated that there are marked differences in the total amount and in the spectrum of different PGs synthesized in different zones of the kidney (Table 1). In the medulla and papilla, PG synthesis occurs mainly in the collecting ducts and interstitial cells. There is also an appreciable rate of PG formation in the kidney cortex, localized mainly in the vascular compartment. On the other hand, PG degradation and metabolism in the kidney prevails in the cortex. In a variety of studies *in vitro*, it has been found that the major PG of the renal medulla and papilla is PGE_2, whereas the formation of 6-keto-$PGF_{1\alpha}$, the stable product of PGI_2, and of $PGF_{2\alpha}$ predominates in the kidney cortex and the outer medulla, respectively (Larsson and Weber, 1978; Whorton *et al.*, 1978). In a study in the rabbit it was demonstrated that there is also an appreciable rate of 6-keto-$PGF_{1\alpha}$ production in the renal medulla (Oliw, 1979), which makes it difficult to consider the formation of PGI_2 as a purely cortical phenomenon (Whorton *et al.*, 1978). The formation of thromboxanes is low in the normal kidney but has been demonstrated in the hydronephrotic kidney of the rabbit on challenge with bradykinin (Morrison *et al.*, 1977). In addition to the difference in the activity of the PG dehydrogenase between the kidney cortex (high activity) and the kidney medulla (low activity) (Larsson and Änggård, 1973), there is also a steep gradient of the enzyme PGE-9-ketoreductase, which, in the rabbit kidney, shows highest activities in the kidney cortex (Stone and Hart, 1975). Thus, the renal PG system is highly compartmentalized (Table 1). As PGs act most probably as local hormones or autacoids, this distribution of the PG system points to different physiological functions of the cortical and medullary PGs. In considering a functional connection between the renal PGs and renin, it is

TABLE 1

Postmortem Accumulation of Prostaglandins in Different Regions of the Normal Rabbit Kidney[a,b]

Region of kidney	PGE_2	$PGF_{2\alpha}$	6-Keto-$PGF_{1\alpha}$	TXB_2
Cortex	0.4	0.4	1.4	N.D.[c]
Medulla	2.4	3.7	2.1	0.2
Papilla	4.2	0.4	3.5	0.2

[a] Values are $\mu g/mg$ tissue. The measurements were performed with gas chromatography/mass spectrometry.
[b] Data from Larsson and Weber (1978) and Oliw (1979).
[c] Not detectable.

important to point out that there are at least two possible ways in which renal PGs could affect renal cortical functions, such as renal vascular resistance or renin secretion. Consequent to the early discovery of high PG formation in the renal medulla it was initially proposed that PGs, formed in the medulla, might be transported by several pathways, such as the tubular fluid or by lymphatics, to the cortex where they could exert their actions (Williams et al., 1977). However, despite the fact that the renal cortex has probably only one-tenth of the capacity of the medulla to produce PGs from arachidonic acid (Larsson and Änggård, 1973), recent studies in the non-filtering kidney make it more likely that it is the PG production in the cortex that affects renal hemodynamics and renin secretion. Renal medullary PGs may operate only by modulating the effects of ADH and aldosterone in the distal tubule, thus acting in concert with the renin–angiotensin system to control sodium, potassium, chloride, and volume balance. Renal cortical PGs may also affect tubular functions in the medulla by their influence on renal blood flow.

4. INFLUENCE OF RENAL PROSTAGLANDINS ON RENIN RELEASE

Many of the experimental conditions known to be associated with an increase in renin secretion have also been shown to lead to the activation of renal PG formation (Table 2). These observations suggested a connection between the PGs and the renin–angiotensin system. Although it has been known since the studies of McGiff and co-workers (1970) that angiotensin can release PGE-like compounds from the kidney, the converse effect, an effect of the PGs on renin secretion, was not known until the work of Larsson and co-workers (1974), demonstrating an increase of plasma renin activity (PRA) following arachidonic acid infusion into the rabbit kidney.

Exogenous PGs as well as changes in intrarenal PG formation influence renin release, renal blood flow, and sodium and volume excretion.

TABLE 2

Experimental Conditions with Parallel Increases of Prostaglandin
and Renin Release from the Kidney

Reduction of renal perfusion pressure
  Renal artery constriction
  Ischemia
  Renal nerve stimulation
  Hemorrhagic hypotension
Increase of renal blood flow (decrease of renal vascular resistance)
  Loop diuretics: furosemide, bumetanide
  Acute unilateral ureteral obstruction
Intrarenal infusion of vasoactive hormones
  Catecholamines
  Bradykinin
Changes in electrolye balance
  Negative NaCl balance
  Negative KCl balance

Following arachidonic acid infusion, there is an increase of total renal blood flow, predominantly in the juxtamedullary cortex (Larsson and Änggård, 1974; Chang *et al.*, 1975). Because of the existing complex interrelationships, it is difficult to delineate the relative importance of PGs and renin in different functional states of the kidney. Both hormonal systems seem to gain importance for the control of renal blood flow, glomerular filtration rate, and systemic blood pressure with increasing deviation from "basal" conditions, e.g., during sodium depletion or, even more, during anesthesia and laparotomy. On the other hand, neither PGs nor the renin–angiotensin system seems to be of major importance for renal vascular resistance or renal blood flow autoregulation in the awake, salt-replete animal (Terragno *et al.*, 1977). It seems that the kidney, by synthesizing PGs, increases renin secretion, but at the same time protects itself from the vasoconstrictor action of angiotensin. These considerations, together with species differences in the renal effects of prostaglandins (Malik, 1978), may explain some of the inconsistent results obtained following inhibition or stimulation of renal PG synthesis on renal blood flow and sodium chloride excretion (for references, see Zins, 1975; Tannenbaum *et al.*, 1975; Kirschenbaum and Stein, 1976; Anderson *et al.*, 1976; Weber *et al.*, 1975a; Kaloyanides *et al.*, 1976; Bolger *et al.*, 1976; Arisz *et al.*, 1976).

4.1. Exogenous Prostaglandins and Renin Release

Previous studies on the effects of exogenous PGs on renin secretion using systematic or intrarenal infusion of PGE_1, PGE_2, PGA_1, and PGA_2

gave inconsistent results. Vander (1968) found no effect of PGE_1 and PGE_2 on PRA in anesthesized dogs. Werning et al. (1971) reported an increase of PRA following high doses of PGE_1, which might have been due to volume depletion. Infusion of PGA_1 or PGA_2 into hyptertensive or normal human subjects also gave inconsistent results (Fichmann et al., 1972; Hornych et al., 1973). In sodium-depleted subjects, PRA increased significantly after PGA_1 infusion (Krakoff et al., 1973), and subsequently Golub et al. (1976) reported that PGA_1 infusion stimulated PRA dose-dependently in normal human volunteers. More recent studies of Yun et al. (1978), Bolger et al. (1977, 1978), and Gerber et al. (1978b) with intrarenal infusion of PGE_1, PGE_2, PGD_2, $PGF_{2\alpha}$, and PGI_2 also failed to clarify which of the PGs influenced renin secretion and by which mechanism. All PGs with the exception of $PGF_{2\alpha}$ increased renin secretion from the kidney but showed different effects on renal plasma or blood flow, glomerular filtration rate, sodium excretion, and urinary volume. These studies provided information on the pharmacological effects of exogenous PGs on renin release. However, exogenous administration of one selected PG probably does not give much meaningful information on the physiological effects of the primary PGs, TXA_2, PGI_2, and the intermediary PG endoperoxides formed and released within renal structures upon stimulation. Furthermore, circulatory levels of PGs are exceedingly low (Dray et al., 1975; Mitchell, 1978) and the existence of the PGs of the A series in the kidney and in the circulation has been repeatedly questioned.

4.2. Effects of Arachidonic-Acid-Stimulated Prostaglandin Synthesis on Renin Release

A more physiological way to study the consequences of an increased intrarenal PG formation on kidney function and renin secretion is through the infusion of the PG precursor arachidonic acid into the renal artery in doses that do not affect systemic hemodynamics or platelet aggregation (Larsson and Änggard, 1974; Chang et al., 1975; Tannenbaum et al., 1975; Silver et al., 1974). By this experimental design, a spectrum of PGs and related compounds that is normally present will be produced at those sites in the kidney where the prerequisite enzymes and cofactors are available, i.e., at their physiological sites of formation.

Intrarenal infusion of nonhypotensive doses of arachidonic acid in rabbits increased both PRA and urinary excretion of prostaglandins (Larsson and Änggård, 1974; Larsson et al., 1974). Similar experiments were performed in rats where arachidonate increased PRA in both normally hydrated and volume-expanded rats (Weber et al., 1975a). In the dog, Bolger et al. (1976) found that arachidonic acid elevated PRA as well as sodium and water excretion.

4.3. Effect of Inhibition of Renal Prostaglandin Formation on Renin Secretion

The possibility of an involvement of PGs in the secretion of renin has also been explored by pharmacological inhibition of PG synthesis in normal conditions and in situations known to be associated with increased renin secretion. Basal PRA has been found to be reduced by different PG synthesis inhibitors such as indomethacin, aspirin, and meclofenamate in rabbits (Larsson *et al.*, 1974; Romero *et al.*, 1976). Indomethacin in therapeutic doses reduces PRA in normal and hypertensive subjects (Rumpf *et al.*, 1975; Patak *et al.*, 1975; Donker *et al.*, 1976; Frölich *et al.*, 1976a,b). The increase of PRA induced by arachidonic acid in rabbits and dogs can be blocked by PG synthesis inhibition (Larsson *et al.*, 1974; Bolger *et al.*, 1976). In the rat, indomethacin treatment reduces the elevation of PRA and urinary PG excretion found after laparotomy (Weber, unpublished observations; Scherer *et al.*, 1978; Schnermann *et al.*, 1979). Renal ischemia either induced by clamping of the renal arteries (Weber *et al.*, 1975b) or occurring in acute renal failure following glycerol or mercuric chloride injection (Torres *et al.*, 1975) is known to release renin. In both these situations, indomethacin was found to suppress the elevation of PRA and the accumulation of intrarenal PG (Larsson *et al.*, 1976; Torres *et al.*, 1975). Indomethacin also suppresses the elevation of PRA seen after stimulation of intrarenal adrenergic receptors either in rabbits after bleeding (Romero *et al.*, 1976) or in man after isoproterenol infusion or after orthostasis (Frölich *et al.*, 1976b,c; Weber *et al.*, 1977b). In contrast, Henrich and co-workers (1978) were unable to demonstrate an effect of PG synthesis inhibition on PRA in hemorrhagic hypotension in dogs, a model which is assumed to be associated with renal ischemia. However, since in the latter experiments there were also significant changes of glomerular filtration rate and renal blood flow, the possibility that accompanying changes in some tubular signal may have obscured an effect of vascular PG formation on renin secretion cannot be excluded. The results mentioned above so far indicate that formation of some PG-cyclooxygenase-derived compound(s) may be of importance in the mechanisms that control renin secretion under a variety of circumstances.

4.4. Effects of Prostaglandins on Renin Release *in Vitro*

The simultaneous synthesis of the various types of prostaglandin products in the kidney and their different, often opposing, effects make it virtually impossible to reach a safe conclusion about the precise function of the PG system in controlling renin release using only studies *in vivo* where the entire PG system is stimulated or inhibited. It was previously reported that PGE_2 stimulated the release of renin from a suspension of rat renal cortical cells, while $PGF_{2\alpha}$ decreased renin release (Dew and Michelakis, 1974). Arachidonic acid, the natural PG endoperoxide PGG_2, and two synthetic stable PG endoperoxide analogues stimulated the release of renin from rabbit renal cortical slices (Weber *et al.*, 1976*b*). PGE_2 had no effect, while $PGF_{2\alpha}$ inhibited renin release in a dose-dependent manner. Arachidonic acid, which was the most potent of the compounds studied, increased renin secretion about fourfold. In all experiments, in which animals were pretreated with either indomethacin or eicosa-5,8,11,14-tetraynoic acid, basal as well as arachidonic-acid-stimulated renin release was inhibited (Fig. 2). Because of the significantly greater effects of C20:4 on renin release, in comparison with the very unstable natural or stable synthetic PG endoperoxides, a role for other PG-endoperoxide-derived metabolites, such as TXA_2 or PGI_2, in influencing renin secretion seems possible. In a subsequent study, it was demonstrated that renal cortical formation of PGI_2 may constitute one major pathway of PG production to increase renin secretion (Whorton *et al.*, 1977).

It is tempting to speculate that a preferential renal metabolism of arachidonate into one of the various PGs mentioned above might be involved in the mechanisms by which renin release is regulated. Such an

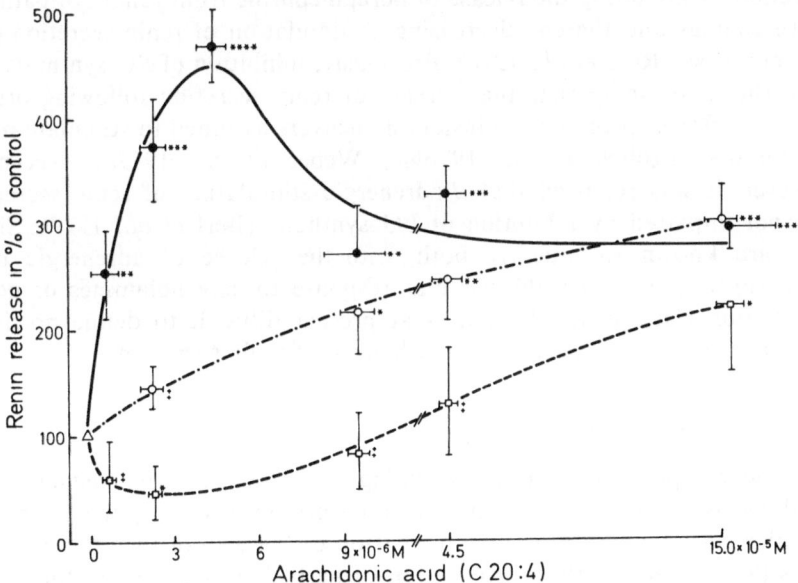

FIGURE 2. Effects of various concentrations of arachidonic acid alone (●——●) and together with PG synthetase inhibitors indomethacin (O—·—O) and eicosa-5,8,11,14-tetraynoic acid (□———□) on renin release in percent of control from slices of rabbit renal cortex. Mean ± SE. [From Weber *et al.* (1967*b*).]

involvement of different PGs in the process of renin release may be a direct one, due to stimulation of the juxtaglomerular cells, or an indirect one, due to an interaction of locally produced PGs with adrenergic transmission, with the response to the stretching of the wall of the afferent arteriole, or with the macula densa signal for renin release.

5. PROSTAGLANDINS AND THE DIFFERENT RECEPTORS FOR RENIN RELEASE

5.1. The Adrenergic Receptor

An important mechanism for renin release is the renal adrenoreceptor. The sympathetic nervous system affects the secretion of renin via the renal nerves and via circulating catecholamines. Sympathetic effects on renin secretion appear to be mediated via both β- and α-adrenergic receptors. Stimulation of the β-receptors causes increased renin secretion. Renal vasoconstriction due to stimulation of α-receptors with a subsequent decrease of perfusion pressure at the site of the afferent arteriole could, indirectly, increase renin secretion consequent to the stimulation of the baroreceptor or the MD mechanism; stimulation of the α-receptor can also decrease renin secretion by inhibiting the release of norepinephrine from renal sympathetic nerve endings and thereby decreasing β-stimulation of renin secretion (for references, see Reid et al., 1978). Previously, inhibition of PG synthesis has been shown to antagonize the increase of renin secretion following orthostasis or after isoproterenol infusion, maneuvers assumed to stimulate renal β-receptors (Frölich et al., 1976b,c; Weber et al., 1977b). Recently, however, it was reported that β-adrenergic stimulation of renin secretion was not impaired by inhibition of PG synthesis (Berl et al., 1979). Since PGs are known to interfere both with the release of adrenergic neurotransmitters and with the vascular response to catecholamines or nerve stimulation (Hedquist, 1976), it is at present difficult to define precisely the role of PGs in the adrenergic mechanism of renin secretion.

5.2. The Baroreceptor Mechanism

The receptor mechanism mediating renin release after reduction of renal perfusion pressure is likely to be a baroreceptor that signals to the JG granular cells changes of stretch or tension of the wall of the afferent arterioles (Tobian et al., 1959). Reduction of perfusion pressure or blood flow to the kidney is followed by the release of both renin and PGs (Skinner et al., 1964; McGiff et al., 1970). It was demonstrated in the nonfiltering dog kidney model, following bilateral adrenalectomy, renal denervation, and continuous propranolol infusion, that a reduction of renal perfusion pressure increased renal venous PRA (Data *et al.*, 1978). Intrarenal infusion of C20:4 increased and inhibition of PG synthesis abolished both the release of renin and the changes of renal vascular resistance under these conditions, suggesting an important role of renal PGs in vascular smooth muscle function (Data *et al.*, 1978; Gerber *et al.*, 1978*a*). Since, in this model, there is no transport of renomedullary PGs to the cortex and since the MD mechanism as well as the adrenergic mechanisms for renin release are interrupted, these results favor the concept that PGs produced in cortical structures are functionally involved in renin secretion following stimulation of the baroreceptor.

5.3. Interactions between Vascular and Tubular Mechanisms of Renin Release

Furosemide and similar loop diuretics cause a rapid increase of renin release 10–15 min after i.v. injection in animal's or man. This is paralleled by an increase of urinary PGs and by a decrease in renal vascular resistance (Williamson *et al.*, 1975; Olsen and Ahnfelt-Rønne, 1976; Romero *et al.*, 1976; Frölich *et al.*, 1976*b*; Weber *et al.*, 1977*b*; Scherer and Weber, 1979). Inhibition of PG synthesis abolishes the evaluation of renin secretion and the hemodynamic changes, whereas sodium and water secretion are affected to a lesser degree, or not at all (Bailie *et al.*, 1975; Weber *et al.*, 1977*b*). The concordance between the increase of PRA, renal flood flow, and urinary PG excretion most probably reflects an increased synthesis of PGs at vascular sites in the kidney (Scherer and Weber 1979). The primary stimulus for the increase of PG formation may be either the furosemide-induced inhibition of (sodium) chloride transport across the distal tubular cells at the site of the MD or a direct effect of furosemide on vascular PG formation.

Acute unilateral ureteral obstruction is associated with an ipsilateral increase of renal blood flow and renin secretion (Vander and Miller, 1964; Vaughan *et al.*, 1971). The excretion of PGs in the obstructed kidney is stimulated (Cadnapaphornchai *et al.*, 1978). Inhibition of PG synthesis prevents the hyperemic response and the increase of renin secretion and hence blood pressure following ureteral obstruction. In this model, it is assumed that either changes in the pressure gradients across vascular/tubular structures or a diminished electrolyte delivery in the distal tubule at the site of the MD triggers renal PG formation and thus decreases renal vascular resistance and increases renin secretion (Eide *et al.*, 1977; Olsen, 1978; Oliw, 1979).

Glomerular filtration rate (GFR) is assumed to be partly controlled by a feedback system in which changes of (sodium) chloride concentration, load, or uptake across the MD segment of the distal tubule are processed in the JGA, causing a change of glomerular arteriolar vasomotor tone. As a result, GFR varies inversely with loop of Henle flow rate. In micropuncture experiments, inhibition of PG synthesis to about 10% of control values attentuates the feedback response observed after changes of loop of Henle flow rate (Schnermann et al., 1979) by about 50%. This diminution of feedback response in GFR could be restored by infusion of PGI_2 into the renal artery (Schnermann and Weber, 1980). The results suggest that PGs may modify the JG feedback system, either directly or by mediating renin secretion, thereby participating in the regulation of GFR. Another possible way for renal PGs to influence GFR would be through an effect on the filtration coefficient, either by affecting the filtration area of the intraglomerular capillaries or by changing the permeability of the filtration barriers (Baylis and Brenner, 1978). Such a mechanism seems attractive, since the production of a variety of PGs has been demonstrated in isolated glomeruli (Folkert and Schlöndorff, 1979). Figure 3 shows the hypothetical role of PGs for the different mechanisms mediating renin secretion from the JGA.

5.4. Sodium Chloride and Potassium Chloride Balance

The predominant role of the renin–angiotensin system is to protect the body against losses of sodium chloride and water. Sodium chloride depletion, as well as a low potassium chloride intake, increases renin secretion and, thereby, the formation of angiotensin. Angiotensin, as well as a high potassium chloride intake, exerts a stimulatory effect on aldosterone secretion, which in turn causes sodium retention and facilitates potassium secretion. Extracellular volume expansion, but also high potassium intake, reduces renin secretion. Thus, a delicate balance, in part complementary and in part antagonistic, exists between the mechanisms that are involved in the regulation of sodium chloride and potassium chloride balance.

The role of PGs in the regulation of sodium chloride excretion is a matter of controversy. A number of studies indicate that renal PGs could have a natriuretic action (for references, see Lee et al., 1976; Tannenbaum et al., 1975; Bolger et al., 1976). The renal hemodynamic effects of PGs could reduce tubular reabsorption and increase urinary excretion of sodium. Other studies, however, have indicated an antinatriuretic role for the renal PGs (Tobian et al., 1974; Kirschenbaum and Stein, 1976). The results of studies of the direct effects of PGs on tubular sodium chloride handling are inconsistent (Fine and Trizna, 1977; Stokes and Kokko, 1977).

A chronic increase of dietary NaCl intake with free access to water induces a decrease of urinary PG excretion in rabbits (Weber et al., 1977a; Scherer et al., 1977; Davila et al., 1978). In addition, the pattern of PG excretion is altered; a marked reduction of PGE_2 excretion is associated with little or no decrease of $PGF_{2\alpha}$ excretion. This was proposed to be the result of a decrease of PG synthesis in association with an increase of PGE_2-9-ketoreductase activity in the kidney (Weber et al., 1977a).

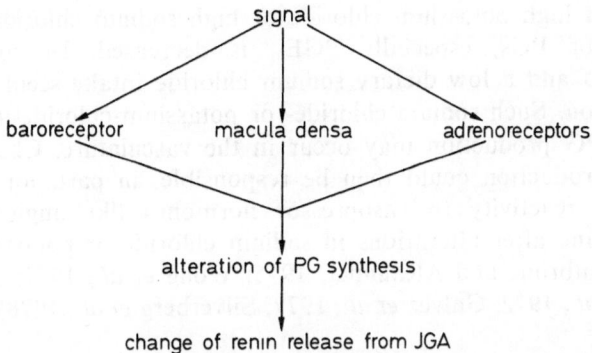

FIGURE 3. Hypothetical interrelation among the different receptors mediating renin release, the renal cortical PG system, and the JGA, despite increased PG synthesis by the kidneys.

Both a reduction of total renal PG synthesis and a relative increase of $PGF_{2\alpha}$ formation have the potential to reduce renin secretion. Reversibly, after a diet with a low sodium chloride content, renal PG synthesis is enhanced with a predominant increase of PGE_2 (Weber *et al.*, 1977*a*; Davila *et al.*, 1978). After restriction of sodium chloride intake, a relative increase of juxtamedullary blood flow has been found (Hollenberg *et al.*, 1970). This change of intrarenal blood flow distribution with low dietary NaCl intake is consistent with an increase of renal PGE synthesis (Larsson and Änggård, 1974).

In man, the effect of renal PGs on salt-intake-related renin release is not very well characterized. In early studies, a high sodium intake was found to reduce immunoreactive PGA in plasma (Zusman *et al.*, 1973). Indomethacin causes a suppression of PRA independent of sodium retention (Frölich *et al.*, 1976*a*). From these findings and from the observation that infusion of PGA_1 stimulates renin release independently of sodium balance (Speckart *et al.*, 1977), a PG–renin interaction not related to sodium balance was suggested (Frölich *et al.*, 1976*a*; Speckart *et al.*, 1977).

In rats on their normal diet with a relatively low potassium content, PGE_2 excretion was found to be significantly higher than $PGF_{2\alpha}$ excretion (Weber *et al.*, 1978*a*). A reduction of this low potassium chloride intake to almost zero in rats had no further effect on PG excretion (Hood and Dunn, 1978). The reverse condition, a high potassium chloride intake, decreased the excretion of PGE_2 and increased that of $PGF_{2\alpha}$ and by these effects reversed the $PGE_2/PGF_{2\alpha}$ ratio (Weber *et al.*, 1978*a*).

The results mentioned above, together with the findings of high PGE levels in hypokalemic man (Gill *et al.*, 1976) and dogs (Galvez *et al.*, 1977) suggest that both sodium chloride balance and potassium chloride balance play a role in the regulation of renal PG production. It seems that in conditions with a high potassium chloride or high sodium chloride intake, the formation of PGs, especially PGE_2, is decreased. In contrast, both hypokalemia and a low dietary sodium chloride intake seem to stimulate PG formation. Such sodium-chloride- or potassium-chloride-intake-related effects on PG production may occur in the vasculature. Changes in vascular PG production could then be responsible, in part, for the changes of vascular reactivity to vasopressor hormones like angiotensin II or norepinephrine after alterations in sodium chloride or potassium chloride balance (Gimbrone and Alexander, 1975; Wong et al., 1977; Limas, 1977; Strewler et al., 1972; Galvez et al., 1977; Silverberg et al., 1978).

6. IMPAIRED PROSTAGLANDIN PRODUCTION AND UNRESPONSIVENESS OF RENIN SECRETION IN ESSENTIAL HYPERTENSION

In an appreciable number of patients with stable, uncomplicated essential hypertension, PRA is suppressed (for references, see Dunn and Tannen, 1974). In addition, by using maneuvers that normally either increase or decrease renin release, investigators have documented a general unresponsiveness of renin secretion in the majority of patients with essential hypertension (Padfield et al., 1975; Thomas et al., 1978; Tuck et al., 1976). Another common feature of patients with essential hypertension is that an increase of renal vascular resistance seems to correlate with a decrease of renin secretion (Schalekamp et al., 1970; Case et al., 1978). The demonstrated primary role of renal cortical PGs in the release of renin, the pronounced vasoactive properties of these compounds, and the possible involvements of the PG-cyclooxygenase-derived products on the function of the juxtaglomerular baroreceptor all point to a defect in the synthesis and/or metabolism of locally produced PGs as a possible cause of both the decrease in renin secretion and the increase of renal vascular resistance in essential hypertension. (Weber et al., 1978b). Renin release, if studied under defined conditions, may be used as a marker of the vasodilating capacity of the renal PGs on the vasculature in the kidney cortex. Thus, the initial increases of PRA and of PGE_2 excretion after furosemide are significantly lower in patients with essential hypertension as compared to controls, whereas $PGF_{2\alpha}$ formation is not different (Abe et al., 1977; Tan et al., 1978; Weber et al., 1978a, 1980).

These results suggest that the reduced response of renin release observed initially after furosemide in essential hypertensive patients is the result of reduced or impaired PG formation at the site of or near the renin-producing structures. Although we cannot appoint PGE_2 as the PG compound responsible for mediating renin secretion, it seems safe to conclude that the reduction in its urinary excretion at initially normal $PGF_{2\alpha}$ formation after furosemide reflects an impairment of renal PG production. The defect may be an alteration in the availability of arachidonic acid or a reduced formation of PG endoperoxides or of endoperoxide-derived compounds able to stimulate renin release and reduce vascular smooth muscle tone. Such alterations in the synthesis or metabolism of renal PGs diminish renin secretion. If they occur at vascular sites in the kidney cortex they will also increase vascular resistance and decrease renal blood flow.

It is possible that the reduction of renin secretion and the changes in PG formation found in essential hypertensive patients reflect an impairment of kidney function, which is secondary to the chronically elevated blood pressure. However, observations in man and in genetically hypertensive rats strengthen the concept that the impaired renal PG synthesis and the unresponsiveness of renin secretion may occur in parallel at an early stage in the development of essential hypertension: (1) Suppression of PRA is observed in most strains of genetically hypertensive rats at an early (sometimes prehypertensive) stage of the disease (Iwai *et al.*, 1973; Bianchi *et al.*, 1975). (2) Suppression of PRA has been documented in a number of normotensive (some years later, hypertensive) offspring of hypertensive parents after a definite simulus that normally increases renin secretion (Fasola *et al.*, 1968). (3) Ahnfelt-Rønne and Arrigoni-Martelli (1978) have found an increased renal production of $PGF_{2\alpha}$ in young, genetically hypertensive rats. (4) A positive correlation between urinary $PGF_{2\alpha}$ excretion and blood pressure was demonstrated in human neonates (Scherer and Weber, 1980).

7. CONCLUSION

Studies both *in vivo* and *in vitro* suggest that PG synthesis in renal cortical structures, possibly in the wall of the afferent arteriole, represents an important step in the mechanisms regulating the secretion of renin. PGs formed in the renal cortex seem to participate also in the control of renal blood flow and GFR. In the rabbit, rat, and man, sodium chloride and potassium chloride intake influence the rate of PG formation and the pathway of PG metabolism in the kidney. Through these relationships, PGs could play a critical role in the regulation of salt and water balance and in blood pressure control.

Because of the close connection between renal PG synthesis and renin secretion, an abnomal production or metabolism of PGs, whether due to genetic or environmental factors, could be involved in the etiology of high- or low-renin states. Thus, the reduced formation of vasodilating prostaglandins could be the common denominator for both the increase in renal vascular resistance and the decrease in renin secretion that have been reported to be associated with essential hypertension.

ACKNOWLEDGMENTS

This study was supported by Deutsche Forschungsgemeinschaft Grant We 681/4. We are grateful to Sabine Havenstein for excellent secretarial help.

REFERENCES

Abe, K., Yasujima, M., Chiba, S., Irokawa, N., Ito, T., and Yoshinaga, K., 1977, Effect of furosemide on urinary excretion of prostaglandin E in normal volunteers and patients with essential hypertension, *Prostaglandins* **14**:513.

Ahnfelt-Rønne, I., and Arrigoni-Martelli, E., 1978, Increased $PGF_{2\alpha}$ synthesis in renal papilla of spontaneously hypertensive rats, *Biochem. Pharmacol.* **27**:2363.

Anderson, R. J., Berl, T., McDonald, K. M., and Schrier, R. W., 1976, Prostaglandins: Effects on blood pressure, renal blood flow, sodium and water excretion, *Kidney Int.* **10**:205.

Änggård, E., and Larsson, C., 1971, The sequence of the early steps in the metabolism of prostaglandin E_1, *Eur. J. Pharmacol.* **14**:66.

Arisz, L., Donker, J. M., Brentjens, J. R. H., and van der Hem, G. K., 1976, The effect of indomethacin on proteinuria and kidney function in the nephrotic syndrome, *Acta Med. Scand.* **199**:121.

Bailie, M. D., Rector, Jr., F. C., and Seldin, D. W., 1971, Angiotensin II in arterial and renal venous plasma and renal lymph in the dog, *J. Clin. Invest.* **50**:119.

Bailie, M. D., Barbour, J. A., and Hook, J. B., 1975, Effect of indomethacin on furosemide-induced changes in renal blood flow, *Proc. Soc. Exp. Biol. Med.* **148**:1173.

Barajas, L., 1970, The ultrastructure of the juxtaglomerular apparatus as disclosed by three-dimensional reconstructions from serial sections: The anatomical relationship between the tubular and vascular components, *J. Ultrastruct. Res.* **33**:116.

Baylis, C., and Brenner, B. M., 1978, Modulation by prostaglandin synthesis inhibitors of the action of exogenous angiotensin II on glomerular ultrafiltration in the rat, *Circ. Res.* **43**:889.

Berl, T., Henrich, W. L., Erickson, A. L., and Schrier, R. W., 1979, Prostaglandins in the β-adrenergic and baroreceptor-mediated secretion of renin, *Am. J. Physiol.* **236**:F472.

Bianchi, G., Baer, P. G., Fox, U., Duzzi, L., Pagetti, D., and Giovannetti, A. M., 1975, Changes in renin, water balance, and sodium balance during development of high blood pressure in genetically hypertensive rats, *Circ. Res.* **36–37**(Suppl. I):153.

Bolger, P. M., Eisner, G. M., Ramwell, P. W., and Slotkoff, L. M., 1976, Effect of prosta-glandin synthesis on renal function and renin in the dog, *Nature* **259**:244.

Bolger, P. M., Eisner, G. M., Terez Shea, P., Ramwell, P. W., and Slotkoff, L. M., 1977, Effects of PGD_2 on canine renal function, *Nature* **267**:628.

Bolger, P. M., Eisner, G. M., Ramwell, P. W., and Slotkoff, L. M., 1978, Renal actions of prostacyclin, *Nature* **271**:467.

Cadnapaphornchai, P., Aisenbrey, G., McDonald, K. M., Burke, T. J., and Schrier, R. W., 1978, Prostaglandin-mediated hyperemia and renin-mediated hypertension during acute ureteral obstruction, *Prostaglandins* **16**:965.

Case, D. B., Casarella, W. J., Laragh, J. H., Fowler, D. L., and Cannon, P. J., 1978, Renal cortical blood flow and angiography in low- and normal-renin essential hypertension, *Kidney Int.* **13**:236.

Chang, L. C. T., Splawinski, J. A., Oates, J. A., and Nies, A. S., 1975, Enhanced renal prostaglandin production in the dog, *Circ. Res.* **36**:204.

Crowshaw, K., 1973, The incorporation of (1-^{14}C) arachidonic acid into the lipids of rabbit renal slices and conversion to prostaglandins E_2 and $F_{2\alpha}$, *Prostaglandins* **3**:607.

Data, J. L., Gerber, J. G., Crump, W. J., Frölich, J. C., Hollifield, J. W., and Nies, A. S., 1978, The prostaglandin system. A role in canine baroreceptor control of renin release, *Circ. Res.* **42**:454.

Davila, D., Davila, T., Oliw, E., and Änggård, E., 1978, The influence of dietary sodium on urinary prostaglandin excretion, *Acta Physiol. Scand.* **103**:100.

Dew, M. E., and Michelakis, A. M., 1974, Effect of prostaglandins on renin release in vitro, *Pharmacologist* **16**:198A.

Donker, A. J. M., Arisz, L., Brentjens, J. R. H., van der Hem, G. K., and Hollemans, H. J. G., 1976, The effect of indomethacin on kidney function and plasma renin activity in man, *Nephron* **17**:288.

Dray, F., Charbonnel, B., and Maclouf, J., 1975, Radioimmunoassay of prostaglandins F_α, E_1 and E_2 in human plasma, *Eur. J. Clin. Invest.* **5**:311.

Dunn, M. J., and Tannen, R. L., 1974, Low-renin hypertension, *Kidney Int.* **5**:317.

Eide, I., Løyning, E., Langard, Ø., and Kiil, F., 1977, Mechanism of renin release during acute ureteral constriction in dogs, *Circ. Res.* **40**:293.

Fasola, A. F., Martz, B. L., and Helmer, O. M., 1968, Plasma renin activity during supine exercise in offspring of hypertensive parents, *J. Appl. Physiol.* **25**:410.

Fichman, M. P., Littenburg, G., Brooker, G., and Horton, R., 1972, Effect of prostaglandin A_1 on renal and adrenal function in man, *Circ. Res.* **30–31**(Suppl. II):19.

Fine, L. G., and Trizna, W., 1977, Influence of prostaglandin on sodium transport of isolated medullary nephron segments, *Am. J. Physiol.* **232**:F383.

Folkert, V. W., and Schlöndorff, D., 1979, Prostaglandin synthesis in isolated glomeruli, *Prostaglandins* **17**:79.

Forssmann, W. G., and Taugner, R., 1977, Studies on the juxtaglomerular apparatus. V. The juxtaglomerular apparatus in Tupaia with special reference to intercellular contacts, *Cell. Tiss. Res.* **177**:291.

Frölich, J. C., Hollifield, J. W., Wilson, J. P., Sweetman, B. J., Seyberth, H. J., and Oates, J. A., 1976a, Suppression of plasma renin activity in man by indomethacin: Independence of sodium retention, *Clin. Res.* **24**:271A.

Frölich, J. C., Hollifield, J. W., Dormois, J. C., Frölich, B. L., Seyberth, H., Michelakis, A. M., Oates, J. A., 1976b, Suppression of plasma renin activity by indomethacin in man, *Circ. Res.* **39**:447.

Frölich, J. C., Hollifield, J. W., and Oates, J. A., 1976c, Effect of indomethacin on isoproterenol induced renin release, *Clin. Res.* **24**:9A.

Galvez, O. G., Bay, W. H., Roberts, B. W., and Ferris, T. F., 1977, The hemodynamic effects of potassium deficiency in the dog, *Circ. Res.* **40**(Suppl. II):11.

Gerber, J. G., Data, J. L., and Nies, A. S., 1978a, Enhanced renal prostaglandin production in the dog. The effect of sodium arachidonate in nonfiltering kidney, *Circ. Res.* **42**:43.

Gerber, J. G., Nies, A. S., Friesinger, G. C., Gerkens, J. F., Branch, R. A., and Oates, J. A., 1978b, The effect of PGI_2 on canine renal function and hemodynamics, *Prostaglandins* **16**:519.

Gill, J. R., Frölich, J. C. Bowden, R. E., Taylor, A. A., Keiser, H. R., Seyberth, H. W., Oates, J. A., and Bartter, F. C., 1976, Bartter's syndrome: A disorder characterized by high urinary prostaglandins and a dependence of hyperreninemia on prostaglandin synthesis, *Am. J. Med.* **161**:43.

Gimbrone, M. A., Jr., and Alexander, R. W., 1975, Angiotensin II stimulation of prostaglandin production in cultured human vascular endothelium, *Science* **189**:219.

Golub, M. S., Speckart, P. F., Zia, P. K., and Horton, R., 1976, The effect of prostaglandin A_1 on renin and aldosterone in man, *Circ. Res.* **39**:574.

Gryglewski, R. J., Korbut, R., and Ocetkiewicz, A., 1978, Generation of prostacyclin by lungs in vivo and its release into the arterial circulation, *Nature* **273**:765.

Hamberg, M., Svensson, J., Samuelsson, B., 1975, Thromboxanes: A new group of biologically active compounds derived from prostaglandin endoperoxides, *Proc. Natl. Acad. Sci.* **72**:2994.

Hedquist, P., 1976, Prostaglandin action on transmitter release at adrenergic neuroeffector junctions, in: *Advances in Prostaglandin and Thromboxane Research*, Vol. 1 (B. Samuelsson and R. Paoletti, eds.), Raven Press, New York, p. 357.

Henrich, W. L. Anderson, R. J., Berns, A. S., McDonald, K. M., Paulsen, P. J., Berl, T., and Schrier, R. W., 1978, The role of renal nerves and prostaglandins in control of renal hemodynamics and plasma renin activity during hypotensive hemorrhage in the dog, *J. Clin. Invest.* **61**:744.

Hollenberg, N. K., Epstein, M., Guttmann, R. D., Conroy, M., Basch, R. I., and Merrill, J. P., 1970, Effect of sodium balance on intrarenal distribution of blood flow in normal man, *J. Appl. Physiol.* **28**:312.

Hood, V. L., and Dunn, M. J., 1978, Urinary excretion of prostaglandin E_2 and prostaglandin $F_{2\alpha}$ in potassium-deficient rats, *Prostaglandins* **15**:273.

Hornych, A., Safar, N., Papanicolaou, N., Meyer, P., and Milliez, P., 1973, Renal and cardiovascular effects of prostaglandin A_2 in hypertensive patients, *Eur. J. Clin. Invest.* **3**:391.

Iwai, J., Dahl, L. K., and Knudsen, K. D., 1973, Genetic influence on the renin–angiotensin system, *Circ. Res.* **32**:678.

Kaloyanides, G. J., Ahrens, R. E., Shepherd, J. A., and DiBona, G. F., 1976, Inhibition of prostaglandin E_2 secretion, Failure to abolish autoregulation in the isolated dog kidney, *Circ. Res.* **38**:67.

Kirschenbaum, M. A., and Stein, J. H., 1976, The effect of inhibition of prostaglandin synthesis on urinary sodium excretion in the conscious dog, *J. Clin. Invest.* **57**:517.

Krakoff, L. R., DeGuia, D., Vlachakis, N., Stricker, J., and Goldstein, M., 1973, Effect of sodium balance on arterial blood pressure and renal responses to prostaglandin A_1 in man, *Circ. Res.* **33**:539.

Larsson, C., and Änggård, E., 1973, Regional differences in the formation and metabolism of prostaglandins in the rabbit kidney, *Eur. J. Pharmacol.* **21**:30.

Larsson, C., and Änggård, E., 1974, Increased juxtamedullary blood flow on stimulation of intrarenal prostaglandin biosynthesis, *Eur. J. Pharmacol.* **25**:326.

Larsson, C., Weber P., and Änggård, E., 1974, Arachidonic increases and indomethacin decreases plasma renin activity in the rabbit, *Eur. J. Pharmacol.* **28**:391.

Larsson, C., Weber, P., and Änggård, E., 1976, Stimulation and inhibition of renal PG biosynthesis: Effects on renal blood flow and on plasma renin activity, *Acta Biol. Med. Germ.* **35**:1195.

Larsson, C., and Weber, P. C., 1978, Renal prostaglandins and renin release, *Acta Biol. Med. Germ.* **37**:857.

Lee, S. C., and Levine, L., 1974, Prostaglandin metabolism. I. Cytoplasmic reduced nicotinamide adenine dinucleotide phosphate-dependent and microsomal reduced nicotinamide adenine dinucleotide-dependent prostaglandin E-9 keoreductase activities in monkey and pigeon tissues, *J. Biol. Chem.* **249**:1369.

Lee, J. G., Covino, B. G., Takman, B. H., and Smith, E. R., 1965, Renomedullary vasodepressor substance, medullin: Isolation, chemical characterization and physiological properties, *Circ. Res.* **17**:57.

Lee, J. B., Patak, R. V., and Mookerje, B. K., 1976, Renal prostaglandins and the regulation of blood pressure and sodium and water homeostasis, *Am. J. Med.* **60**:798.

Limas, C. L., 1977, Selective stimulation of venous prostaglandin E-9-ketoreductase by bradykinin, *Biochim. Biophys. Acta* **498**:306.

McGiff, J., Crowshaw, K., Terragno, N. A., and Lonigro, A. J., 1970, Release of a prostaglandin-like substance into renal venous blood in response to angiotensin II, *Circ. Res.* **27**(Suppl. I):121.

Malik, K. U., 1978, Prostaglandins—Modulation of adrenergic nervous system, *Fed. Proc. Fed. Am. Soc. Exp. Biol.* **37**:203.

Mandal, A. K., Muehrcke, R. C., Epstein, M., and Volini, F. I., 1967, Relationship of the renomedullary interstitial cells to experimental hypertension, *J. Lab. Clin. Med.* **70**:872.

Mitchell, M. D., 1978, A sensitive radioimmunoassay for 6-keto-prostaglandin $F_{1\alpha}$: Preliminary observations on circulating concentrations, *Prostaglandins and Medicine* **1**:13.

Moncada, S., Gryglewski, R., Bunting, S., and Vane, J. R., 1976, An enzyme isolated from arteries transforms prostaglandin endoperoxides to an unstable substance that inhibits platelet aggregation, *Nature* **263**:663.

Morgan, T., and Davis, J. M., 1975, Renin secretion at the individual nephron level, *Pflügers Arch. Ges. Physiol.* **359**:23.

Morrison, A. R., Nishikawa, K., and Needleman, P., 1977, Unmasking of thromboxane A_2 synthesis by ureteral obstruction in the rabbit kidney, *Nature* **267**:259.

Nissen, H. M., 1968, On lipid droplets in renal interstitial cells. II. A histological study on the number of droplets in salt-depletion and acute salt-repletion, *Z. Zellforsch.* **85**:483.

Oliw, E., 1979, Prostaglandins and kidney function. An experimental study in the rabbit, *Acta Physiol. Scand. Suppl.* **461**:7.

Olsen, U. B., 1978, The effect of ureteral occlusion and renal venous constriction on kidney kallikrein–kinin and prostaglandin systems in dogs, *Acta Physiol. Scand.* **104**:443.

Olsen, U. B., and Ahnfelt-Ronne, I., 1976, Bumetanide induced increase of renal blood flow in conscious dogs and its relation to local renal hormones (PGE, kallikrein and renin), *Acta Pharmacol. Toxicol.* **38**:219.

Pace-Asciak, C. R., and Rangaraj, G., 1977, Distribution of prostaglandin biosynthetic pathways in several rat tissues. Formation of 6-keto-prostaglandin $F_{1\alpha}$, *Biochim. Biophys. Acta* **486**:579.

Padfield, P. L., Allison, M. E. M., Brown, J. J., Lever, A. F., Luke, R. G., Robertson, C. C., Robertson, J. I. S., and Tree, M., 1975, Effect of intravenous frusemide on plasma renin concentration: Suppression of response in hypertension, *Clin. Sci. Mol. Med.* **49**:353.

Patak, R. V., Mookerje, B. K., Bentzel, C. J., Hysert, P. E., Babej, M., and Lee, J. B., 1975, Antagonism of the effects of furosemide by indomethacin in normal and hypertensive man, *Prostaglandins* **10**:649.

Reid, A., Morris, B. J., and Ganong, W. F., 1978, The renin–angiotensin system, *Annu. Rev. Physiol.* **40**:377.

Romero, J. C., Dunlap, C. L., and Strong, C. G., 1976, The effect of indomethacin and other anti-inflammatory drugs on the renin–angiotensin system, *J. Clin. Invest.* **58**:282.

Rumpf, K. W., Frenzel, S., Lowitz, H. D., and Scheler, F., 1975, The effect of indomethacin on plasma renin activity in man under normal conditions and after stimulation of the renin–angiotensin system, *Prostaglandins* **10**:641.

Schalekamp, M. A. D. H., Schalekamp-Kuyken, M. P. A., and Birkenhäger, W. H., 1970, Abnormal renal haemodynamics and renin suppression in hypertensive patients, *Clin. Sci.* **38**:101.

Scherer, B., and Weber, P. C., 1979, Time-dependent changes in prostaglandin excretion in response to frusemide in man, *Clin. Sci.* **56**:77.

Scherer, B., and Weber, P. C., 1980, Urinary prostaglandins (PG) in the newborn: Relationship to U_{osm}, U_{K^+} and blood pressure, in: *Advances in Prostaglandin and Thromboxane Research*, Vol. 7 (B. Samuelsson, P. W. Ramwell, and R. Paoletti, eds.), Raven Press, New York, p. 1033.

Scherer, B., Siess, W., and Weber, P. C., 1977, Radioimmunological and biological measurement of prostaglandins in rabbit urine: Decrease in PGE_2 excretion at high NaCl intake, *Prostaglandins* **13**:1127.

Scherer, B., Schnermann, J., Sofroniev, M., and Weber, P. C., 1978, Prostaglandin (PG) analysis in urine of humans and rats by different radioimmunoassays: Effect on PG-excretion by PG-synthetase inhibitors, laparotomy and furosemide, *Prostaglandins* **15**:255.

Schnermann, J., Schubert, G., Hermle, M., Herbst, R., Stowe, N. T., Yarimizu, S., and Weber, P. C., 1979, The effect of inhibition of prostaglandin synthesis on tubuloglomerular feedback in the rat kidney, *Pflügers Arch.* **379**:269.

Schnermann, J., and Weber, P. C., 1980, A role of renal prostaglandins (PG's) in the regulation of glomerular filtration rate (GFR) in rat kidneys, in: *Advances in Prostaglandin and Thromboxane Research*, Vol. 7 (B. Samuelsson, P. W. Ramwell, and R. Paoletti, eds.), Raven Press, New York, p. 1047.

Silver, M. J., Hoch, W., Kocsis, J. J., Ingermann, C. M., and Smith, J. B., 1974, Arachidonic acid causes sudden death in rabbits, *Science* **183**:1085.

Silverberg, A. B., Mennes, P. A., and Cryer, P. E., 1978, Resistance to endogenous norepinephrine in Bartter's syndrome, *Am. J. Med.* **64**:231.

Skinner, S. ..., McCubbin, J. W., and Page, I. H., 1964, Control of renin secretion, *Circ. Res.* **15**:64.

Smith, W. L., and Bell, T. G., 1978, Immunohistochemical localization of the prostaglandin-forming cyclooxygenase in the mammalian renal cortex, *Prostaglandins* **15**:715A.

Smith, W. L., and Wilkin, G. P., 1977, Immunochemistry of prostaglandin endoperoxide-forming cyclooxygenases: The detection of the cyclooxygenases in rat, rabbit, and guinea pig kidneys by immunofluorescence, *Prostaglandins* **13**:873.

Speckart, P., Zia, P., Zipser, R., and Horton, R., 1977, The effect of sodium restriction and prostaglandin inhibition on the renin angiotensin system in man, *J. Clin. Endocrinol. Metab.* **44**:832.

Stokes, J. B., and Kokko, J. P., 1977, Inhibition of sodium transport by prostaglandin E_2 across the insolated, perfused rabbit collecting tubule, *J. Clin. Invest.* **59**:1099.

Stone, K. J., and Hart, M., 1975, Prostaglandin-$E_2$9-ketoreductase in rabbit kidney, *Prostaglandins* **10**:273.

Strewler, G. J., Hinrichs, K. J., Guiod, L. R., and Hollenberg, N. K., 1972, Sodium intake and vascular smooth muscle responsiveness to norepinephrine and angiotensin in the rabbit, *Circ. Res.* **31**:758.

Tan, S. Y., Sweet, P., and Mulrow, P. J., 1978, Impaired normal production of prostaglandin E_2: A newly identified lesion in human essential hypertension, *Prostaglandins* **15**:139.

Tannenbaum, J., Splawinski, J. A., Oates, J. A., and Nies, A. S., 1975, Enhanced renal prostaglandin production in the dog, I. Effects on renal function, *Circ. Res.* **36**:197.

Terragno, N. A., Terragno, D. A., and McGiff, J., 1977, Contribution of prostaglandins to the renal circulation in conscious, anesthetized, and laparotomized dogs, *Circ. Res.* **40**:590.

Thomas, G. W., Ledingham, J. G. G., Beilin, L. J., Stott, A. N., and Yeates, K. M., 1978, Reduced renin activity in essential hypertension: A reappraisal, *Kidney Int.* **13**:513.

Tobian, L., Tomboulian, A., and Janecek, J., 1959, Effect of high perfusion pressures on the granulation of juxtaglomerular cells in an isolated kidney, *J. Clin. Invest.* **38**:605.

Tobian, L., O'Donnel, M., and Smith, P., 1974, Intrarenal prostaglandin levels during normal and high sodium intake, *Circ. Res.* **35**(Suppl. I):83.

Torres, V. E., Strong, C. G., Romero, J. C., and Wilson, D. M., 1975, Indomethacin enhancement of glycerol-induced acute renal failure in rabbits, *Kidney Int.* **7**:170.

Tuck, M. L., Williams, G. H. Dluhy, R. G., Greenfield, M., and Moore, T. J., 1976, A delayed suppression of the renin–aldosterone axis following saline infusion in human hypertension, *Circ. Res.* **39**:711.

Vander, A. J., 1968, Direct effects of prostaglandin on renal function and renin release in anesthetized dog, *Am. J. Physiol.* **214**:218.

Vander, A. J., and Miller, R., 1964, Control of renin secretion in the anesthized dog, *Am. J. Physiol.* **207**:537.

Vaughan, Jr., E. D., Shenasky II, J. H., and Gillenwater, J. Y., 1971, Mechanism of acute hemodynamic response to ureteral occlusion, *Invest. Urol.* **9**:109.

Weber, P., Holzgreve, H., Stephan, R., and Herbst, R., 1975a, Plasma renin activity and renal sodium and water excretion following infusion of arachidonic acid in rats, *Eur. J. Pharmacol.* **34**:299.

Weber, P., Held, E., Uhlich, E., and Eigler, J. O. C., 1975b, Reaction constants of renin in juxtaglomerular apparatus and plasma renin activity after renal ischemia and hemorrhage, *Kidney Int.* **7**:331.

Weber, P. C., Larsson, C., Änggård, E., Hamberg, M., Corey, E. J., Nicolaou, K. C., and Samuelsson, B., 1976b, Stimulation of renin release from rabbit renal cortex by arachidonic acid and prostaglandin endoperoxides, *Circ. Res.* **39**:868.

Weber, P. C., Larsson, C., and Scherer, B., 1977a, Prostaglandin E$_2$-9-ketoreductase as a mediator of salt intake-related prostaglandin–renin interaction, *Nature* **266**:65.

Weber, P. C., Scherer, B., and Larsson, C., 1977b, Increase of free arachidonic acid by furosemide in man as the cause of prostaglandin and renin release, *Eur. J. Pharmacol.* **41**:329.

Weber, P. C., Scherer, B., and Schnermann, J., 1978a, Effect of sodium and potassium chloride loading on urinary prostaglandin excretion in the rat, *Clin. Res.* **26**:478A.

Weber, P. C., Scherer, B., Lange, H.-H., Held, E., and Schnermann, J., 1978b, Renal prostaglandins and renin release: Relationship to regulation of electrolyte excretion and blood pressure, *Proceedings of the VIIth International Congress of Nephrology*, Montreal, Karger, Basel, pp. 99–106.

Weber, P. C., Scherer, B., Siess, W., and Held, E., 1980, Reduction of renal prostaglandin (PG) E formation in essential hypertension, in: *Advances in Prostaglandin and Thromboxane Research*, Vol. 7 (B. Samuelsson, P. W. Ramwell, and R. Paoletti, eds.), Raven Press, New York, p. 1145.

Werning, C., Vetter, W., Weidmann, P., Schweikert, H. U., Stiel, D., and Siegenthaler, W., 1971, Effect of prostaglandin E$_1$ on renin in the dog, *Am. J. Physiol.* **220**:852.

Whorton, A. R., Misono, K., Hollifield, J., Frölich, J. C., Inagani, T., and Oates, J. A., 1977, Prostaglandins and renin release: I. Stimulation of renin release from rabbit renal cortical slices by PGI$_2$, *Prostaglandins* **14**:1095.

Whorton, A. R., Smigel, M., Oates, J. A., and Frölich, J. C., 1978, Regional differences in prostacyclin formation by the kidney: Prostacyclin is a major prostaglandin of renal cortex, *Biochim. Biophys. Acta* **529**:176.

Williams, W. M., Frölich, J. C., Nies, A. S., and Oates, J. A., 1977, Urinary prostaglandins: Site of entry into renal tubular fluid, *Kidney Int.* **11**:256.

Williamson, H. E., Bourland, W. A., Marchand, G. R., Farley, D. B., and van Orden, D. E., 1975, Furosemide induced release of prostaglandin E to increase renal blood flow, *Proc. Soc. Exp. Biol. Med.* **150**:104.

Wong, P.Y.-K., Terragno, D. A., Terragno, N. A., and McGiff, J. C., 1977, Dual effects of
    bradykinin on prostaglandin metabolism: Relationship to the dissimilar vascular actions
    of kinins, *Prostaglandins* **13**:1113.
Yun, J. C. H., Kelly, G. D., Bartter, F. C., and Smith, G. W., 1978, Role of prostaglandins in
    the control of renin secretion in the dog (II), *Life Sci.* **23**:945.
Zins, G. R., 1975, Renal prostaglandins, *Am. J. Med.* **58**:14.
Zusman, R. M., Spector, D., Caldwell, B. V., Speroff, L., Schneider, G., and Mulrow, P. J.,
    1973, Effect of chronic sodium loading and sodium restriction on plasma prostaglandin A,
    E and F concentrations in normal humans, *J. Clin. Invest.* **52**:1093.

Index